Fourth Edition

Experimental Pharmaceutical Chemistry

for BPharm and DPharm Courses

As per the syllabus prescibed by Pharmacy Council of India

Anees Ahmad Siddiqui

M Pharm, PhD

Professor and Head
Department of Pharmaceutical Chemistry
School of Pharmaceutical Education and Research (SPER)
Jamia Hamdard, New Delhi

Seemi Siddiqui

M Pharm, PhD

Ex-Vice Principal
International Institute of Pharmaceutical Sciences
Sonipat, Haryana

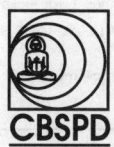

CBSPD

CBS Publishers & Distributors Pvt Ltd

New Delhi • Bengaluru • Chennai • Kochi • Kolkata • Lucknow • Mumbai
Gujarat • Hyderabad • Jharkhand • Nagpur • Patna • Pune • Uttarakhand

Fourth Edition

Experimental Pharmaceutical Chemistry

for B Pharm and D Pharm Courses

As per the syllabus prescribed by Pharmacy Council of India

ISBN: 978-81-948986-6-5

Fourth Edition: 2021
  Reprint: 2023, **2026**
First Edition: 2005
  Reprint: 2007
Second Edition: 2008
Third Edition: 2013

Published by **Satish Kumar Jain** and produced by **Varun Jain** for

CBS Publishers & Distributors Pvt Ltd

4819/XI Prahlad Street, 24 Ansari Road, Daryaganj, New Delhi 110 002, India
Ph: 011-23289259, 23266838
  Website: www.cbspd.com
  e-mail: delhi@cbspd.com

Corporate Office: 204 FIE, Industrial Area, Patparganj, Delhi 110 092
Ph: 011-4934 4934   Fax: 011-4934 4935   e-mail: publishing@cbspd.com; publicity@cbspd.com

Branches

- **Bengaluru:** Seema House 2975, 17th Cross, K.R. Road, Banasankari 2nd Stage, Bengaluru 560 070, Karnataka, India
  Ph: +91-80-26771678/79   Fax: +91-80-26771680   e-mail: bangalore@cbspd.com

- **Chennai:** 18/8B, Subbarayan Street, Shenoy Nagar, Chennai 600 030, Tamil Nadu, India
  Ph: +91-44-42032115, 26681266   e-mail: chennai@cbspd.com

- **Kochi:** 42/1325, 1326, Power House Road, opposite KSEB, Power House, Ernakulam 682 018, Kochi, Kerala, India
  Ph: +91-484-4059061-65   Fax: +91-484-4059065   e-mail: kochi@cbspd.com

- **Kolkata:** 147, Hind Ceramics Compound, 1st Floor, Nilgunj Road, Belghoria, Kolkata 700 056, West Bengal, India
  Ph: +91-33-25633055-56   e-mail: kolkata@cbspd.com

- **Lucknow:** Basement, Khushnuma Complex, 7-Meerabai Marg (behind Jawahar Bhawan), Lucknow 226 001, UP, India
  Ph: +91-522-4000032   e-mail: tiwari.lucknow@cbspd.com

- **Mumbai:** PWD Shed. Gala No. 25/26, Ramchandra Bhatt Marg, Next to JJ Hospital Gate No. 2, Opposite Union Bank of India Noorbaug Mumbai 400 009, Maharashtra, India
  Ph: +91-22-66661880/89   e-mail: mumbai@cbspd.com

Representatives

- **Gujarat**   • **Hyderabad**   • **Jharkhand**   • **Nagpur**   • **Patna**   • **Pune**   • **Uttarakhand**

For trade terms please contact customercare@cbspd.com

For general enquiries please contact info@cbspd.com

Printed at: SRK Graphics, Delhi, India

Preface to the Fourth Edition

The third edition of the book *Experimental Pharmaceutical Chemistry* was launched considering the valuable suggestions of our readers and to stay updated in the field. The fourth edition is compiled to include the practicals mentioned in the new PCI syllabus. In this edition, there is a complete coverage of practical exercises included in the new PCI syllabus which is mandatory for the B Pharm course. It is written at a level intended for students whose professional goals do not include a mastery of chemistry but for whom an understanding of the principles of chemistry and their practical ramification is a necessity.

Key changes in the fourth edition

In the compilation of the fourth edition, we have been guided by the experienced reviewers who represent the diversity of higher education experiences, including two years diploma and four years B Pharm courses.

There are twenty chapters. Each chapter is compiled as per the syllabus prescribed by PCI, mandatory to be included in various universities/colleges in India. Chapter 4, electroanalytical methods to determine the normality of a solution, is new a inclusion as per PCI syllabus. Chapter 5, qualitative inorganic analysis, is divided into three parts. Part I includes the identification tests for inorganic drugs. Part II consists of tests for purity. Part III consists of systematic analysis of cations and anions, illustrated with easily understandable schemes and tables to see the various qualitative tests at a glance. Chapter 6 illustrates the preparation of some inorganic pharmaceuticals like alum as per inclusion in PCI syllabus. The students will also find new exercises like assay of chlorpheniramine maleate, frusemide, dapsone, chloroquine, phenobarbitone, atropine, etc. in Chapter 7 (volumetric analysis) to cover the PCI syllabus. In Chapter 15, some new preparations are included. For example, preparations of tolbutamide, phenothiazine, salicylic acid, benzoic acids, *para*-iodobenzoic acid, 5-nitrosalicylic acid, etc. are new entries to explain some named reactions. Chapter 16 is assigned for the extraction procedures for isolation of particular constituents. The new Chapter 18 consists of some practical exercises based on spectroscopical methods. Two exercises are added in Chapter 17 based on determination of partition coefficient of drug. The practical exercise—separation of plant pigments by column chromatography is added in Chapter 20.

The typographic mistakes prevailing in the previous editions are rectified. We hope the present edition will be more useful to the students as well as to the teachers.

We are thankful to the faculty members especially Prof S Bawa, Dr Shaquiquzzaman and Prof Nagarajan, from KIET, Ghaziabad, for their suggestions.

We are also thankful to Mr S K Jain and Mr Varun Jain, CBS Publishers & Distributors, for bringing out this edition.

Anees Ahmad Siddiqui
Seemi Siddiqui

Preface to the First Edition

The science has no value without experimental work. The experimental work or practical chemistry is concerned with the determination of physical constant, performance of qualitative tests, derivatization, synthesis, quantitative chemistry, limit tests, etc. The present book entitled "Experimental Pharmaceutical Chemistry" is compiled to fulfil the requirements of undergraduate students of pharmacy course after the success of practical pharmaceutical chemistry book. The present book is divided into sixteen chapters; each chapter is written in a simple language. Chemical reactions are mentioned at appropriate place to make the subject simple and understandable. The exercises related to synthetic methods, extraction procedures, volumetric and gravimetric assays, qualitative organic analysis, chromatographic procedures, physical analysis, pharmaceutical chemistry of natural products etc. are designed to fulfil the need of the recently introduced syllabus of various universities. The synthetic methods are divided into single step, two steps and three steps for the convenience.

Method of preparation of reagents and solution is enclosed to make the practical work much easier. The methods of recording experiments are presented in the Appendix-I, Appendix-II and Appendix-III for the easiness of students. Detailed alphabetical index is given at the end of the book for cross reference.

It is hoped that the present edition will satisfy all the requirements of undergraduate students as well as teachers of pharmacy course concerning with pharmaceutical chemistry practicals.

We acknowledge to Shri Satish Kumar Jain and Vinod Kumar Jain of M/s CBS Publisher & Distributors for encouraging us and bringing out this book. We have special thanks to Mr Mohd. Islam Ansari of our department who with their vast experience gave a constructive suggestions in bringing out this edition. Thanks also due to valuable suggestion for inclusion of Chromato-graphic procedures and re-setting of text as per requirement to Mr. Ashok Khusnoor. Our greatest debt of gratitude is due to Mrs Rafat Siddiqui for sharing us to complete the present edition.

All constructive criticism and comments on this book from students and teachers are most welcome and shall form the basis for future editions.

Anees Ahmad Siddiqui
Seemi Siddiqui

Contents

Chapter 19   Quantitative Organic Analysis

356

Chapter 20   Chromatography

370

Thin layer chromatography (TLC)   *370*

Paper chromatography   *375*

Introduction

APPARATUS AND BASIC TECHNIQUES

The cleaning of glassware, equipment and bench is necessary before starting a chemistry experiment. The bench should be kept clean, free from any solid or liquid chemicals. Glassware are first washed with a detergent and then rinsed with distilled water before use. The outer surface may be dried with a cloth or filter paper. All the apparatus used in a particular experiment should be kept together on the bench to avoid confusion in determining duplicate experiments. Excess of apparatus, which are not in use, should be removed from the bench. All the solutions, precipitates and filtrates should be labelled to avoid confusion and covered to prevent contamination of the contents. Reagent bottles must be transferred on the reagent shelves immediately after use. Experimental observations must be recorded in a stiff covered notebook containing an index page and remaining one-sided line pages. The record must be concluded with calculations and the results.

GLASSWARE

Graduated Apparatus

Graduated flasks, burettes and pipettes are the most commonly used apparatus in volumetric analysis. All these glassware must be perfectly free from greasy matter to get exact results. Many detergents are available for cleaning the glass apparatus. Saturated solution of powdered sodium/potassium dichromate in concentrated sulphuric is also used for cleaning purpose. It is generally referred as 'chromic acid', cleaning mixture. It possesses powerful oxidizing and solvent properties. To prepare this, dissolve 5 g of sodium dichromate in 5 ml of water and then add sufficient concentrated sulphuric acid slowly with constant stirring to make up the volume 100 ml. The temperature will rise to 70–80°C. The mixture is allowed to cool to about 40°C and then transfer to a dry, glass stoppered bottle.

(i) Volumetric Flask

A volumetric flask (Fig. 1.1) is flat-bottomed, pear-shaped apparatus with long narrow neck. A thin line mark around the neck indicates the volume which the flask holds at a certain definite temperature, usually 20°C. The capacity and temperature are clearly marked on the flask. Both the front and the back of the mark should be seen as a single line to avoid errors due to parallax while making the final adjustment. The lower edge of the miniscus should tangential to the graduation mark. A small change in the volume is detected easily in the long narrow neck.

Volumetric flasks are available in the capacities of 1, 2, 5, 10, 20, 50, 100, 200, 250, 500, 1000, 2000, 5000 cm^3. The standard solutions are obtained for analysis with the help of pipette in different analytical techniques.

(ii) Pipettes

Pipettes are of two type:

(i) *Transfer pipettes*, which have one mark and withdraw a small and constant volume of the solutions.

(ii) *Measuring or graduated pipettes*, which are graduated and used to deliver various small volumes.

The transfer pipette is made up of a cylindrical bulb joined at both ends to narrower tubing. A calibration mark is present around the upper tube while the lower delivery tube is made to a fine tip. This type of pipette is used to deliver pre-determined variable volume of liquids. The transfer pipette are constructed with the capacities of 1, 2, 5, 10, 20, 25, 50 and 100 cm^3. The pipettes of the capacities of 10, 25, and 50 cm^3 are frequently used in macro work.

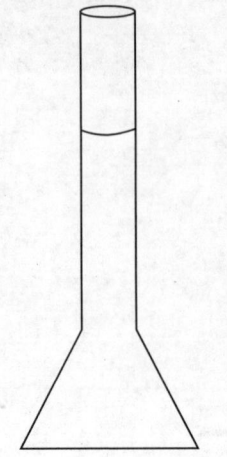

Fig. 1.1: Volumetric flask

Before using, the pipettes are first rinsed with the liquid to be used, then filled with liquid by suction to about 2–3 cm above the mark and upper end of the pipette is closed with the tip of the finger. The liquid is allowed to run out slowly by slightly relaxing the pressure of the finger and rotating the pipette until the bottom of the meniscus just reached the graduation mark. The pipette is held vertically to fix the mark at the same level as the eye. The adhering drops at the tip are removed by stroking against a glass surface. Then the liquid is transferred into a flask keeping the tip of the pipette in contact with the wall of the flask. When all the solution is transferred, the upper end is closed with the tip of finger and the cylindrical bulb is closed with the fingers of other hand to discharge the last drop of the jet.

Corrosive or toxic liquids are drawn in the pipette with the help of rubber or plastic bulb with glass ball valves operated between finger and thumb. A piston-control is also attached to the suction end of the pipette.

Graduated pipettes are made up of straight, narrow tubes with no central bulbs. They deliver a measured volume from a top zero to a selected graduation mark or to the jet, i.e. the zero is at the set.

(iii) Burettes

Burettes are long cylindrical tubes with uniform bore throughout the graduated length, a narrow lower end with a glass stopcock and a jet. When in use, a burette must be firmly supported on a stand with a burette holder. The stopcock should be lubricated to prevent sticking or freezing and ensure smoothness in action. Vaseline may be used as a lubricant.

Before using, the burette is thoroughly cleaned with a cleansing agent, rinsed well with distilled water, the stopcock is lubricated and fixed in a burette holder. The solution is filled with the help of a small funnel up to zero mark. The liquid is discharged from a burette into a conical flask. The flask is gently rotated with the right hand for mixing the contents well.

Purified water

Purified distilled water is used in analytical operations. Highly purifed water is obtained by allowing tap water to percolate through a mixture of ion-exchange resins. A strong acid resin will remove cations from the water and replace them by hydrogen ions, and a strong base resin will remove anions by hydroxyl ions. Various commercial unit are available for the preparation of de-ionized water.

Wash bottles

A wash bottle is a flat-bottomed flask fitted up to withdraw a fine stream of distilled water. The thumb is kept over the tube and water is blown out.

A polythene wash bottle is cheap, fitted with a plastic cap and a plastic jet and has flexible sides. Pressure is applied by squeezing and jet of water is controlled.

Filtration apparatus

A conical funnel fitted with a filter paper is usually used for filtration. The funnel should have an angle nearly 60° and a long stem.

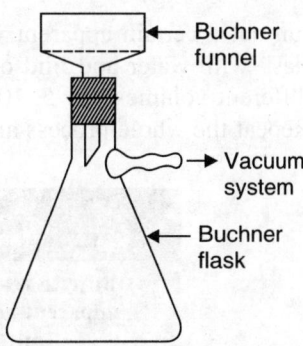

Fig. 1.2: Filtration assembly

Sintered glass crucibles are made of resistance glass and have porous disc fused into body of the crucible. The filter disc is made up of various pore diameters as indicated by numbers from 0 to 5. The numbers 3 and 4 are used for gravimetric analysis. The number '0' has largest pore size while number '5' has smallest pore size.

Buchner funnel and Buchner flask are used to filter large quantity of material. The Buchner flask consists of thick-walled conical flask (Fig. 1.2) with a short side-arm for connection to a water pump. Into the neck of the flask is fitted the Buchner funnel which is pierced by a number of small holes. Before filtration, a good quality of filter paper is placed in the funnel and moistened with a few drops of liquid to be filtered.

CALIBRATION OF PIPETTES, BURETTES AND GRADUATED FLASKS

The convenient unit to measure the large volume of liquid is 'litre'. The litre and millilitre are sufficiently precise for the requirements of titrimetric analysis.

The capacity of a glass vessel varies with temperature. Therefore, the temperature of the experiment should be recorded.

If high degree of accuracy is to be required, the correctness of all measuring apparatus must be tested. The process of testing is usually accomplished by comparing the actual weight of water contained in the apparatus with its apparatus volume. The weight of the water taken at a specified temperature will occupy only a definite volume at that temperature. The volumes of water for its definite weights at different specified temperatures may be known with the help of density table.

(i) Pipette

Weigh an empty weighing bottle or a small conical flask. Fill the pipette to the mark with distilled water. Deliver the contents into the weighing bottle and reweigh. Repeat the process three times. Find out the temperature of water and with the help of density table calculate the volumes of observed weights of water. Tabulate the result as in Table1.1 and find out the correction constant of the pipette for that temperature.

(ii) Burette

Fill a clean burette vertically clamped with distilled water. Record the temperature of this water which is same as that of room temperature. Adjust the level of the water to zero and carefully

Table 1.1 (temperature of water = 20°C, 1 ml = 0.9982 g)						
Apparatus volume (ml)	Weight of empty bottle (g)	Weight of bottle + water (g)	Weight of water only (ml)	Real volume of water (ml)	Diff.	Mean
1. 20	35.5	55.5	20.0	20.04	+0.04	
2. 20	-do-	55.52	20.02	20.05	+0.05	+0.05 ml
3. 20	-do-	55.52	20.02	20.05	+0.05	

run out a certain apparent volume into the flask which has been weighed earlier. Weigh the flask with water and find out the weight of water by difference. Carry out this process with different volumes, say 5, 10, 15, 20 ml, etc. taking always the zero mark as the starting point. Repeat the whole process and tabulate the result as in Table 1.2.

Table 1.2 (temperature of water = 20°C, 1 ml = 0.9982 g)			
Burette readings apparent volume (ml)	Weight of water delivered (g)	True volume (ml)	Correction at each mark (ml)
1. 0.0 – 15.00 = 15.00	15.04	15.07	+ –0.07
2. 15.00 – 30.00 = 15.00	15.00	15.02	+ –0.02
3. 30.00 – 50.00 = 20.00	19.95	19.98	+ –0.02

The apparent volume should be substracted from the true volume and a plus correction should be added to and a minus correction should be substracted from the corresponding burette reading.

(iii) Graduated Flask

The procedure of standardizing a measuring flask is practically same as that applied to pipette. It is only necessary to weigh the water delivered by or contained in the flask, as the case may be. Sometimes, the measuring flasks are also standardized in reference to a standardized flask knowing exactly the difference of volumes with the help of other standard apparatus such as a burette or a pipette.

DRYING OF ORGANIC SOLUTIONS

The process of synthesizing and isolating an organic compound often results in an organic compound or solution contaminated with traces of water. For instance, in aqueous extractions some water will be transferred into the organic phase because of the partial miscibility of the organic phase and water. Also, many reactions themselves are performed in an aqueous solution. This water must be removed before the required compound can be properly characterized.

The following two methods for drying the organic solutions are commonly used:

• Saturated aqueous sodium chloride
• Solid drying agents

These two methods are described below.

1. Saturated Aqueous Sodium Chloride Solution

The bulk of the water can often be removed by shaking or "washing" the organic layer with saturated aqueous sodium chloride (also called brine). The salt water works to pull the water from the organic layer to the water layer. This is because the concentrated salt solution wants to become more dilute and because salts have a stronger attraction to water than to organic solvent. Traces of water are removed by treating the organic solution with a drying agent.

Procedure

 (i) Place the organic solution in a separatory funnel. The organic solvent might be methylene chloride, diethyl ether, hexanes, etc., as long as it is not, of course, water.
 (ii) Add an amount of saturated aqueous sodium chloride, less than or equal to the amount of organic solution you have.
(iii) Stopper the funnel and shake as in an extraction. Allow the layers to separate. The rules as to which layer is on top are the same as for extraction. Since there is a lot of salt dissolved in the water, the density of the saturated aqueous sodium chloride solution is 1.2 g/ml.

2. Solid Drying Agents

Some anhydrous inorganic salts like calcium chloride ($CaCl_2$), calcium sulphate ($CaSO_4$), magnesium sulphate ($MgSO_4$), potassium carbonate (K_2CO_3), sodium sulphate (Na_2SO_4), etc., which readily takes up water to become hydrated, are used routinely for drying organic solvents.

Of the five drying agents in the above table, magnesium sulphate is a fine powder and the rest are of a larger particle size. Calcium chloride, magnesium sulphate, and sodium sulphate are the three most commonly used drying agents.

Procedure

 (i) Add a smaller amount of the solid drying agent directly to the organic solution. Swirl the solution.
 (ii) Observe the drying agent; if it is all clumped together, add more.
(iii) Continue swirling and observing the solution for 5–15 minutes, adding more drying agent only until a fresh addition no longer forms clumps.

Each drying agent adopt a slightly different appearance when "clumped" on absorbing water and practice will make you better at judging whether the inorganic salt is wet or dry. There is no set "rule" as to how much drying agent needs to be added. The amount required depends on the amount of water in the solvent solution which you are drying, and this amount varies from experiment to experiment. Use as much as it takes to dry the solution. In most cases, drying process is completed in 20 minutes. When drying is complete, you need to remove the dried organic solution from the drying agent. There are several methods by which you can do this.

You can filter the solution by gravity filtration. If the powder is quite fine (as when using magnesium sulphate) or if the volume is large, gravity filtration is the method of choice. If the drying agent is of larger particle size (e.g. sodium sulphate or calcium chloride), decanting is the method of choice. An alternative to decanting is to remove the liquid from the drying agent simply by drawing it off with a pipet attached with rubber bulb. Squeeze the bulb of the pipet, carefully and slowly draw liquid into the pipet, leaving the solid drying agent behind.

Note: Sodium hydroxide (solid) is also used for drying the organic solvent. For example, pyridine becomes moisture free on distillation under anhydrous condition after adding NaOH pellets.

Limit Tests

Every pharmaceutical substance contains some impurities varying in proportion. These impurities are different in nature. These are either highly toxic or incompatible in nature. Hence, Indian pharmacopoeia has fixed a limit of these impurities, mainly based on their toxic effects. To check the limit, some official tests, called limit tests, are carried out.

Limit tests involve the comparison of opalescence, turbidity or colour with fixed standards (having known amount of impurities). The extent of opalescence, turbidity and colour is affected by the presence of other impurities present in the substance, variation in time and method of performance of the tests. Generally an aqueous solution of substance is prepared. Sometimes a solution of the substance is prepared by dissolving in an acid or, if the solution is alkaline, it is neutralized with nitric acid or hydrochloric acid. Generally, limit tests are carried out in Nessler cylinder which is cylindrical tube having 50 ml mark.

LIMIT TEST FOR CHLORIDE

Theoretical Concept

It involves the reaction of silver nitrate with soluble chlorides to form the precipitate of silver chloride which is insoluble in dilute nitric acid. The extent of precipitate depends upon the amount of silver chloride formed or amount of chloride ions present in the substance. The opalescence produced is compared with a standard opalescence from standard solution containing fixed amount of chloride under the same experimental conditions.

$$NaCl + AgNO_3 \xrightarrow{\text{dil } HNO_3} \underset{\text{White precipitate}}{AgCl\downarrow + NaNO_3}$$

Procedure

Standard Opalescence

Place standard chloride solution (25 ppm, 1 ml) and dilute nitric acid (10 ml) in a Nesslar cylinder. Dilute to 50 ml with water and add 0.1M silver nitrate solution (1 ml). Stir immediately with glass rod and allow to stand for 5 minutes.

Test Opalescence

Dissolve the specified quantity of the substance or prepare a solution as directed in monograph and transfer in a Nessler cylinder. Add dilute nitric acid (10 ml) except when it is used in the preparation of solution. Dilute to 50 ml with water and add 0.1M silver nitrate solution (1 ml). Stir immediately with glass rod and allow to stand for 5 minutes.

Observe the opalescence in both the solutions (views transversely). The opalescence produced should not be greater than the standard opalescence.

Chloride standard solution (25 ppm Cl⁻)

Dilute 5 volumes of 0.0824% w/v NaCl solution to 100 volumes with water.

Chloride standard solution (5 ppm Cl⁻)

Dilute 1 volume of 0.0824% w/v NaCl solution to 100 volumes with water.

LIMIT TEST FOR SULPHATE

Theoretical Concept

Limit test for sulphate is based on the reaction between barium chloride and soluble sulphate in acidic solution. The turbidity formed in the test solution is compared with the standard turbidity obtained by the fixed quantity of the sulphate under the same experimental conditions.

$$BaCl_2 + Na_2SO_4 \longrightarrow BaSO_4\downarrow + 2NaCl$$
White precipitate

Note: Addition of acetic acid, used as a acidifying agent in place of hydrochloric acid, is recommended in recent Indian pharmacopoeia.

Procedure

Test Solution Opalescence

To a 25% w/v barium chloride solution (1.0 ml) in a Nessler cylinder, add ethanolic sulphate standard solution (10 ppm SO₄, 1.5 ml), mix and allow to stand for 1 minute. Add solution of test substance (15 ml) prepared as directed in the individual monograph or a solution of the specified quantity of substance being examined in water (15 ml) and 5M acetic acid solution (0.15 ml). Add sufficient water to produce 50 ml, stir immediately with a glass rod and allow to stand for 5 minutes.

Standard Opalescence

Adopt the same procedure by taking standard sulphate solution (10 ppm SO₄⁻, 15 ml).

The opalescence produced by the test solutions should not be greater than standard opalescence when viewed transversely. Test solution contain a small amount of potassium sulphate to increase the sensitivity of test. Any sulphate ion impurity in test substance will produce barium sulphate in excess of already dissolved amount, causing turbidity. To prevent supersaturation of barium sulphate which may occur, the small amount of ethanol is added.

Ethanolic standard sulphate solution (10 ppm SO₄)

Dilute 1 volume of 0.181% w/v K₂SO₄ solution in ethanol (30%) to 100 volumes with ethanol (30%).

LIMIT TEST FOR IRON

Theoretical Concept

The limit test for iron depends on the reaction of iron in ammonical solution in the presence of citric acid with thioglycollic acid to form ferrous thioglycolate.The ammonical ferrous thioglycolate solution is pink to deep reddish purple colour depending on concentration of iron. The intensity of colour is compared with standard intensity, obtained from fixed concentration of iron. Iron may be precipitated as ferrous or ferric hydroxide on reaction with ammonia solution. The precipitate may interfere with the intensity of colour. Citric acid is added to prevent the precipitation of iron as hydroxide by forming complex with iron which is not precipitated by ammonia solution.

$$2HSCH_2COOH + \text{Ferrous or Ferric ion} \longrightarrow Fe(HSCH_2COO)_2 + 2H^+$$
Thioglycolic acid   Ferrous thioglycolate

Thioglycolic acid also reduces the ferric (if present as impurity) into ferrous which forms the coloured ferrous thioglycolate.

Procedure

Standard Colour

Dilute standard iron solution (20 ppm Fe, 2 ml) with water (40 ml) in a Nessler cylinder. Add 20% w/v solution of iron free citric acid (2 ml) and thioglycollic acid (0.1 ml), mix, make alkaline with iron free ammonia solution, dilute to 50 ml with water and allow to stand for 5 minutes.

Test Colour

Dissolve the specified quantity of the substance in water (40 ml) or use of this solution (10 ml) as prescribed in the monograph. Add 20% w/v solution of iron free citric acid (2 ml) and thioglycollic acid (0.1 ml), mix, make alkaline with iron free ammonia solution, dilute to 50 ml with water and allow to stand for five minutes.

The intensity of colour in the test solution should not be more than standard colour.

Standard Iron Solution (20 ppm Fe)

Dilute one volume of a 0.1726% w/v ferric ammonium sulphate in 0.05M sulphuric acid to 10 volumes with water.

Standard Iron Solution (10 ppm Fe)

Dilute 7.022 g of ferrous ammonium sulphate in water containing 25 ml of 1M sulphuric acid and add sufficient water to produce 100 ml. Dilute 1 volume to 100 volumes with water.

LIMIT TEST FOR HEAVY METALS

The test for heavy metals is designed to determine the content of metallic impurities that are coloured by sulphide ion, under the specified conditions. The limit for heavy metals is indicated in the individual monographs in terms of part of lead per million parts of the substance (by weight) as determined by visual comparison of the colour produced by the substance with that of the control prepared from standard lead solution.

The amount of heavy metals is determined by one of the following methods directed in the individual monograph.

The methods used for limit test for heavy metals are classified as methods A, B, C and D depending on behaviour of inorganic substances.

The method A is used for substances that yield clear, colourless solutions under the specified test condition. Method B is used for substances that do not yield clear, colourless solutions under the test conditions specified for Method A, or for substances which, by virtue of their complex nature, interfere with the precipitation of metals by sulphide ion or for fixed and volatile oils. Method C is used for substances that yield clear, colourless solutions with sodium hydroxide solution. Method D is used for non-colour-forming and/or water-soluble substances, which are tested by colour comparison with sulphide ion. Sulphide ion source in this method is generated by adding glycerol to thioacetamide solution.

Method A

Procedure

Standard Colour

Take standard lead solution (20 ppm Pb) (1 ml) in 50 ml Nessler cylinder dilute with water to 25 ml and then add either dilute acetic acid sp. or dilute ammonia solution sp. to adjust a pH between 3.0 and 4.0. Dilute with water to about 35 ml, and mix. Add freshly prepared hydrogen sulphide solution (10 ml), mix, dilute with water to 50 ml, allow to stand for 5 minutes and view downwards over a white surface.

Test Colour

Into a 50 ml Nessler cylinder, take the test solution (25 ml) prepared as directed, in the individual monograph and then add either dilute acetic acid sp. or ammonia solution Sp. to adjust a pH between 3.0 and 4.0. Dilute with water to about 35 ml and mix. Add freshly prepared hydrogen sulphide solution (10 ml), mix dilute with water to 50 ml, allow to stand for five minutes and view downwards over a white surface.

The colour produced in the test solution should not be darker than that produced in the standard solution.

Method B

Standard Colour

Proceed as directed under Method A.

Test Colour

Take the specified quantity of substance as mentioned in individual monograph. Ignite carefully after adding sufficient sulphuric acid. To the charred mass, add nitric acid (2 ml) and sulphuric acid (5 drops) and heat until white fumes are no longer evolved. Ignite the contents preferably in muffle furnance at 500–600°C until carbon is completely burnt off. Cool down, digest the mass with hydrochloric acid for 15 minutes. Evaporate the content to dryness, moist the content with sufficient HCl and then digest with H_2O for 2 minutes. Add ammonia solution to make alkaline to litmus paper, and then dilute to 25 ml. Add acetic acid to maintain pH between 3 and 4. Filter and add water to filtrate to make 35 ml and mix. Add freshly prepared hydrogen sulphide solution (10 ml), mix, dilute with water to 50 ml, allow to stand for 5 minutes and view downwards over a white surface.

The colour produced in the test solution should not be darker than the colour of the standard solution.

Method C

Procedure

Standard Colour

Into a 50 ml Nessler cylinder, take standard lead solution (20 ppm Pb) (1 ml), dilute sodium hydroxide solution (5 ml) and then dilute with water to 50 ml and mix. Add 5 drops of sodium sulphide solution, mix, allow to stand for 5 minutes and view downwards over a white surface.

Test Colour

Into a 50 ml Nessler cylinder, take the test solution (25 ml) as prepared mentioned hydroxide in the individual monograph or the specified quantity dissolved in a mixture of water (20 ml) and dilute sodium hydroxide solution (5 ml). Dilute to 50 ml with water and mix. Add 5 drops of sodium sulphide solution, mix, allow to stand for 5 minutes and view downwards over a white surface.

The colour produced in the test solution should not be darker than the colour of the standard solution.

Method D

Standard Colour

Into a small Nessler cylinder, pipette 10 ml of either lead standard solution (1 ppm Pb) or lead standard solution (2 ppm) and add the test solution (2 ml). Mix and carry out the same procedure as done in test colour.

Test Colour

Prepare the solution of substance as directed in individual monograph and pipette out 10 ml into a small Nessler cylinder. Add acetate buffer (2 ml) pH 3.5, mix, add thioacetamide (1.2 ml) reagent, allow to stand for 2 minutes and view downward over a white surface.

The colour produced in the test solution should not be more intense than that produced with the standard solution.

Lead Nitrate Stock Solution

Dissolve lead nitrate (0.1589 g) in water (100 ml) to which has been added nitric acid (1 ml), then dilute with water to 1000.0 ml.

Standard Lead Solution

On the day of use, dilute lead nitrate stock solution (10 ml) with water to 100 ml. Each ml of standard lead solution contains the equivalent of 10 µg of lead.

Lead standard solution (100 ppm Pb)

Dilute one volume of standard lead solution (0.1% Pb) to 10 volumes with water.

Lead standard solution (10 ppm Pb)

Dilute one volume of lead standard solution (100 ppm) to 10 volumes with water.

Lead standard solution (20 ppm Pb)

Dilute one volume of lead standard solution (100 ppm) to 5 volumes with water.

This solution must be prepared and stored in a polyethylene or glass container free from soluble lead salts.

Lead standard solution (2 ppm Pb)

Dilute 1 volume of standard lead solution (20 ppm) to 10 volumes with water.

LIMIT TEST FOR LEAD

Theoretical Concept

Lead is a toxic substance present in pharmaceutical preparations. The main sources of this impurity are sulphuric acid (prepared by lead chamber process) and the lead apparatus used in the manufacture of pharmaceutical substance. The limit for lead is indicated in the individual monograph in terms of ppm, Pb per million parts (by weight) of substance being examined. The I.P. and U.S.P. method is based on the reaction between lead and dithizone (diphenyl-thiocarbazone). In chloroform solution, dithizone extracts lead from an alkaline aqueous solution as lead dithizonate which has red colour in chloroform solution. Since dithizone itself imparts a green colour in chloroform, the resultant colour of dithizone and lead dithizone is violet. The colour produced by a given amount of the sample is compared with that produced by a known volume of a standard solution of lead. If the colour is intense than that produced by the standard, it contains lead in excess of prescribed limit. For the test, the lead present as impurity is separated by extracting an alkaline solution of the substance with dithizone extraction solution which removes all the lead in the form of its complex in chloroform layer.

$$Pb + 2S=C\begin{array}{c} NH-NH-C_6H_5 \\ NH-NH-C_6H_5 \end{array}$$

Diphenyl thiocarbazone (dithizone) (green colour)

Lead dithizonate (violet colour)

Method

Transfer the volume of the prepared test solution as directed in the individual monograph to a separator and unless otherwise directed in monograph, add ammonium citrate solution (6 ml) and hydroxylamine hydrochloride solution (2 ml). Add two drops of phenol red solution and make the alkaline by adding sufficient quantity of ammonia solution. Cool down the solution if necessary and add potassium cyanide solution (2 ml). Immediately, extract the solution with several quantities of dithizone extraction solution (each 5 ml), draining off each extract into another separating funnel until dithizone extraction solution retain its green colour. Shake the combined dithizone solution for 30 seconds with 1% w/v solution of nitric acid (30 ml) and discard the chloroform layer. Add dithizone standard solution (5 ml) to the acid layer and ammonia-cyanide solution (4 ml) and shake for 30 seconds. The colour of chloroform layer should not be more intense than that of standard obtained by treating in the same manner a volume of lead standard solution (1 ppm Pb) equivalent to the amount of lead permitted in the substance being examined.

All reagents used for the test should have as low a content of lead as practicable. All reagent solutions should be stored in containers of borosilicate glass. Glassware should be rinsed thoroughly with warm dilute nitric acid, followed by water.

Standard Dithizone Solution

Dissolve diphenyl thiocarbazone (30 mg) in chloroform (1000 ml). Store the solution in glass stoppered lead free bottle, protected from light and in a refrigerator.

Dilute Standard Lead Solution

Dilute standard lead solution (10.0 ml) (as prepared in heavy metals) with sufficient 1% v/v solution of nitric acid to produce 100 ml. Each ml of this solution contains 1 µg of lead per ml.

Special Reagents

1. **Ammonia-cyanide solution sp.:** Dissolve 2 g of *potassium cyanide* in 15 ml of *strong ammonia solution* and dilute with *water* to 100 ml.
2. **Ammonium citrate solution sp.:** Dissolve 40 g of *citric acid* in 90 ml of *water*. Add two drops of *phenol red solution*, then add slowly *strong ammonia solution* until the solution acquires a reddish colour. Remove any lead present by extracting the solution with 30 ml of *dithizone extraction solution* until the dithizone solution retains its orange green colour.
3. **Hydroxylamine hydrochloride solution sp.:** Dissolve 20 g of *hydroxylamine hydrochloride* in sufficient *water* to produce about 65 ml. Transfer to a separator, add five drops of *thymol blue solution*, add *strong ammonia solution* until the solution becomes yellow. Add 10 ml of a 4% w/v solution of *sodium diethyl-dithiocarbamate* and allow to stand for 5 minutes. Extract with successive quantities, each of 10 ml, of *chloroform* until a 5 ml portion of the extract does not assume a yellow colour when shaken with *dilute copper sulphate solution*. Add *dilute hydrochloric acid* until the solution is pink and then dilute with sufficient *water* to produce 100 ml.
4. **Potassium cyanide solution sp.:** Dissolve 50 g of *potassium cyanide* in sufficient *water* to produce 100 ml. Remove the lead from this solution by extraction with successive quantities, each of 20 ml, of *dithizone extraction solution* until the dithizone solution retains its orange-green colour. Extract any dithizone remaining in the cyanide solution by shaking with *chloroform*. Dilute the cyanide solution with sufficient *water* to produce a solution containing 10 g of potassium cyanide in each 100 ml.

LIMIT TEST FOR ARSENIC

The IP prescribes limit test for arsenic as presence of arsenic in drugs even in traces is not desirable due to its toxic nature. The limit for arsenic is indicated in the individual monograph in terms of ppm, e.g. parts of arsenic per million part (by weight) of substance being examined. The Indian Pharmacopoeia has recommended the **Gutzeit method**.

Theoretical Concept

The Gutzeit test of arsenic is based on the fact that arsenic in the arsenious state can be readily reduced to arsine (AsH_3) gas which on passing over mercuric chloride paper develops a yellow to brown stain, the intensity of which are proportional to the amount of arsenic. The test intensity is compared from intensity of standard stain. The standard stain is prepared from a definite amount of arsenic. Reduction of the arsenic to arsine, both in the test sample and the standard, is done by the combined action of zinc, hydrochloric acid, stannous chloride and potassium iodide. The arsine is carried over along with hydrogen to the mercuric chloride or bromide paper supported in the test apparatus. The rate of evolution of hydrogen is controlled which is dependent on the quantity and surface area of zinc, concentration of hydrochloric acid, salt in the reaction mixture, temperature and dimension of the apparatus. Rapid evolution produces a long and diffuse stain while a short and intense colour is developed by a slow evolution.

Chemically, the arsenic impurity is converted in acidic medium into arsenious acid or arsenic acid depending upon the valency state of arsenic:

$$As^{3+} \longrightarrow H_3AsO_3$$
Trivalent   Arsenious acid

$$As^{5+} \longrightarrow H_3AsO_4$$
Pentavalent   Arsenic acid

This solution is reacted with a reducing agent like stannous chloride or sulphurous acid to convert the pentavalent arsenic acid into the trivalent arsenious acid which is converted into gaseous arsenious hydride (arsine gas) with the help of nascent hydrogen produced by the action of zinc with hydrochloric acid.

$$H_3AsO_4 \longrightarrow H_3AsO_3 \xrightarrow{Zn + HCl} AsH_3\uparrow + 3H_2O$$
Arsenic acid   Arsenious acid   Arsine

Arsine gas is carried out through the tube with the help of hydrogen to the mercuric chloride paper. Reaction of arsine with mercuric chloride produces a yellow coloured stain. The intensity of the colour is dependent on the quantity of arsenic.

$$2AsH_3\uparrow + HgCl_2 \longrightarrow Hg\begin{array}{c} As\,H_2 \\ \diagdown \\ As\,H_2 \end{array} + 2HCl$$
Yellow colour

Note: *The reagent used in the limit test for arsenic is designated as 'AsT' reagent. It means, these reagents are free from arsenic.*

Apparatus

The apparatus (Fig. 2.1) consists of a 100 ml bottle or conical flask closed with a rubber or ground glass stopper through which passes a glass tube (about 20 cm × 5 mm). The lower part of the tube is drawn to an internal diameter of 1.0 mm, and 15 mm from its tip is a lateral orifice 2 to 3 mm in diameter. When the tube is in position in the stopper the lateral orifice should be at least 3 mm below the lower surface of the stopper. The upper end of the tube has a perfectly flat surface at right angles to the axis of the tube. A second glass tube of the same internal diameter and 30 mm long, with a similar flat surface, is placed in contact with the first and is held in position by two spiral springs or clips. Into the lower tube insert 50 to 60 mg of *lead acetate cotton*, loosely packed, or a small plug of cotton and a rolled piece of *lead acetate paper* weighing 50 to 60 mg. Between the flat surfaces of the tubes place a disc or a small square of *mercuric chloride paper* large enough to cover the orifice of the tube (15 × 15 mm).

Lead acetate is used to trap the H_2S gas which otherwise give the same yellow stain on reaction with mercuric chloride paper.

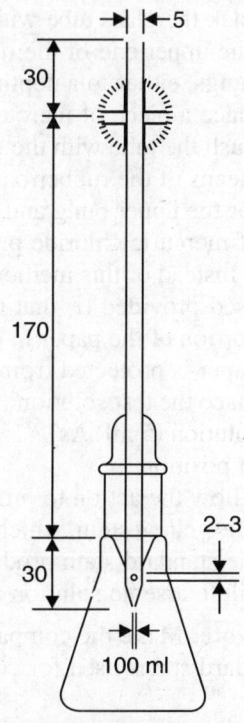

(Dimensions in mm)

Fig. 2.1: Apparatus for limit test for arsenic

Procedure

It consists of preparation of standard and test stain.

Standard Stain

Carry out the same procedure by taking the arsenic standard solution (10 ppm, As 1 ml) diluted to 50 ml with water.

Test Stain

Into a bottle or conical flask, introduce the test solution as directed in the individual monograph, add 1M KI solution (5 ml) and zinc AsT (10 g).

Immediately assemble the apparatus and immerse the flask in a water bath at a temperature such that a uniform evolution of gas is maintained. After 40 minutes, compare the intensity of stain with standard stain. After 40 minutes the yellow stain on the mercuric chloride paper is not more than that obtained by treating in the same manner 1.0 ml of arsenic standard solution (10 ppm As) diluted to 50 ml with water.

General Method of Testing

By a variable method of procedure, suitable to the particular needs of each substance, a solution is prepared from the substance being examined which may or may not contain that substance, but contains the whole of the arsenic (if any) originally present in that substance. This solution, referred to as the 'test solution', is used in the actual test.

Stepwise Procedure

1. Pack the glass tube with cotton wool, previously moistened with lead acetate solution.
2. The upper end of the tube is then inserted into the narrow end of one of the pair of rubber bungs, either to a depth of about 10 mm when the tube has a rounded off end, of the bung.
3. Place a piece of mercuric chloride paper in a flat condition on the top of the bung and the flush the tube with the larger end of the bung and place the other bung over it and secure by means of the rubber band or spring clip in such a manner that the borings of the two bungs (or the upper bung and the glass tube) meet to form a true tube, interrupted by a diaphragm of mercuric chloride paper.

   Instead of this method of attaching the mercuric chloride papar, any other method may be used provided (i) that the whole of the evolved gas passes through the paper; (ii) that the portion of the paper in contact with the gas is a circle, 6.5 mm in diameter; and (iii) that the paper is protected from sunlight during the test.
4. Place the test solution (prepared as specified) in wide mouthed bottle, add potassium iodide solution (5 ml) AsT (1 g) and zinc AsT (10 g) to it and place the prepared glass tube quickly in position.
5. Allow the action to proceed for 40 minutes.
6. The yellow stain, which is produced on the mercuric chloride paper if arsenic is present with the standard stain produced by operating in a similar manner with the known quantities of dilute arsenic solution AsT.

   Note: Make the comparison of the stains immediately after the completion of the test. The standard stains used for comparison should be freshly prepared.

Notes:

1. The action may be accelerated by placing the apparatus on a warm surface, care being taken that the mercuric chloride paper remains dry throughout the test.

2. The most suitable temperature for carrying out the test is generally about 40°C, but because the rate of evolution of the gas varies somewhat with different batches of zinc AsT, the temperature may be adjusted to obtain a regular, but not violent, evolution of gas.

3. The tube must be washed with hydrochloric acid AsT, rinsed with water, and dried between successive tests.

4. The stain may be preserved by dipping in hot melted paraffin or placing over phosphorus pentaoxide protected from light. Potassium iodide blackens the stains and makes the comparison easier.

5. Lead acetate papers are used to trap any hydrogen sulphide evolved together with arsine. Hydrogen sulphide reacts with mercuric chloride paper developing a dark stain, thus interfering with the formation of the required mercuric arsenide stain. Metallic zinc may contain traces of sulphide which on reaction with the acid yields hydrogen sulphide.

6. KI facilitates the release of nascent hydrogen from the reaction of zinc metal with HCl solution.

Standard arsenic solution (1.0 ppm As)

Dilute one volume of standard arsenic solution (10 ppm, As) to 10 volumes with water.

Arsenic standard solution (10 ppm As)

Dissolve arsenic trioxide (0.330 g) in 2M NaOH solution (5 ml) and dilute to 250.0 ml with water. Dilute 1 volume of this solution to 100 volumes with water.

Mercuric Chloride Paper

Smooth white paper not less than 25 mm in width, soaked in a saturated solution of mercuric chloride, pressed to remove superfluous solution and dried at about 60°C in the dark. The grade of the filter paper is such that the weight is between 65 and 120 g per sq mm, the thickness in mm of 400 papers is approximately equal to the weight in 'g' per sq m.

Note: Mercuric chloride should be stored in stoppered bottle in the dark. Paper which has been exposed to sunlight or to the vapours of ammonia afford a lighter stain or no stain at all when employed in the limit test for arsenic.

Stannated Hydrochloric Acid AsT

Stannous chloride solution AsT	1 ml
Hydrochloric acid AsT	100 ml

Potassium Iodide AsT

Potassium iodide which complies with the following additional test: Dissolve the substance (1 gm) in hydrochloric acid solution AsT (25 ml) and water (35 ml), add 2 drops of stannous chloride solution AsT and apply the general test, no visible stain is produced.

Standard Stains

Solutions are prepared by adding to 50 ml of water, 10 ml of stannated hydrochloric acid AsT and quantities of dilute arsenic solution AsT varying from 0.2 to 1 ml. The resulting solutions, when treated as described in the General test yield stains on the mercuric chloride paper referred to as the standard stain.

PREPARATION OF THE TEST SOLUTION

In the various methods of preparing the test solution, the quantities are so arranged, unless otherwise stated, that when the stain produced from the solution to be examined is not deeper than the standard stain obtained from 1 ml of arsenic standard solution (10 ppm) diluted to 50 ml with water, the proportion of arsenic present does not exceed the permitted limit.

MODIFICATION OF THE GENERAL TESTING METHOD FOR ARSENIC

Some substances require special treatment for performing limit test for arsenic. All the arsenic present in the sample should be present in the final solution in a readily reducible form and the interfering substances should be removed from test sample.

CARBONATES, HYDROXIDES AND OXIDES

Treatment of carbonates with hydrochloric acid produces carbon dioxide and some hydrochloric acid gas with effervescence and the reaction is exothermic. Oxides and hydroxides on treatment with hydrochloric acid from hydrogen gas with effervescence and evolution of heat. Arsenious chloride ($AsCl_3$) is evolved with hydrochloric acid. If a sample of these substances is treated with hydrochloric acid as such, a part of arsenic may be lost as $AsCl_3$. Therefore, carbonates, oxides and hydroxides are first treated with excess of brominated hydrochloric acid. The bromine oxidizes arsenious to arsenic to the pentavalent form which is not volatile with hydrochloric acid. To perform the test, the arsenic should again be reduced to arsenious state by removing excess of bromine with a few drops of stannous chloride solution.

Sodium Carbonate, Anhydrous, AsT

Anhydrous sodium carbonate should complied the following additional test: Dissolve anhydrous sodium carbonate AsT (5 g) in water (50 ml) and then add brominated hydrochloric acid solution AsT (20 ml) to it. Remove the excess of bromine with a few drops of Stannous chloride solution AsT, and apply the General test. There should be no visible stain.

ORGANIC COMPOUNDS

Most of the organic compounds are insoluble in acid as well as in water. When gas is evolved in the liquid containing such compounds, undesirable frothing occurs. Therefore, any such organic compound should be removed by igniting with anhydrous sodium carbonate before performing the test. Some organic compounds are destroyed be wet oxidation with nitric and sulphuric acids.

Ammonium Oxalate AsT

Ammonium oxalate should complied with the following additional test: Heat ammonium oxalate (5 g) with water (15 ml), nitric acid solution AsT (5 ml), and sulphuric acid solution AsT (10 ml) in a narrow-necked, round-bottomed flask until frothing ceases, cool and apply the General test. There should be no visible stain.

NITRIC ACID AND NITRATES

Nitric acid and nitrates prevent the reduction of arsenic which are removed by heating the substance with concentrated sulphuric acid and evaporating nitric acid off. Arsenic is left in the sulphuric acid. The remaining traces of nitric acid are removed by diluting residual sulphuric acid with water and re-evaporating the mixture. Now the nitrosylsulphuric acid formed during first evaporation is decomposed and the sulphuric acid becomes free from nitric acid. Solution of ferric chloride also contains some nitric acid which is also removed by the similar treatment.

Nitric Acid AsT

Nitric acid should complied the following additional test: Heat nitric acid solution AsT (20 ml) in a porcelain dish with sulphuric acid AsT (2 ml) until white fumes are given off. Cool, add water (2 ml) to it and again heat until white fumes are given off. Cool, add water (50 ml) and stannated hydrochloric acid AsT (10 ml) to it and apply the General test. There should be no visible stain.

BORIC ACID AND BORAX

Boric acid is slightly soluble in hydrochloric acid, but it is dissolved along with citric acid. Borax is converted into boric acid on treatment with hydrochloric acid. Therefore, citric acid is added to dissolve boric acid and borax before addition of stannated hydrochloric acid.

AMMONIA SOLUTION

Solutions are heated on a water bath to remove the free ammonia. Arsenic is left as ammonium arsenate and arsenite in the solution which are acidified with brominated hydrochloric acid and stannous chloride is added.

LIQUID GLUCOSE AND POTASSIUM ACID TARTARATE

Liquid glucose often contains traces of sulphur dioxide as preservative while sulphite are present in potassium acid tartarate. These substances are treated with brominated hydrochloric acid to oxidize the sulphurous acid. Excess of bromine is removed by adding a few drops of stannous chloride solution.

HYPOPHOSPHORUS ACID

Reduction of hypophosphorus acid yields phosphine which interacts with mercuric halide papers. Hence, it is oxidized to phosphoric acid by treating with potassium chlorate and hydrochloric acid. Excess of chloride formed by the reaction of chlorate and hydrochloric acid is removed by boiling and then by treating with stannous chloride.

OXIDIZING AGENTS

The oxidizing agents such as potassium chlorate should be completely reduced, otherwise, whole of the hydrogen will be utilized to reduce the substance and arsine would not be evolved.

Potassium Chlorate AsT

Potassium chlorate should complied the following additional test: Mix the substance (5 g) with cold water (20 ml) and then add hydrochloric acid solution AsT (22 ml) ; when the first reaction has subsided, heat gently to expel chlorine, remove the last traces with a few drops of stannous chloride solution AsT; add water (20 ml) and apply the General test. There should be no visible stain.

COMPOUNDS OF COPPER, BISMUTH, ANTIMONY AND IRON

Copper deposits on zinc forming a zinc–copper mixture which interfere in the steady evolution of hydrogen and all the arsenic will not convert into arsine. Bismuth deposits on zinc forming a solid sponge-like mass preventing evolution of hydrogen. Antimony compounds form antimony hydride with nascent hydrogen which produces a dark stain on mercuric chloride paper interfering with the stain developed due to arsine. Iron also reduces the rate of evolution of hydrogen and arsenic is not reduced completely to arsine.

Copper, bismuth and iron salts are treated with dilute hydrochloride acid (205) and distilled. Whole of the arsenic in the substance distills in the first 75% distillate. Sufficient stannous chloride is added to reduce ferric salts to ferrous state.

A double distillation is required to perform the test of antimony compounds since antimony is slightly volatile in hydrochloric acid.

SULPHUR

Sulphur is present as arsenic sulphide which is soluble in ammonium sulphide and ammonia. Therefore, digest sulphur with ammonia to form ammonium polysulphides in which arsenic sulphide is soluble. Filter the mixture to separate undissolved sulphur and discard the filtrate. Treat the residue containing arsenic and some sulphur with anhydrous sodium carbonate and water. Sodium polysulphide is formed in which arsenic sulphide is soluble. Boil the solution and add bromine to oxidize arsenic to arsenate and sulphide to sulphate. Acidify the solution, boil and treat with stannous chloride to perform the General tests.

Titrimetric Analysis

Titrimetric analysis is the quantitative chemical analysis, performed by determining the volume of a solution of accurately known concentration required to react quantitatively with the solutions of substance to be analysed. The solution of known strength is called a **standard solution** which is usually taken in burette. The process of addition of a standard solution to a solution (to be analysed) until the reaction is just complete is called *titration*, and the substance to be analysed is called a *titrant*. The point at which the reaction is completed is called the *equivalent point* or *end point* which is detected by addition of an *indicator*. On completion of this reaction, the indicator gives a clear visual colour change in the liquid being titrated.

Standard solution

A standard solution contains a known weight of the reagent in a definite volume of solvent. The concentration of standard solution is generally expressed either in terms of molarity or normality.

Molarity (M)

A molar solution contains *1 g molecular weight of substance per litre of solution.* For example, 1M HCl solution contains 36.5 g of HCl in one litre solution. The strength of molar solutions are independent of the reaction.

Normality

A normal solution is a solution which contains one *gram equivalent of substance per litre of solution.* For example, 1N HCl solution contains one equivalent weight (36.5 g) of HCl and 1N H_2SO_4 solution contains 49 g of H_2SO_4. The strength of the solutions are designated as: two normal (2N), half normal (0.5N or N/2), decinormal (0.1N or N/10) and centinormal (0.01N or N/100).

Equivalent weight

The equivalent weight of an acid or base is that weight of it which contain 1.008 g of replacable hydrogen or its equivalent, such as hydroxyl group. The equivalent weights of hydrochloric acid (HCl) and sodium hydroxide (NaOH) are equal of their molecular weights (36.5 and 40 mol. wt.).

Sulphuric acid (H_2SO_4) and oxalic acid, $(COOH)_2$ contain two replacable hydrogens, therefore, their equivalent weights are equal to half of their respective molecular weights.

The equivalent weight of a base is that mass of it which contains one replacable hydroxyl group, i.e. 17.008 g equivalent to 1.008 g of hydrogen. The equivalents of sodium hydroxide and potassium hydroxide are the same to the molecular weight 1 mole (M) = 1 equivalent (N); calcium hydroxide and barium hydroxide are half a mole (1.0N = 0.5M).

In oxidation-reduction titrations, the equivalent weight is that weight which combines with 1.008 g of available hydrogen or 8.008 g of available oxygen for use in the oxidation or reduction reaction under consideration.

In precipitation reaction, as in argentimetry, the equivalent weight is defined as that weight of substance which contains or combines with 1 g atom of a univalent metal.

CALCULATION OF EQUIVALENT WEIGHT

Acid and Base

1. Hydrochloric Acid

HCl = H

Therefore, $(1 + 35.45) = 36.45$ g HCl $\equiv$ 1000 ml of 1.0N solution

2. Sodium Carbonate

$$Na_2CO_3 + 2HCl \rightarrow 2NaCl + H_2O + CO_2$$

Therefore, $Na_2CO_3 \equiv 2HCl \equiv 2H$ (replaceable hydrogens)

$(2 \times 23 + 12 + 3 \times 16) = 106$ g of $Na_2CO_3 = 2000$ ml N HCl

or   53 g $Na_2CO_3 = 1000$ ml of 1.0N solution

Oxidizing and Reducing Agents

1. Sodium Acid Oxalate

The equivalent weight varies with the reaction under consideration:

(i) **As a Neutralizing Agent**

$$NaHC_2O_4 + NaOH \rightarrow Na_2C_2O_4 + H_2O$$

Therefore, $NaHC_2O_4 \equiv NaOH \equiv H$

$(23 + 1 + 24 + 64) = 112$ g $NaHC_2O_4 = 1000$ ml of 1.0N NaOH solution

(ii) **As a Reducing Agent** $C_2O_4^- \longrightarrow 2CO_2 + 2e$

In the above reaction, there is a loss of two electrons.

$(23 + 1 + 24 + 64) = 112$ g $NaHC_2O_4$

One half mole, $112/2 = 56$ g, is the equivalent weight of anhydrous sodium acid oxalate.

2. Potassium Permanganate

The equivalent weight varies with the pH of the reaction media.

(i) **In acidic media** $MnO_4^- + 8H^+ + 5e \longrightarrow Mn^{++} + H_2O$

For oxidation, it consume 5 electrons.

Therefore, the equivalent weight of the $KMnO_4$ is one-fifth of the molecular weight or

$\dfrac{158}{5} = 31.6$ or 32 g.

(ii) In neutral or faintly alkaline media Mn^{+7} changes into Mn^{+4}; there is gain of 3 electrons. For oxidation, it consumes three electron. Therefore, the equivalent weight of the $KMnO_4$ is one-third of the molecular weight or $\dfrac{158}{3} = 52.66$ or 53 g.

(iii) In highly basic media, there is involvement of one electron only; so equivalent weight = $\dfrac{158}{1} = 158.$ Therefore, the equivalent weight of $KMnO_4$ is equal to molecular weight.

EQUIVALENCE OF STANDARD SOLUTIONS

If an acid 'A' of volume V_A is titrated against a base 'B' of volume V_B to neutrality, then since the two solutions contain the same number of gram equivalents at end point,

$$V_A \times normality_A = V_B \times normality_B$$

If the normality of one solution is known, the equivalent volumes of two solutions are determined by titration, and the normality of the second solution can be determined.

PREPARATION OF STANDARD SOLUTIONS

Primary Standard

If a chemical compound is available in pure state (primary standard), weigh an exact equivalent amount, dissolve in water and make up to volume. The compounds, which are not available in pure state (secondary standard), e.g. caustic soda, mineral acids, iodine, potassium permanganate,

Table 3.1: Equivalent weights of some acids/bases and oxidizing agents/reducing agents

Compound	Molecular weight	Acidity/Basicity/loss or gain of electrons	Equivalent weight
Hydrochloric acid	36.46	1	36.46
Nitric acid	63.01	1	63.01
Sulphuric acid	98.07	2	49.03
Acetic acid	60.05	1	60.05
Boric acid	61.83	3	20.61
Sodium hydroxide	40.0	1	40.00
Potassium hydroxide	56.11	1	56.11
Sodium carbonate	105.99	2	53.00
Sodium bicarbonate	84.01	1	84.01
Potassium carbonate	138.21	2	69.10
Potassium bicarbonate	100.12	1	100.12
Potassium permanganate	158.03	5	31.61
Potassium dichromate	294.18	6	49.03
Iodine	253.8	2	126.90
Oxalic acid (anhydrous)	90.0	2	45.00
Oxalic acid (dihydrate)	126.07	2	63.03
Ferrous sulphate (anhydrous)	152.0	1	152.00
Ferrous sulphate (heptahydrate)	278.0	1	278.00
Ferrous ammonium sulphate	392.13	1	392.13
Sodium thiosulphate (pentahydrate)	248.17	1	248.17

* in acidic medium

etc. are prepared a little more concentrated than are required, diluted with distilled water until the desired normality is obtained. These secondary standard solutions must be standardized. The compound available in highly pure form and suitable for the preparation of standard solutions are sodium carbonate, sodium tetraborate, sodium oxalate, sodium chloride, potassium chloride, potassium bromate, potassium iodate, potassium dichromate, arsenic (III) oxide, benzoic acid, succinic acid and potassium hydrogen phthalate.

When the reagent is not available in the pure form, e.g. most alkali solutions, some inorganic acids, deliquescent substances, etc., solutions of the approximate normality required are first prepared. These solution are then standardized by titrating against a solution of a pure substance of known concentration (standard solution/primary standard).

Factors

The standard solutions are only approximately 1N, 0.5N and 0.1, etc. The relationship of the exact strength of such a solution to the nominal normality of the solution is then indicated by a factor, defined as the number of millimeters of exactly 1N, 0.5N, etc., solutions which are equivalent to 1 ml of the solution of the same nominal normality. It is the number by which the actual volume of the solution of approximate strength must be multiplied to obtain the equivalent volume of a standard solution of exact normality. For example:

Factor in Standardization of approximate 1N H_2SO_4 by 1N Na_2CO_3

If 20 ml of N Na_2CO_3 solution is neutralized by 19.40 ml of 1N H_2SO_4,

Then 19.40 ml of $H_2SO_4 \equiv$ 20 ml N Na_2CO_3

Therefore, 1 ml N $H_2SO_4 \equiv \dfrac{20}{19.40}$ ml N $\equiv$ 1.031 ml N Na_2CO_3 solution

Therefore, the strength of the H_2SO_4 solution is N (1.031). The factor of the solution is 1.031 and all volumes of this solution when multiplies by 1.031 will be the equipment volume of normal solution.

REACTIONS IN TITRIMETRIC ANALYSIS

Two types of reactions are involved in titrimetric analysis:

(a) Those in which there is no change in oxidation state, these are dependent upon the combination of ions.
(b) Oxidation-reduction reactions in which a change of oxidation state is involved.

Generally, these two types of reactions are divided into four main classes:

(a) Acidimetry and alkalimetry or neutralization reaction
(b) Complex formation reactions
(c) Precipitation reactions
(d) Oxidation-reduction reactions.

ACIDIMETRY AND ALKALIMETRY OR NEUTRALIZATION REACTION

A neutralization reaction involves the titration of free bases with a standard acid (acidimetry) or the titration of free acid with a standard base (alkalimetry). These reactions include the combination of hydrogen and hydroxide ion to form water. The point at which this is reached is called the **equivalence point or theoretical end-point.** If both the acid and base are strong electrolytes, the resultant solution will be neutral and have a pH of 7. If either the acid or the base is a weak electrolyte, the salt will be hydrolyzed to only some extent and the solutions at the equivalence point will be either slightly alkaline or slightly acidic.

The acid base indicators give different colours, depending on the hydrogen-ion concentration of the solution, and the position of the colour-change interval in the pH scale varies widely with different indicators.

In aqueous medium/solution, an acid is dissociated into hydrogen ion and an anion (Cl^-, HSO_4^-, NO_3^-, etc.).

$$HCl \rightleftharpoons H^+ + Cl^- \rightleftharpoons H_3O^+$$

The hydrogen ion combines with water to give hydronium ion (H_3O^+).

An alkali on dissociation in water gives hydroxyl ions,

$$NaOH \rightleftharpoons Na^+ + OH^-$$

The neutralization reaction is the reaction between an acid and a base to give a salt. (also the solution is electrically neutral)

$$HCl + NaOH \longrightarrow NaCl + H_2O$$

Preparation of Indicator Solutions

In most cases, 70–90% ethanol is used to prepare indicator solution. However, if indicator is water soluble (like sodium salt), water may also be used.

- *Methyl orange*: Dissolve methyl orange (0.5 g) (free acid) in 1 litre of water and filter, if necessary. When methyl orange is in the salt form, dissolve sodium salt (0.5 g) in 1 litre of water, add 0.1M HCl (15 ml) and filter, if necessary.
- *Methyl red*: Dissolve free acid (1 g) in 1 litre of hot water or in 600 ml of ethanol and dilute with sufficient water to make up 1 litre.
- *Phenolphthalein*: Dissolve the reagent (5 g) in 500 ml of ethanol and add water (500 ml) with constant stirring. Filter off the precipitate if formed.
- *Thymolphthalein*: Dissolve a reagent (0.5 g) in 600 ml of ethanol and add sufficient water to make up 1 litre.
- *1-Naphthalein*: Dissolve a indicator (0.1 g) in 500 ml of ethanol and dilute with sufficient water to make up 1 litre.
- *Quinaldine red*: Dissolve 1 g in 100 ml of 80% ethanol.
- *Methyl yellow, Neutral red, and Congo red:* Dissolve a indicator (1.0 g) in 1 litre of 80% ethanol. Congo Red may also be dissolved in water.
- *4-Niitrophenol:* Dissolve 2 g of the reagent in 1 litre of water.
- *Alizarin yellow R:* Dissolve the indicator (0.5 g) in 1 litre of 80% ethanol.
- *Tropaeolin:* Dissolve 1 g of the solid in 1 litre of water.
- *Mixed indicator:* Mixed indicators are used to get sharp colour change over narrow and selected range of pH by the use of suitable mixture of indicators. For example, a mixture of equal parts of neutral red (0.1% in ethanol) and methylene blue gives a sharp colour change from violet-blue to green at pH 7. This indicator is used in the titration of acetic acid with ammonia solution or vice versa. A mixture of phenolphthalein (3 parts of a 0.1% aqueous solution of the sodium salt) and cresol red (1 part of a 0.1% aqueous solution of the sodium salt) changes its colour from yellow to violet at pH 8.3 and is recommended for the titration of carbonate to the hydrogen carbonate stage.

Preparation and standardization of 1N H₂SO₄ solution

Add slowly, with stirring sulphuric acid (30 ml) to about 1000 ml of water. Allow to cool to 25°C.

Sulphuric acid is a dibasic acid so 1000 ml of 1N H_2SO_4 solution should contain 98.08/2 = 49.04 g or 1 equivalent of sulphuric acid. Sulphuric acid has percentage purity of about 95% w/v and specific gravity of about 1.83 at 25°C. According to this, 30 ml of the concentrated sulphuric acid should contain about 30 × 1.83 × 95 = 52.15 g of H_2SO_4.

Note: Alternate method: Concentrated sulphuric acid which is usually available is a 36N solution. For preparation of 1N H₂SO₄, transfer this acid (about 28 ml) into 600 ml of water dropwise into 1 litre flask. Make up the volume to 1.0 litre to make 1N H₂SO₄ solution.

$$N_1V_1 = N_2V_2$$

$$36 \times V_1 = 1.0 \times 1000$$

$$V_1 = \frac{1.0 \times 1000}{36} = 27.77 \text{ ml}$$

For standardization, weigh accurately about 1.5 g of anhydrous sodium carbonate previously heated in a nickel crucible at 270°C for 1 hr to remove any trace of water. Cool in a desiccator, weigh, dissolve in 100 ml of water, add 0.1 ml of methyl orange indicator and titrate with sulphuric acid solution until the solution becomes pink. Heat the solution to boiling, cool and continue the titration. Heat again to boiling and titrate further as necessary until the faint pink column persists, uneffected by continued boiling.

The normality of sulphuric acid is calculated as follows:

$$N = \frac{\text{Weight of sodium carbonate (g)}}{\text{Volume of H}_2\text{SO}_4 \text{ solution consumed} \times 0.053}$$

where 0.053 is the milliequivalent weight of sodium carbonate.

Sodium carbonate contain varying amount of moisture and sodium bicarbonate. Hence, it is heated to evaporate off the moisture and convert the $NaHCO_3$ into Na_2CO_3.

$$2NaHCO_3 \longrightarrow Na_2CO_3 + H_2O + CO_2\uparrow$$

The titrated solution is boiled to expell out the CO_2 which may cause hinderance in observing the end point.

The reaction involved in the titration of sulphuric acid with sodium carbonate, is

$$H_2SO_4 + Na_2CO_3 \longrightarrow Na_2SO_4 + CO_2 + H_2O$$

Note: Alternatively, 1N sulphuric acid solution can be standardized by titrating with 1N sodium carbonate solution by using methyl orange as indicator. The 1N sodium carbonate solution is prepared by dissolving 53 g of sodium carbonate in 1 litre of water. The normality is calculated out by applying the formula.

$$N_1V_1 = N_2V_2$$

$$(Na_2CO_3) = (\text{Approximate 1N H}_2SO_4 \text{ solution})$$

$$N_2 = \frac{N_1V_1}{V_2}$$

Preparation and Standardization of 1N HCl Solution

Concentrated hydrochloric acid is roughly a 11N solution. For preparation of 1N HCl solution, transfer this acid (about 90 ml) into 1 litre flask and dilute it to 1000 ml with water. Shake it thoroughly before standardization.

$$N_1 V_1 = N_2 V_2$$
$$11 \times V_1 = 1.0 \times 1000$$
$$V_1 = \frac{1.0 \times 1000}{11} = 90.9 \text{ ml}$$

Note: It can also be prepared by weight method. Hydrochloric acid is a monobasic acid so 1000 ml of 1N HCl solution should contain 36.5 g of acid or 1 equivalent weight of HCl. It has percentage purity of 36.6% and specific gravity of about 1.14 at 25°C temperature. Accordingly, 90 ml of the concentrated HCl contain $90 \times 1.14 \times 36.5 = 37.44$ g of HCl.

For standardization, same procedure may be followed as in standardization of sulphuric acid.

Preparation and Standardization of 1N NaOH Solution

Dissolve 40 g of NaOH in sufficient carbon dioxide free water to produce 1000 ml.

The 40 g of NaOH is equivalent to 1 g equivalent weight of sodium hydroxide. This quantity is required to prepare 1000 ml of 1N solution. But more than 1 equivalent, 40.0 g of NaOH is weighed out due to its hygroscopic nature.

For standardization, weigh accurately about 5 g of potassium hydrogen phthalate, previously powdered and dried at 120°C for 2 hours and dissolve in 75 ml of CO_2 free water; add 0.1 ml of phenolphthalein solution and titrate with NaOH solution until permanent pink colour appears.

According to IP method, sodium hydroxide is standardized by titration against primary standard potassium hydrogen phthalate.

$$C_6H_4(COOH)(COOK) + NaOH \longrightarrow C_6H_4(COONa)(COOK) + H_2O$$

Potassium hydrogen phthalate

$$\text{Normality of NaOH} = \frac{\text{Weight of } KHC_8H_4O_4 \text{ (g)}}{\text{Volume of NaOH consumed} \times 0.20423}$$

where 0.20423 is the milliequivalent weight of potassium hydrogen phthalate.

Note: Sodium hydroxide can also be standardized by titration against primary standards like succinic acid, oxalic acid, benzoic acid, or standardized hydrochloric acid.

COMPLEX FORMATION REACTIONS

Complexometric titrations involving complex formation reactions, have found important applications in analysis of pharmaceuticals especially for metal ion such as Al, Ca, Mg, Zn, etc.

Complexometric titrations involve the reaction in which simple metal ion is transformed into a complex ion by addition of a complexing agent. The complexing agent is an electron donating group or ion, which by its ability to form one or more covalent bond with the metal ion to form a complex. The complexes have different property from those of free metal ion. The bonds are either ordinary covalent bond (in which both the metal and ligand contribute one electron) or coordinate bond (in which both electrons are contributed by the ligand).

Complex involving simple ligands that is those forming only one bond, are described as coordination compounds. Ligands having more than one electron donating group are called chelating agents. The ethylenediaminetetra-acetic acid (EDTA) is a best example of chelating agents widely used in complexometric titration (Fig. 2.1). Ethylene diamine, dimethylglyoxime and salicylaldoxime are other complex forming agents.

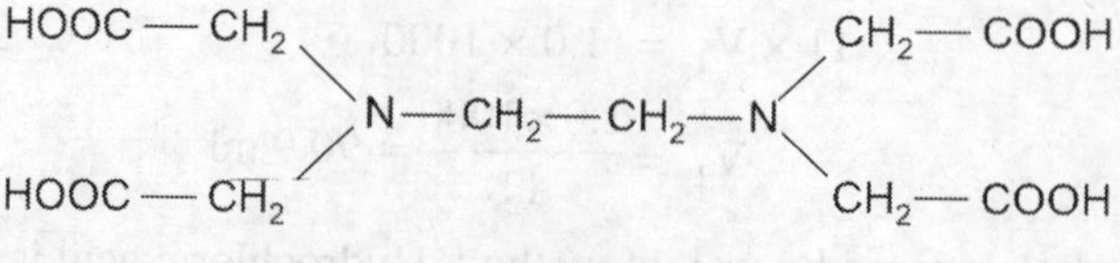

EDTA

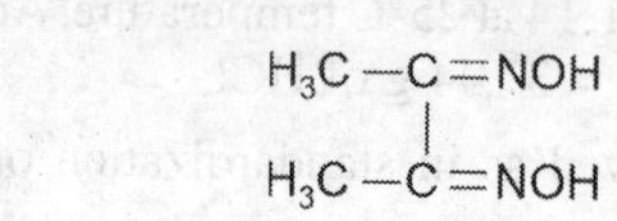

Dimethylglyoxime 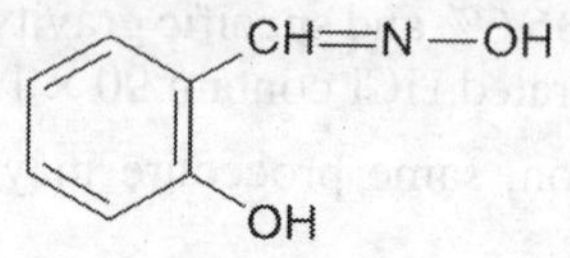   Salicylaldoxime

Fig. 3.1: Complex forming agents

Stability of Complexes

The stability of complex is driving factor for complexometric titration. The general equation for the formation of 1 : 1 chelate complex, MX is:

$$M + X \rightleftharpoons MX$$

where M is the metal and X is the chelating ion. The stability constant is:

$$K = \frac{[MX]}{[M][X]}$$

End Point Detection

The end point of complexometric titration is detected by metallic indicator, designated as pM. The pM indicator is a dye which is capable of acting as chelating agent to give dye-metal complex. This complex is different in colour from the dye itself and has lower stability constant than the chelate-metal complex. The colour of the solution remains that of dye complex until the end point when a equivalent amount of disodium salt of EDTA (complexing agent) is added. As soon as there is a slight excess of EDTA salt, the metal dye complex decomposes to produce free dye. This is accomplished by change in colour. The colour of dye and of metal complex vary with the pH, therefore it is also essential to buffer the solution to maintain the required pH.

The end point of complexometric titrations can also be determined by some physical methods like potentiometric, amperometric, conductometric, etc.

pM INDICATORS

Murexide

Murexide is ammonium purpurate which is used for the titration of calcium at pH 12. Calcium is bound in an eight-membered ring in the murexide chelate which is less stable in comparison to five and six membered ring chelates. Since magnesium–murexide is less stable then the calcium complex, calcium can be titrated in the presence of magnesium as in water analysis.

Murexide (violet at pH 12)   Calcium murexide complex

Copper, cobalt and cerium from yellow complexes with murexide in alkaline solution. They give clear colour changes when titrated with sodium edetate.

Mordant Black 2 (Eriochrome Black T)

This indicator is blue at about pH 10 and most of its complexes are reddish. Below pH 6.3 and above pH 11.5, the dye itself is reddish. The titration is carried out in the presence of a buffer at pH 10.

Blue (pH 10)   Pink $+ 2H^+$

Magnesium, calcium, cadmium, zinc, manganese, lead and mercury are titrated directly using this indicator. Cobalt, nickel, copper, aluminium, silver, titanium and platinum form more stable complexes with the dye than with the edetate. Therefore, the dye cannot be used as an indicator.

Catechol Violet

The catechols form weak, highly-coloured complexes in neutral, acid and alkaline solutions. All these complexes are blue coloured in alkaline solution. In this solution, clear end points are shown with magnesium, manganese, iron, cobalt, nickel, zinc, cadmium and calcium.

Catechol violet
(Blue colour at pH 10)

Xylenol Orange

This is an acid-base indicator having the same characteristics as cresol red. It is used to titrate metal whose edetate complexes are stable in acid solution, e.g. bismuth, thorium, lead, lanthanum, cadmium and mercury. The stability of the complexes varies with pH.

Methyl Thymol Blue

It is derived from thymol blue and used for titration of bismuth in strongly acid solution and for lead, zinc, cadmium, mercury and cobalt in weakly acid solution.

Alizarin Fluorine Blue

It is used in acidic solution at pH 4.3 for the titration of lead (Pb^{2+}), zinc (Zn^{2+}), cobalt (Co^{2+}), mercury (Hg^{2+}) and copper (Cu^{2+}) when the colour changes from red to yellow. It is also used in the determination of fluorine in some synthetic drugs.

Alizarin fluorine blue
(3,4-Dihydroxy-2-anthraquinoyl methyl iminodiacetic acid)

Sodium Alizarine sulphonate (alizarin red)

It yields a bluish-red colour with aluminium and thorium ions at pH 4 and a yellow in the absence of these ions. It is used to determine fluorine in triamcinolone by titration with standard thorium nitrate solution.

Sodium alizarine sulphonate
(yellow colour)

Diphenylcarbazone

It is used an indicator for determination of mercury in methyl thiouracil.

$$C_6H_5N = NCONHC_6H_5$$
Diphenylcarbazone

Tiron

It forms a blue colour with ferric iron between pH 2 and 5, a violet colour between pH 5.7 and 7 and a red complex in alkaline solution.

Tiron
(1,3-Benzene disulphonic acid,
4,5-dihydroxy disodium salt)

Types of EDTA Titrations

A. Direct titration

The metallic ions are directly titrated with standard EDTA solution, by using a metallic indicator. The estimation of calcium gluconate is an example of direct titration.

B. Back titration

In thus, an excess of standard EDTA solution is added. The resulting solution is buffered to desired pH and the excess of EDTA is back titrated with standard metal ion solution by using metallic indicator. The determination of calcium phosphate is example of back titration. The EDTA (excess) is added to the calcium phosphate solution and the resulting solution is buffered to pH 10 by adding ammonia buffer and then titrated with standard $ZnCl_2$ solution by using mordant black II as indicator.

C. Replacement titration

In this titration, metal may be determined by the displacement of an equivalent amount of magnesium or zinc from a less staple edetate complex. For example, the calcium in sodium calcium edetate is determined by titration with standard lead nitrate solution.

D. Alkalimetric titration

In this method, protons from disodium edetate are displaced by a heavy metal and acidity produced due to the liberated protons is titrated with standard alkali solution.

PREPARATION AND STANDARDIZATION OF 0.1M DISODIUM EDETATE SOLUTION

Dissolve 37.2 g of disodium edetate in sufficient water to produce 1000 ml.

The disodium salt of ethylenediaminetetra-acetic acid is preferred due to purity reason. EDTA titrant solutions are generally stored in polyethylene or borosilicate glass containers.

For standardization, dissolve granulated zinc (0.8 g) in dilute hydrochloric acid (12 ml) and bromine water (0.1 ml) by gentle warming. Boil to remove excess of bromine, cool and add sufficient water to produce 200 ml. Pipette 20 ml of the resulting solution into a flask and neutralize with 2M sodium hydroxide solution. Dilute the solution with water (150 ml), and add sufficient ammonia buffer to maintain the pH to 10. Add mordant black II mixture (50 mg) and titrate with disodium edetate until the solution turns blue.

The standardization of 0.1M disodium edetate solution is based on titration of the prepared disodium edetate solution with a standard zinc chloride solution prepared from a known weight of granulated zinc.

Bromine solution is added to ensure oxidation of trace impurity of trace iron (II) to iron (III), which forms a much less stable edetate complex than iron (II).

$$Zn + 2HCl \longrightarrow ZnCl_2 + H_2\uparrow$$

$$ZnCl_2 + C_{10}H_{14}N_2Na_2O_8 \longrightarrow C_{10}H_{14}N_2O_8Zn + 2NaCl$$

A suitable buffer solution and indicator are added to the metal ion solution and the solution titrated with standard disodium edetate until the indicator just changes colour.

Ammonia buffer

Dissolve 70 g of ammonium chloride in 570 ml concentrated ammonia solution and dilute to 1 litre with distilled water.

Factor: Each ml of 0.1M disodium edetate is equivalent to 0.000654 g of zinc.

PRECIPITATION REACTIONS

It involves the formation of precipitates by the titrants as in silver nitrate titration. Most precipitation reactions involve the silver cation, Ag^+. Silver chloride precipitation is rapid and quantitative.

Silver Nitrate Titration (Direct and Indirect method)

In a direct method, silver nitrate solution is run into a solution of sodium chloride (to be analysed), a precipitates of silver chloride are formed:

$$NaCl + AgNO_3 \longrightarrow AgCl \downarrow + NaNO_3$$
$$K_2CrO_4 + 2AgNO_3 \longrightarrow Ag_2Cr_2O_4 \downarrow + 2KNO_3$$
(Red colour)

   At the end point, due to complete precipitation of chloride as silver chloride, a slight excess of silver nitrate react with potassium chromate (indicator) to give a precipitates of red coloured silver chromate.

   In the indirect method, accurately measured excess of standard silver nitrate solution is added to a solution of the halide, for the complete precipitation of halide as silver halide. The excess of silver nitrate is then back titrated with ammonium thiocyanate. At the end point, a slight excess of ammonium thiocyanate reacts with ferric alum to give red colour due to formation of ferric ferrithiocyanate:

$$AgNO_3 + NH_4SCN \longrightarrow AgSCN \downarrow + NH_4NO_3$$
$$2Fe^{3+} + 6SCN^- \rightleftharpoons Fe^{3+}[Fe(SCN)_6]^{3-}$$
(Red colour)

Preparation and standardization of 0.1N AgNO₃ solution

Dissolve silver nitrate (17.0 g) in sufficient water to produce 1000 ml.

   Silver nitrate AR has a purity of 99.9% so standard solution can be prepared by direct weighing. However, commercial grade silver nitrate need standardization.

   For standardization, weigh accurately NaCl (about 0.1 g), previously dried at 110°C for 2 hours and dissolve in water (5 ml). Add acetic acid (5 ml), methanol (50 ml) and eosin solution (0.15 ml). Stir and titrate with 0.1N AgNO₃ solution until change in colour.

   It is an IP official method; standardization is done by direct titration with sodium chloride by using adsorption indicator—eosin. Acetic acid is used to get the sharp end point. At the end point, pink colour appears due to adsorption of indicator—eosin (Fig. 3.2). Sodium chloride is slightly hygroscopic so it is dried before use.

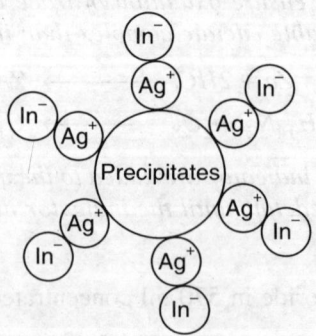

Fig. 3.2: Adsorption of indicator (In⁻) at the end point

$$AgNO_3 + NaCl \longrightarrow AgCl\downarrow + NaNO_3$$

$$AgNO_3 \equiv NaCl \equiv H$$

169.89 g $AgNO_3 \equiv 58.45$ g NaCl $\equiv 1000$ ml N of $AgNO_3$ solution

Therefore, 0.01699 g $AgNO_3 \equiv 0.005845$ g NaCl $\equiv 1$ ml 0.1N $AgNO_3$ solution.

Preparation and standardization of 0.1N NH₄SCN solution

Dissolve ammonium thiocyanate (7.612 g) in sufficient water and then dilute with water to produce 1000 ml.

For standardization, pipette out 20 ml of 0.1N $AgNO_3$ solution into a glass stoppered flask, dilute with 50 ml of water, add 2 ml of HNO_3 and 2 ml of ferric ammonium sulphate (indicator) solution and titrate with ammonium thiocyanate solution till red brown coloured precipitate appears.

Ammonium thiocyanate is available as deliquescent solid so standardized by direct titration against silver nitrate, using ferric alum as indicator.

OXIDATION-REDUCTION REACTIONS

Oxidation and reduction reactions can be defined in terms of loss or gain of electrons. Reactions in which electrons are transferred from one species to another are called oxidation-reduction (redox) reactions. When one species loses electrons by oxidation process another species simultaneously gains electrons by reduction process in chemical reactions. Consider, e.g. the displacement of Br^- from a bromide salt by chlorine:

$$Cl_2 + 2Br^- \longrightarrow 2Cl^- + Br_2\uparrow$$

Each Cl atom in Cl_2 molecule is reduced as it gain one electron to become Cl^- ion.

$$Cl^\circ + 1e^- \longrightarrow Cl^- \text{ (Reduction)}$$

The oxidation number of Cl decreases from 0 to –1. At the same time a Br^- ion is oxidized to a Br atom as it loses one electron. The oxidation number of Br increases from –1 to 0.

$$Br^- \longrightarrow Br^\circ + 1e^- \text{ (Oxidation)}$$

When two half reactions are added together and balanced, 2Cl atom in Cl_2 gain 2 electrons and $2Br^-$ ion lose 2 electrons to form a Br_2 molecule and $2Cl^-$ ions. Cl_2 acts as an oxidizing agent because it accept electrons from $2Br^-$ ions and causes the Br^- ion to be oxidized, the Br^- ions act as reducing agent because they lose their electrons to Cl_2 and causes the Cl_2 to be reduced.

The more complex redox reaction between $KMnO_4$ and $(COOH)_2$ is:

$$2KMnO_4 + 5(COOH)_2 + 3H_2SO_4 \longrightarrow 10CO_2 + 2MnSO_4 + K_2SO_4 + 8H_2O$$

We can separate this equation into two half cell reactions.

$$2MnO_4^- + 16H^+ + 10e^- \longrightarrow 2Mn^{2+} + 8H_2O \text{ (Reduction)}$$

$$5(COOH)_2 \longrightarrow 10CO_2 + 10H^+ + 10e^- \text{ (Oxidation)}$$

Note, in the half cell equation, that the number of electrons gained (10) is equal to the number of electron lost (10), you will use the stiochiometry of the balanced equation to calculate the molarity of the $KMnO_4$ solution. The calculated molarity of the $KMnO_4$ will then be used to calculate the molarity of unknown oxalic acid solution. Molarity is the most commonly used concentration term when analyst is interested in the amount of materials involved in a chemical reaction in solution. Molarity (M) is defined as the number of moles of solute per litre of solution. The number of moles is calculated by dividing the mass in g of the sample by the gram formula weight (GFW). One GFW is the same as one mole.

$$M = \frac{\text{number moles (solute)}}{\text{number litres (solution)}}$$

$$\text{Number moles} = \frac{\text{number moles (solute)}}{\text{GFW}}$$

For example, in a 0.150M $(COOH)_2$, there are 0.150 moles of $(COOH)_2$ in one litre of this solution. The following factors may then be used in chemical calculations.

$$\frac{0.150 \text{ mol } (COOH)_2}{1 \text{ L solution}} \quad \text{or} \quad \frac{1 \text{ L solution}}{0.150 \text{ mol } (COOH)_2}$$

For a chemical reaction that take place in solution, the volume and the molarity of one reactant and the volume of second reactant can be used together with the stiochiometry of the equation to find out the molarity of the second reactant needed to completely react with the first reactant.

A concentration term, normally (N) is used in certain disciplines. Normality is the number of gram equivalent weights (GEW) of solute in a litre of solution. One gram equivalent weight (GEW) is also called one equivalent.

$$N = \frac{\text{number GEW solute}}{\text{number litres solution}} \quad \text{or} \quad \frac{\text{number equivalent solution}}{\text{number litres solution}}$$

$$\text{Number GEW} = \frac{\text{number grams}}{\text{GEW}}$$

One GEW of an oxidizing agent (OA) or reducing agent (RA) is the amount of that agent which gains or loses 1 mole of electrons. One mole of $KMnO_4$ gains 5 moles of electron when it react completely as shown above.

$$\overset{+7}{Mn}O_4^- + 5e^- \longrightarrow \overset{+2}{Mn}^{2+} \quad (5 \text{ electrons change/mole } MnO_4^-)$$

Therefore, the GEW of $KMnO_4$ will be one fifth its GFW since that is the weight of $KMnO_4$ which will gain one mole of electron.

The two C's in mole of $(COOH)_2$ lose 2 moles of electron when $(COOH)_2$ reacts completely. Therefore, the GEW of $(COOH)_2$ will be one half of its GFW since that is the weight of $(COOH)_2$ which will lose one mole of electron.

$$\overset{+3}{(CO}OH)_2 \longrightarrow 2\overset{+4}{C}O_2 + 2e^- \quad (2 \text{ electrons change/mole } (COOH)_2)$$

The usefulness of normality lies in the fact that one GEW or one equivalent of oxidizing agent reacts exactly with GEW or one equivalent of reducing agent. This leads to a simple relationship that the normality of the oxidizing agent times its volume is equal to the normality of the reducing agent times its volume.

$$N_{OA} \times V_{OA} = N_{RA} \times V_{RA}$$

The normality of a solution is related to the molarity of that solution through equation:

$$N = M \times \text{no. of electron lost or gained by reactant}$$

How to calculate equivalent weight of oxidizing/reducing agents

The equivalent weight of an oxidizing or reducing agent is calculated by the no. of electrons gain or lost by one mole during redox reaction.

In a redox reaction, permanganate ion is converted to manganous ion by the gain of 5 electrons. Therefore, its equivalent weight is one fifth of its molecular weight, 158/5 = 31.6

$$MnO_4^- + 8H^+ + 5e^- \longrightarrow Mn^{2+} + 4H_2O$$

Potassium dichromate gains 6 electrons. Hence, its equivalent weight is one sixth of the molecular weight.

$$Cr_2O_7^{2-} + 14H^+ + 6e^- \rightarrow 2Cr^{3+} + 7H_2O$$

Similarly, potassium iodate gains 6 electrons, so its equivalent weight is one-sixth of molecular weight.

$$IO_3^- + 6H^+ + 6e \longrightarrow I^- + 3H_2O$$

Two thiosulphate ($S_2O_3^{2-}$) ions are transformed to tetrathionate ($S_2O_6^{2-}$) ion in the redox reaction by the loss of two electrons. Therefore, the equivalent weight of sodium thiosulphate ($Na_2S_2O_3.5H_2O$) is equal to its molecular weight, 248.17.

$$2S_2O_3^{2-} \longrightarrow S_4O_6^{2-} + 2e^-$$

Acidified $KMnO_4$ oxidizes oxalic acid to carbon dioxide. In other words the oxalate ion is oxidized to carbon dioxide with the loss of two electrons.

$$(COOH)_2.2H_2O + [O] \longrightarrow 2CO_2 + 3H_2O$$

The equivalent of oxalic acid is half of its molecular weight, 126.07/2 = 63.035.

Indicators used in redox titrations

The oxidized or reduced form acts as a self-indicator. Acidified solution of $KMnO_4$ has deep purple colour. A permanent pink colour is appeared at the end point when $KMnO_4$ is used as titrant. Ceric sulphate (yellow) and iodine (brown) are reduced to colourless ions at the end point.

Potassium ferricyanide is used as an external indicator in the titration of ferrous ion by potassium dichromate. There is formation of deep prussian blue colour with potassium ferricyanide due to the presence of ferrous ions. At the end point, only ferric ion is present and this does not give a colour with potassium ferricyanide.

In the standardization of sodium thiosulphate by iodometric titration, iodine is liberated. Therefore, starch mucilage is used as an indicator. Starch combines with iodine to form a blue colour.

Diphenylamine, sodium diphenylaminosulphonate, diphenylbenzidine and ferroin are also used as indicators in redox titration.

POTASSIUM PERMANGANATE TITRATION

Potassium pemanganate is used as an oxidizing substance as indicated by the following equation:

$$MnO_4^- + 8H^+ + 5e^- \longrightarrow Mn^{2+} + 4H_2O$$

Therefore, $KMnO_4 \equiv 5e^-$

158.0 g $KMnO_4 \equiv 5000$ ml N

3.160 g $KMnO_4 \equiv 1000$ ml 0.1N $KMnO_4$ solution

Preparation and standardization of 0.1N of KMnO$_4$ Solution

Weigh the KMnO$_4$ (about 3.2 g), transfer to a 250 ml beaker containing cold water and stir thoroughly breaking up the crystals with a glass rod. Boil the solution for 10 minutes, stopper the flask and keep it for 24 hours and then filter the solution through a small plug of glass wool in a funnel into a 1 litre graduated flask. Add more water to make the solution up to the graduation mark and mix with thorough shaking.

Organic matter present in the water are oxidized with the formation of MnO$_2$ during 24 hours. The precipitate of manganese dioxide is filtered out, otherwise it catalyze the formation of more MnO$_2$.

$$4KMnO_4 + 2H_2O \longrightarrow 4KOH + 4MnO_2 + 3O_2$$

For standardization, weigh accurately sodium oxalate (0.2 g), previously dried at 110°C to constant weight. Dissolve in water, transfer into 1 litre graduated flask and make up to the volume. Pipette out this solution (20 ml). Add dilute sulphuric acid (10 ml), warm to about 60°C and titrate with KMnO$_4$ solution till permanent a pink colour persists for about 10 seconds.

Note: Formation of a brown colour during the titration is caused by insufficient acid or using too high temperature or by the use of a dirty flask.

$$\text{Normality of KMnO}_4 \text{ solution} = \frac{\text{Weight of sodium oxalate (g)}}{\text{Volume of KMnO}_4 \text{ solution consumed (ml)} \times 0.067}$$

where 0.067 is the milliequivalent weight of sodium oxalate.

Sodium oxalate is best standard for standardization due to its availability in pure state. Sufficient acid is added to maintain the hydrogen ion concentration during titration. KMnO$_4$ oxidize sodium oxalate into CO$_2$ and at the end point, a slight excess of KMnO$_4$ imparts pink colour.

$$MnO_4^- + 8H^+ + 5e \longrightarrow Mn^{2+} + 4H_2O$$
$$(Oxalate)\ C_2O_4^- \longrightarrow 2CO_2 + 2e$$

The complete reaction with sodium oxalate may thus be represented as:

$$2KMnO_4 + 5Na_2C_2O_4 + 14H_2SO_4 \rightarrow 2MnSO_4 + 2KHSO_4 + 10NaHSO_4 + 10CO_2 + 8H_2O$$

According to IP official method, a potassium permanganate solution is standardized by iodometric method.

Take 0.1N potassium permanganate solution (20 ml), add KI (2 g) in iodine flask, acidify with 1M H$_2$SO$_4$ solution (10 ml) and then titrate the liberated iodine with 0.1N sodium thiosulphate solution using starch mucilage as indicator. The indicator is added toward the end of titration (when slight yellow colour appears).

Potassium permanganate oxidizes the KI into iodine in acidic media. The liberated iodine is titrated with standard thiosulphate solution till yellow colour appears. At this stage, starch mucilage indicator is added. The resulting blue colour is discharged on continuing the titration at the end point.

$$KMnO_4 + 5KI + 4H_2SO_4 \longrightarrow 3K_2SO_4 + MnSO_4 + 3I_2\uparrow + 4H_2O$$
$$I_2 + Na_2S_2O_3 \longrightarrow Na_2S_4O_6 + NaI$$
$$\text{Sodium}$$
$$\text{tetrathionate}$$

Note: *The yellow colour indicates the presence of less iodine which gives blue colour with starch mucilage indicator. This blue colour is discharged on addition of sodium thiosulphate* *solution. The starch mucilage indicator forms stable blue colour with excess of iodine which is not discharged on adding sodium thiosulphate solution.*

CERIC SULPHATE TITRATION

Solution of ceric sulphate in dilute sulphuric acid is a strong oxidizing agent and has many advantages over potassium permanganate, e.g.

(i) The solution is stable on boiling.

(ii) The cerous ion is colourless and does not cause any hindrance in detecting end point.

(iii) Ceric (Ce^{3+}) on reduction gives Ce^{4+} (Cerum). There is no intermediate product while permanganate can be reduced to any of several oxidation states.

(iv) *o*-phenanthroline ion (ferrous) complex is a satisfactory indicator in the titration with ceric sulphate.

Preparation and standardization of 0.1N ceric sulphate solution

Place ceric ammonium nitrate (59 g) in a beaker, add sulphuric acid (30 ml) to it and cautiously add water, in 20 ml portion until solution is complete. Allow to stand for 24 hours, filter through a fine porosity sintered glass crucible, dilute with water to make up 1 litre.

For standardization, dissolve an accurately weighed quantity (about 0.2 g) of As_2O_3 in sodium hydroxide solution (25 ml). Add water (about 100 ml), dilute sulphuric acid (10 ml), 2 drops of each of *o*-phenanthroline test solution and osmium tetraoxide. Titrate slowly with approximate 0.1N ceric sulphate solution till pink colour changes to a pale blue.

Factor: Each ml of 0.1N ceric sulphate solution is equivalent to 0.00494 g of As_2O_3.

Sodium hydroxide is used to solubilise the arsenic trioxide. Ceric sulphate oxidizes the arsenite to arsenate. The traces of osmium tetroxide is added to catalyze the reaction with ceric ion and arsenite ion otherwise it is a slow reaction.

$$As_2O_3 + 6NaOH \longrightarrow 2Na_3AsO_3 + 3H_2O$$

$$2Ce(SO_4)_2 + 2Na_3AsO_3 + H_2O \longrightarrow Ce_2(SO_4)_3 + 2Na_3AsO_4 + H_2SO_4$$

Normality of ceric sulphate is calculated as follows:

$$N = \frac{\text{Weight of } As_2O_3 \text{ (g)}}{\text{ml of ceric sulphate solution consumed} \times 0.0494}$$

where 0.0494 is the milliequivalent weight of As_2O_3.

o-Phenanthroline test solution (1.5% w/v)

Dissolve *o*-phenanthroline (0.15 g) in a solution of ferrous sulphate solution (10 ml).

o-phenanthroline form red coloured complex with ferrous ion. Strong oxidizing agent, e.g. ceric sulphate convert the ferrous complex into light blue coloured ferric complex.

1,10-Phenanthroline

$$C_{12}H_8N_2 + Fe^{++} \longrightarrow [Fe(C_{12}H_8N_2)_3]^{2+} \rightleftharpoons [Fe(C_{12}H_8N_2)_3]^{3+} + e^-$$

| *o*-Phenanthroline (colourless) | *o*-Phenanthroline ferrous complex (red) | *o*-Phenanthroline ferric complex (blue) |

TITRATION OF IODINE

In the titration of iodine in aqueous solution, the following reaction involves:

$$I_2 + 2e^- \longrightarrow 2I^-$$

Therefore, $I_2 = 2e^-$

126.9 g $I_2 \equiv 1000$ ml N

12.69 g $I_2 \equiv 1000$ ml 0.1N iodine solution

Preparation and Standardization of 0.1N Iodine Solution

Weigh iodine (about 3.2 g) and transfer to a beaker containing potassium iodide (7.5 g) and water (100 ml). Dissolve, transfer to a 250 ml graduated flask and adjust to volume with water.

Iodine is practically insoluble in water. It dissolves in solution of potassium iodide due to polyiodide formation, KI_3, which behaves in solution as free iodine.

Note: Iodine is volatile and standard solutions should be stored in tightly stoppered glass bottles.

For standardization, dissolve accurately weighed As_2O_3 (about 150 mg) in 20 ml of 1.0N NaOH solution by warming if necessary. Dilute with water (40 ml), add 2 drop of methyl orange and add sufficient quantity of dilute HCl solution until yellow colour changes to pink.

As_2O_3 (primary standard) is insoluble in water but solubilized in NaOH due to formation of sodium arsenite

$$As_2O_3 + 6NaOH \longrightarrow 2Na_3AsO_3 + 3H_2O$$
$$\text{Sodium arsenite}$$

The excess of sodium hydroxide is neutralized by adding dilute HCl using methyl orange as indicators otherwise hypoiodite, NaIO or similar compound forms.

$$2NaOH + I_2 \longrightarrow NaIO + NaI + H_2O$$
$$\text{Sodium hypoiodite}$$

Then, add sodium bicarbonate (2 g), dilute it with water (50 ml), add starch mucilage indicator (3 ml) and titrate with 0.1N iodine solution until permanent blue colour is produced.

Iodine oxidize arsenite into arsenate.

$$H_3AsO_3 + H_2O + I_2 \rightleftharpoons H_3AsO_4 + 2HI$$

Due to strong reducing properties of HI, the oxidation with iodine is a reversible reaction. The reaction proceeds to the right by removal of hydroiodic acid by reaction with $NaHCO_3$. Sodium hydroxide or sodium carbonate cannot be used due to their reactivity with iodine. Sodium bicarbonate does not react with iodine but if an excess of iodine is added, it may react slightly.

The overall reaction is

$$Na_3AsO_3 + I_2 + 2NaHCO_3 \longrightarrow Na_3AsO_4 + NaI + 2CO_2 + H_2O$$
$$\text{Sodium arsenite} \qquad\qquad\qquad\qquad \text{Sodium arsenate}$$

Finally, normality of iodine is calculated as follows:

$$N = \frac{\text{weight of } As_2O_3 \text{ (g)}}{\text{ml of iodine consumed} \times 0.0494}$$

where 0.0494 is the milliequivalent weight of As_2O_3

Note: *Alternatively, iodine solution can be standardized by titration with standardized sodium thiosulphate solution.*

Iodine–Sodium Thiosulphate Titration

Sodium thiosulphate is oxidized to sodium tetrathionate by iodine.

$$2S_2O_3^{2-} \longrightarrow S_4O_6^{2-} + 2e^-$$
$$I_2 + 2e^- \longrightarrow 2I^-$$

Therefore, $2S_2O_3 = I_2 = 2e^-$

$$2 \times 248.2 \text{ g Na}_2S_2O_3.5H_2O = 2000 \text{ ml N}$$
$$24.82 \text{ g Na}_2S_2O_3.5H_2O = 1000 \text{ ml } 0.1N \text{ iodine solution}$$

Preparation and Standardization of 0.1N sodium thiosulphate solution

Dissolve sodium thiosulphate (about 25 g) and sodium carbonate (0.20 g) in 1000 ml of recently boiled and cooled water.

Water is boiled for the sterilization purposes as solution may deteriorate due to bacterial action. Boiling also expels CO_2 which if present as carbonic acid may cause hydrolysis and decomposition of sodium thiosulphate.

$$Na_2S_2O_3 + 2H_2CO_3 \longrightarrow 2NaHCO_3 + H_2S_2O_3$$
$$H_2S_2O_3 \longrightarrow H_2SO_3 + S\downarrow$$

The sodium carbonate act as preservative to prevent the acid catalyzed hydrolysis.

For standardization, dissolve potassium bromate (0.2 g) in water and make up the volume to 250 ml. Take 50 ml of this solution in iodine flask, add KI (2 g) and acidify it with 2M HCl solution (3 ml). Titrate the liberated iodine with standard sodium thiosulphate solution, using starch mucilage as indicator. Starch mucilage is added toward the end of titration.

According to IP official method, sodium thiosulphate is standardized by iodometric method. The reaction between potassium bromate and potassium iodide in presence of hydrochloric acid yield the iodine. The liberated iodine is titrated with approximately prepared sodium thiosulphate solution till yellow colour appears.

$$KBrO_3 + 6KI + 6HCl \longrightarrow 6KCl + KBr + 3I_2 + 3H_2O$$

At this stage, starch mucilage indicator is added and titration is continued till the disappearance of blue colour.

$$I_2 + Na_2S_2O_3 \longrightarrow Na_2S_4O_6 + 2NaI$$

Note: *Sodium thiosulphate can also standardized by titration against potassium dichromate or potassium iodate using same above principle.*

TITRATION OF BROMINE

This titration is used to determine percentage of phenol. For quantitative estimation, phenol is treated with excess of 0.1N bromine solution.

Phenol   Tribromophenol

The excess of bromine not consumed in the reaction react with KI to liberate an equivalent amount of iodine. The liberated iodine is determined by titration with sodium thiosulphate solution.

$$Br_2 + 2I^- \longrightarrow 2Br + I_2\uparrow$$

Therefore, $C_6H_5OH \equiv 3Br_2 \equiv 3I_2 \equiv 6e^-$

Each ml of 0.1N Br_2 solution = 0.01568 g of C_6H_5OH

A solution of bromine is not stable. Therefore, a solution containing potassium bromide and potassium bromate is used. This solution liberates an equivalent amount of bromine on acidification.

$$BrO_3^- + 5Br^- + 6H^+ \longrightarrow 3Br_2 + 3H_2O$$

Preparation and standardization of 0.1N bromine solution

Dissolve $KBrO_3$ (3 g) and KBr (15 g) in sufficient water to produce 1000 ml.

For standardization, pipette out 25 ml of this solution in iodine flask and dilute with water. Add hydrochloric acid (5 ml), stopper iodine flask and dilute with more quantity of water. Then add 20% potassium iodide solution (5 ml), restopper, shake the flask, allow it to stand for 5 minutes. Titrate the liberated iodine with 0.1N $Na_2S_2O_3$ solution using starch mucilage as indicator.

The bromine solution cannot be used due to its volatile nature. Hence, solution of potassium bromate and potassium bromide in water is used. The equivalent amount of bromine is liberated when KBr and $KBrO_3$ react in acidified solution.

$$5KBr + KBrO_3 + 6HCl \longrightarrow 6KCl + 3Br_2\uparrow + 3H_2O$$

The liberated bromine oxidises potassium iodide to liberate an equivalent amount of iodine.

$$2KI + Br_2 \longrightarrow 2KBr + I_2\uparrow$$

The free iodine is titrated with the sodium thiosulphate. From the volume of sodium thiosulphate consumed, the normality of bromine is calculated out.

TITRATION IN NON-AQUEOUS SOLVENTS

Substances with very weak acidic or very weak basic property do not give sharp end point in aqueous solution and can often be titrated in non-aqueous solvents. The water behaves as both a weak acid and a weak base, thus in aqueous environment, it can compete effectively with very weak acids and bases with regard to proton donation and acceptance, as shown below:

$$H_2O + H^+ \rightleftharpoons H_3O^+ \text{ competes with weak base, } RNH_2 + H^+ \rightleftharpoons RNH_3^+$$

or $$H_2O \rightleftharpoons H^+ + OH^- \text{ competes with } ROH \rightleftharpoons RO^- + H^+.$$

This competition makes the endpoint difficult to detect.

According to the Lowry-Bronsted theory, an acid (HB) is a proton donor and a base (B) is a proton acceptor, i.e. a substance which tends to combine with a proton. When the acid dissociates, it yields a proton together with the conjugate base B^- of the acid.

$$\underset{\text{Acid}}{HB} \rightleftharpoons \underset{\text{Proton}}{H^+} + \underset{\text{Base}}{B^-}$$

A base B combines with a proton to form the conjugate acid HB of the base B. For every base, there is a conjugate acid and *vice versa*. Based on Lowry-Bronsted concept, the weak bases are titrated by dissolving in an aprotic solvents or acidic solvents. The acidic solvent increases the basic property of weak base. Similarly, the weak acids are titrated in an aprotic solvent or basic solvent, the basic solvent, e.g. DMF increases the acidity of the weak acid.

Sometimes, non-aqueous titrations are opted due to solubility of drug in non-aqueous solvents.

Types of Solvents

Aprotic Solvents

These are chemically inert organic solvents like benzene and chloroform. They have a low dielectric constant, do not react with either acids or bases and do not ionize like other compounds. Picric acid forms a colourless solution in benzene which becomes yellow on adding aniline since the acid does not dissociate in benzene solution and in the presence of the base aniline, it acts as an acid.

Protophilic Solvents

These are basic in character and form solvated protons on reaction with acids.

$$HB + \text{basic solvent} \longrightarrow \text{Solvated proton} + B^-$$

A weakly basic solvent has less tendency to accept a proton than a strongly basic one. Similarly, a weak acid has less tendency to donate protons than a strong acid. For example, the strong acid like perchloric acid exhibits more strongly acidic properties than a weak acid such as acetic acid when dissolved in a weakly basic solvent. All acids tend to become equal in strength when dissolved in strongly basic solvents due to the greater affinity of strong bases for protons. This is termed *levelling effect*. Strong bases are levelling solvents for acids; weak bases are differentiating solvents for acids.

Protogenic Solvents

These are acidic substances, e.g. hydrochloric acid. They exert a levelling effect on bases.

Amphoteric Solvents

These solvents have both protophilic and protogenic properties, e.g. water, acetic acid and alcohols. The dissociation of acetic acid, which is frequently used as a solvent for titration of basic substances, is shown in the equation below:

$$CH_3COOH \rightleftharpoons CH_3COO^- + H^+$$

If a strong acid like perchloric acid is added in acetic acid, the acetic acid behaves as a base and combines with protons donated by the perchloric acid to form an 'Onium' ions which acts as a strongly acidic solution due to donating nature of proton to a base.

$$HClO_4 \rightleftharpoons ClO_4^- + H^+$$
$$CH_3COOH + H^+ \rightleftharpoons CH_3COOH_2^+$$
Onium ion

When a weak base, e.g. pyridine, is dissolved in acetic acid, the acid exhibits its levelling effect and increases the basic properties of the pyridine. Therefore, it is useful to titrate a solution of a weak base in acetic acid with acetous perchloric acid to obtain a sharp end point. Titrations of these compounds in aqueous solution are not successful.

$$HClO_4 + CH_3COOH \rightleftharpoons CH_3COOH_2^+ + ClO_4^-$$
$$C_5H_5N + CH_3COOH \rightleftharpoons C_6H_5N^+H + CH_3COO^-$$
$$CH_3COOH_2^+ + CH_3COO^- \rightleftharpoons 2CH_3COOH$$

Therefore, $\qquad HClO_4 + C_5H_5N \rightleftharpoons C_6H_5N^+H + ClO_4^-$

Titration of weak bases

Alkali metals, alkaline earth metals, amines and pyridine due to their weak basic properties are titrated with perchloric acids.

Preparation and standardization of 0.1M or 0.1N perchloric acid solution

Mix perchloric acid (8.5 ml) with anhydrous glacial acid (500 ml) and acetic anhydride (25 ml). Cool down and then add sufficient quantity of anhydrous glacial acetic acid to produce 1000 ml. Allow the prepared solution to stand for one day for the excess of acetic anhydride to be combined and determine the percentage of water. If the water content exceeds 0.05%, add more acetic anhydride. If the solution contain no titrable water, add sufficient water to obtain a content of water between 0.02% and 0.05%. Allow the solution to stand for one day and titrate the water content.

Perchloric acid is available as 70–72% mixture with water, having specific gravity of about 1.6. It undergoes spontaneous explosive decomposition. For this reason, it is handled in the form of solution. Acetic anhydride is added to react with water present in perchloric acid (nearly 30% v/v).

For standardization, weigh accurately potassium hydrogen phthalate (about 0.35 g), previously dried at 120°C for 2 hours and dissolve in anhydrous glacial acetic acid (50 ml). Add crystal violet solution (0.1 ml) and titrate with perchloric acid solution until the violet colour changes to emerald green. Perform a blank determination and make any necessary correction.

Factor: Each ml of 0.1N $HClO_4$ = 0.02042 g of potassium hydrogen phthalate.

Non-aqueous solvents show greater coefficients of expansion than water. A small temperature variation can result in significant errors unless suitable correction factors are used. Therefore, standardization and titration should be carried out at the same temperature. If there is a temperature difference, the volume of titrant may be corrected by applying the following formula:

$$V_a = V_b [1 + 0.001 (t_1 - t_2)]$$

where, V_a = corrected volume of titrant
V_b = volume of titrant measured
t_1 = temperature of which titrant was standardized
t_2 = temperature of which titration was carried.

Titration of weak acids

Weak acids are titrated by standard sodium methoxide solution in basic (protophilic) solvent or aprotic solvent.

Preparation and standardization of 0.1M Sodium Methoxide Solution

Cool down anhydrous methanol (150 ml) in ice-cold water and add freshly cut sodium metal (about 2.5 g) in portions. When the metal has dissolved, add sufficient amount of toluene, previously dried over sodium wire, to produce 1000 ml.

The dissolution of sodium metal should be made carefully due to exothermic reaction.

$$Na° + CH_3OH \longrightarrow CH_3ONa + H°\uparrow$$

Carbon dioxide and moisture should be excluded to avoid their reaction with sodium methoxide. Turbidity may appear due to this reaction.

$$H_2O + CH_3ONa \longrightarrow CH_3OH + NaOH$$
$$H_2CO_3 + 2CH_3ONa \longrightarrow 2CH_3OH + Na_2CO_3$$

For standardization, dissolve accurately weighed benzoic acid (0.4 g) in dimethylformamide (DMF) (80 ml), add thymolphthalein indicator (0.15 ml) and titrate with sodium methoxide solution to a blue colour end point.

Sodium methoxide is standardized by primary standard benzoic acid in DMF which enhances its acidity. The reaction are as follows:

$$C_6H_5COOH + HCON(CH_3)_2 \rightleftharpoons HCON^+H(CH_3)_2 + C_6H_5COO^-$$
$$\text{DMF}$$

$$CH_3ONa \rightleftharpoons CH_3O^- + Na^+$$

$$HCON^+H(CH_3)_2 + CH_3O^- \longrightarrow HCON(CH_3)_2 + CH_3OH$$

Overall reaction is

$$C_6H_5COOH + CH_3ONa \rightleftharpoons C_6H_5COONa + CH_3OH$$

Factor: Each ml of 0.1M sodium methoxide is equivalent to 0.01221 g of benzoic acid.

Indicators used in non-aqueous titrations

Indicators used in non-aqueous titrations along with their colour change are given in Table 3.2.

Indicator	Colour change (basic)	Colour change (neutral)	Colour change (acidic)
1. Crystal violet (0.5% in glacial acetic acid)	Violet	Blue-green	Yellowish green
2. Naphtholbenzein (0.2% in glacial acetic acid)	Blue or blue green	Orange	Dark green
3. Oracet blue (0.5% in glacial acetic acid)	Blue	Purple	Pink
4. Quinaldine red (0.1% in methanol)	Magenta	—	Almost colourless

Table 3.2: Indicators used in non-aqueous titrations

SODIUM NITRITE TITRATIONS

When aromatic primary amines are reacted with sodium nitrite in acid solution at low temperature (0–5°C), diazonium salts are formed.

$$\underset{\text{Aniline}}{C_6H_5NH_2} + NaNO_2 + HCl \xrightarrow{0-5^\circ C} \underset{\text{Diazonium salt}}{C_6H_5N_2^+Cl^-} + NaCl + 2H_2O$$

Under controlled conditions, the reaction is quantitative and used for determination of free aromatic amines like sulphanilamide and other sulpha drugs. The presence of a small excess of nitrous acid indicates the end point which is detected using starch–iodide paper as an external indicator.

$$KI + HCl \longrightarrow HI + KCl$$

$$2HI + 2HNO_2 \longrightarrow I_2 + 2NO + 2H_2O$$

The liberated iodine reacts with starch to impart a blue colour.

The end point may also be detected electrometrically.

ESTIMATION OF SODIUM AMINOSALICYLATE

Treatment of sodium aminosalicylate ($C_7H_6NNaO_3$) with sodium nitrite forms a diazonium salt.

Sodium aminosalicylate   Diazotised sodium aminosalicylate

$$175.2 \text{ g of } C_7H_6NNaO_3 \equiv NaNO_2 \equiv 1000 \text{ ml 1M or 1N } NaNO_2$$

or $0.01752 \text{ g of } C_7H_6NNaO_3 \equiv 1 \text{ ml } 0.1M \text{ or } 0.1N \text{ } NaNO_2 \text{ solution}$

Procedure

Weigh accurately sodium aminosalicylate (about 0.25 g) and dissolve in glacial acetic acid (50 ml), warm gently, if necessary. Add cold water (175 ml) and cool below 10°C, add hydrochloric acid (10 ml) and slowly titrate with 0.1M sodium nitrite at a temperature below 10°C until a drop of the solution immediately gives a blue colour when drawn quickly by means of a fine rod across the surface of a starch iodide paper. The titration is completed when the end point is reproducible after the titrated solution has been allowed to stand for 5 minutes.

The end point may also be determined by electrometric method.

Preparation and standardization of 0.1M or 0.1N NaNO₂ solution

Dissolve sodium nitrite (7.5 g) in sufficient water to make 1000 ml.

For standardization, weigh accurately sulphanilamide (about 0.5 g) previously dried at 105°C for three hours. Add water (50 ml) and HCl (5 ml) and stir well until dissolved. Maintain the temperature below 10°C and titrate slowly with sodium nitrite solution, with stirring until glass rod dipped into the titrated solution produces an immediate blue colour when touched to starch iodide paper. The end point should be reproducible after the mixture has been allowed to stand for 1 minute.

Factor: Each ml of 0.1M or 0.1N NaNO₂ solution = 0.01722 g of sulphanilamide.

Standardization reactions are identical with the assay method given in Chapter 7.

Electroanalytical Methods to Determine Normality of Solution

In electroanalytical methods of instrumental analysis, analyst measures voltage (potential) and /or current signals. There are various types of methods but commonly used methods are listed here.

- **Potentiometry:** There is a measurement of electrical potential in chemical analysis.
- **Conductometry:** There is a measurement of electrolytic conductivity to monitor a progress of chemical reaction
- **Coulombmetry:** It involves determination of the amount of matter transformed during an electrolysis reaction by measuring the amount of electricity (in coulombs) consumed or produced.
- **Electrogravimetry:** This method used to separate and quantify ions of a substance, usually a metal.
- **Voltammetry (polarography/amperometry):** In this, the information about an analyte is obtained by measuring the current as the potential is varied.

CONDUCTOMETRIC TITRATIONS

Experimental overview

Conductometry is a measurement of electrolytic conductivity to monitor a progress of chemical reaction. The principle of conductometric titration is based on the fact that during the titration, one of the ions is replaced by the other and invariably these two ions differ in the ionic conductivity with the result that conductivity of the solution varies during the course of titration. The equivalence point may be located graphically by plotting the change in conductance as a function of the volume of titrant added in titration curve. The unit of conductance is Siemens per meter (S/m) or micro siemens per centimeter.

Typical Conductometric Titration Curves

Some typical conductometric titration curves are:

1. **Strong acid with a strong base, e.g. HCl with NaOH:** Initially, before NaOH is added, the conductance is high due to the presence of highly mobile hydrogen ions. On addition of base, the conductance falls due to the replacement of hydrogen ions by the added cation as H^+ ions react with OH^- ions to form undissociated water. This decrease in the conductance continues till the equivalence point. At the equivalence point, the solution contains only NaCl. After the equivalence point, the conductance increases due to the large conductivity of OH^- ions (Fig. 4.1a).

2. **Weak acid with a strong base, e.g. acetic acid with NaOH:** Initially, the conductance is low due to the feeble ionization of acetic acid. On the addition of base, there is decrease in conductance not only due to the replacement of H^+ by Na^+ but also suppresses the dissociation of acetic acid due to common ion acetate. But very soon, the conductance increases on adding NaOH as NaOH neutralizes the un-dissociated CH_3COOH to CH_3COONa which is the strong electrolyte. This increase in conductance continues raise up to the equivalence point. The graph near the equivalence point is curved due the hydrolysis of salt CH_3COONa. Beyond the equivalence point, conductance increases more rapidly with the addition of NaOH due to the highly conducting OH^- ions (Fig. 4.1b).

3. **Strong acid with a weak base, e.g. sulphuric acid with dilute ammonia:** Initially, the conductance is high and then it decreases due to the replacement of H^+. But after the endpoint has been reached the graph becomes almost horizontal, since the excess aqueous ammonia is not appreciably ionised in the presence of ammonium sulphate (Fig. 4.1c).

4. **Weak acid with a weak base:** The nature of curve before the equivalence point is similar to the curve obtained by titrating weak acid against strong base. After the equivalence point, conductance virtually remains same as the weak base which is being added is feebly ionized and, therefore, is not much conducting (Fig. 4.1d).

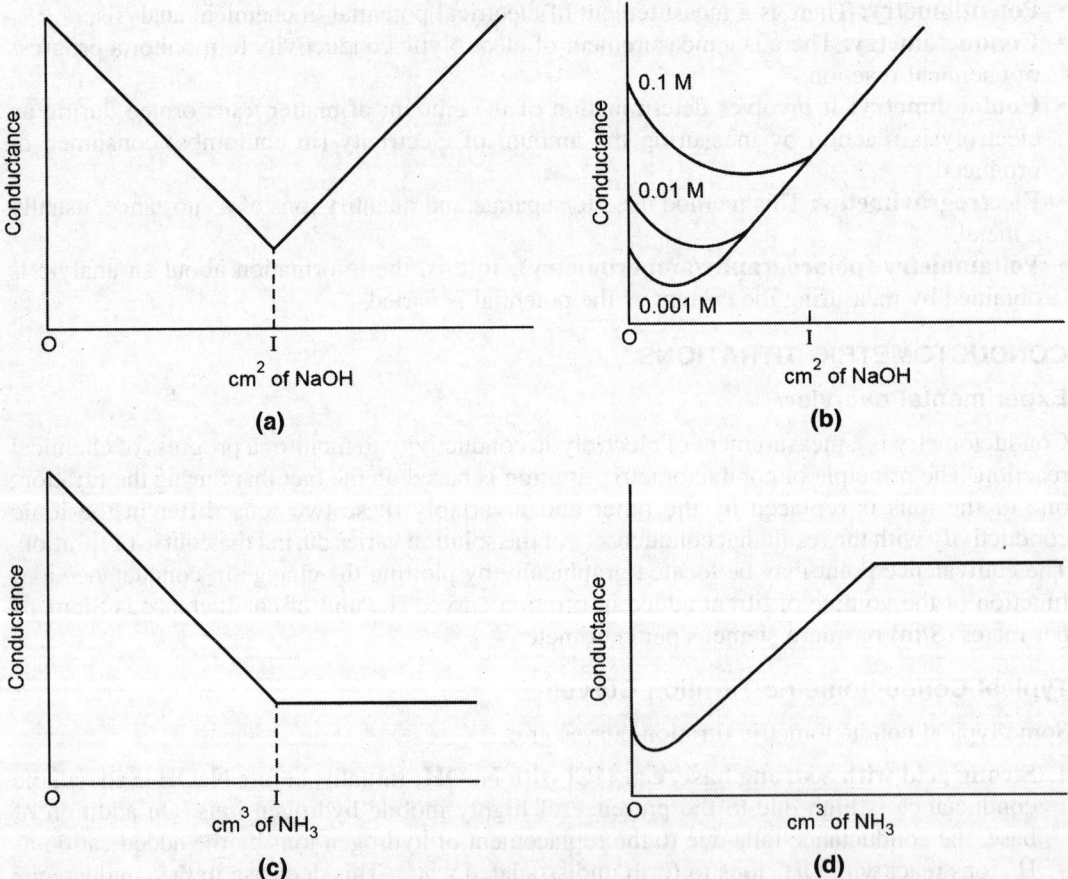

Fig. 4.1: Titrations curves of some conductometric titrations. (a) Strong acid with a strong base, e.g. HCl with NaOH; (b) Weak acid with a strong base, e.g. acetic acid with NaOH; (c) Strong acid with a weak base, e.g. sulphuric acid with dilute ammonia solution; (d) Weak acid (acetic acid) with a weak base (NH_4OH).

In order to reduce the influence of errors in the conductometric titration to a minimum, the angle between the two branches of the titration curve should be as small as possible. If the angle is very obtuse, a small error in the conductance data can cause a large deviation. The following approximate rules will be found useful.

- The smaller the conductivity of the ion which replaces the reacting ion, the more accurate will be the result. Thus, it is preferable to titrate a silver salt with lithium chloride rather than with HCl. Generally, cations should be titrated with lithium salts and anions with acetates as these ions have low conductivity.
- The larger the conductivity of the anion of the reagent which reacts with the cation to be determined, or *vice versa*, the more acute is the angle of titration curve.
- The titration of a slightly ionized salt does not give good results, since the conductivity increases continuously from the commencement. Hence, the salt present in the cell should be virtually completely dissociated; for a similar reason; the added reagent should also be as strong electrolyte.
- Throughout a titration the volume of the solution is always increasing, unless the conductance is corrected for this effect, non-linear titration curves result. The correction can be accomplished by multiplying the observed conductance either by total volume $(V + V')$ or by the factor $(V + V')/V$, where V is the initial volume of solution and V' is the total volume of the reagent added. The correction presupposes that the conductivity is a linear function of dilution, this is true only to a first approximation.
- In the interest of keeping V small, the reagent for the conductometric titration is ordinarily several times more concentrated than the solution being titrated (at least 10–20 times). A microburette may then be used for the volumetric measurement.

The main advantages to the conductometric titration are its applicability to very dilute, and coloured solutions and to system that involve relative incomplete reactions.

Experiment 4.1: Conductometric titration of a strong acid with a strong base

Principle

Before NaOH is added, the conductance is high due to the presence of highly mobile hydrogen ions. When the base is added, the conductance falls due to the replacement of hydrogen ions by the added cation as H^+ ions react with OH^- ions to form un-dissociated water. This decrease in the conductance continues till the equivalence point. At the equivalence point, the solution contains only NaCl. After the equivalence point, the conductance increases due to the large conductivity of OH^- ions. The titration curve which resembles the one shown in Fig. 4.1 will be obtained. The point of intersection of the two lines gives the point of neutralization, i.e. equivalence point.

Requirements

Apparatus

Conductometer, conductance cell, burette, pipette, beaker (100 cm^3), standard flask (100 cm^3), glass rod, burette stand with clamp.

Chemicals

Hydrochloric acid and sodium hydroxide.

Solutions provided

0.1M sodium hydroxide solution (which was standardised with standard oxalic acid or potassium hydrogen phthalate) and ~0.01M HCl solution.

Procedure

1. Take 30 ml of HCl (~0.01M) solution in a 100 ml beaker with the conductance cell.
2. Take NaOH solution in the burette.
3. Connect the conductometer to the mains and to the conductance cell. Switch on the instrument keeping the meter switch at 'CAL'.
4. Calibrate the meter keeping the selector knob at '20 ms' by rotating the 'sensitivity knob' till the meter reads 1.0.
5. Shift the meter switch to 'Read'. Read the conductance of the solution (keep the stirrer above the solution). Record this value in Observation Table 1.
6. Make additions of NaOH from the burette as given in Observation Table 1. After each addition, stir the solution well and read the conductance, keeping the stirrer above the solution. Enter all the conductance values in Observation Table 1.
7. Plot conductance versus volume of NaOH added on a graph sheet.
8. Determine the end point from the graph (Fig. 4.1a).

Observations

Observation Table 1: Conductometric titration of a strong acid (HCl) with a strong base (NaOH)

Volume of NaOH added (ml)	Conductance (mS)
0.00	
0.40	
0.80	
1.20	
1.60	
2.00 and so on	

Calculations

Estimation of the strength of a given HCl solution: ?

Molarity of standard NaOH solution = M_1 (0.1M)

Volume of NaOH solution used from plotted curve = V_1 ml

Volume of HCl taken = V_2 (30 ml)

Molarity of HCl = M_2

Molarity equation for the titration of HCl and NaOH can be written as

$$M_1V_1 \text{ (NaOH)} = M_2V_2 \text{ (HCl)}$$

Molarity of HCl = M_1V_1/V_2

Results

Molarity of HCl =

Precautions

1. After switching on the instrument (conductometer), it should be allowed to stabilize prior starting the experiment.
2. The conductance cell must always be dipped either in solution or in distilled water.

3. The platinum electrodes of the conductance cell must be completely immersed in the solution during the measurement of conductance.
4. There should be no air bubble between the two electrodes.
5. The titrant must be at least ten times more concentrate than the analyte.

Experiment 4.2: Conductometric determination of acetic acid with NaOH

Principle

This experiment is also based on the same principle as the previous experiment. In this experiment, acetic acid is a weak acid. When it is titrated with a strong base like NaOH, initially the conductance is low due to the feeble ionization of acetic acid. On the addition of base, there is decrease in conductance not only due to the replacement of H^+ by Na^+ but also suppresses the dissociation of acetic acid due to common ion acetate. But very soon, the conductance increases on adding NaOH as NaOH neutralizes the un-dissociated CH_3COOH to CH_3COONa which is the strong electrolyte. This increase in conductance continues raise up to the equivalence point. The graph near the equivalence point is curved due the hydrolysis of salt CH3COONa. Beyond the equivalence point, conductance increases more rapidly with the addition of NaOH due to the highly conducting OH^- ions. You will get a titration curve which resembles the one shown in Fig. 4.1. The point of intersection of the two lines gives the point of neutralization, i.e. equivalence point.

Requirements

Apparatus

Same as given in previous experiment

Chemicals

Acetic acid solution and sodium hydroxide.

Solutions provided

1. 0.1M sodium hydroxide solution (standardized with either standard oxalic acid or potassium hydrogen phthalate).
2. Acetic acid solution.

Procedure

1. Pipette out 30 ml of acetic acid solution in a 50 ml beaker and dip the conductivity cell into it.
2. Take NaOH solution in the burette.
3. Connect the conductometer to the mains and to the conductance cell. Switch on the instrument keeping the meter switch at 'CAL'.
4. Calibrate the meter keeping the selector knob at '20 ms' by rotating the 'sensitivity' knob till the meter reads 1.0.
5. Shift the meter switch to 'Read'. Read the conductance of the solution. Record this value in the Observation Table 2.
6. Make additions of NaOH from the burette as given in Observation Table 2. After each addition, stir the solution well and read the conductance. Enter all the conductance data in Observation Table 2.
7. Plot conductance versus volume of NaOH on a graph sheet and calculate the volume (V_1 ml) of standard NaOH used in the titration.

Observations

Observation Table 2: Conductometric titration of a given acetic acid solution with a strong base (NaOH)

Volume of 0.1M NaOH added (ml)	Conductance (mS)
0.00	
0.30	
0.60 and so on	

Calculations

Molarilty of acetic acid solution (M_2) = ?
Molarity of standard NaOH solution = M_1
Volume of NaOH solution used from (from the graph) = V_1 ml
Volume of the acetic acid solution taken = V_2 (30 ml)
Molarity equation for the titration of acetic acid solution) and NaOH can be written as

$$M_1V_1 \ (NaOH) = M_2V_2 \ (CH_3OOH)$$

Molarity of the acetic acid solution, $M_2 = M_1V_1/V_2$

Result

The molarity of acetic acid solution = ... M

Experiment 4.3: Conductometric titration of a mixture of a strong acid (HCI) and weak acid (CH₃COOH) with a strong base

Principle

This experiment is also based on the same principle as the previous Experiment 4.2. When a mixture of a strong acid and a weak acid is titrated with a strong base or a weak base, a titration curve similar to Fig. 4.2 is obtained. In this curve there are two break points. The first break point corresponds to the neutralization of strong acid. When the strong acid has been completely neutralized only then the weak acid starts neutralizing. The second break point corresponds to the neutralization of weak acid and after that the conductance increases due to the excess of OH^- ions in case of a strong base as the titrant. However, when the titrant is a weak base, it remains almost constant after the end point.

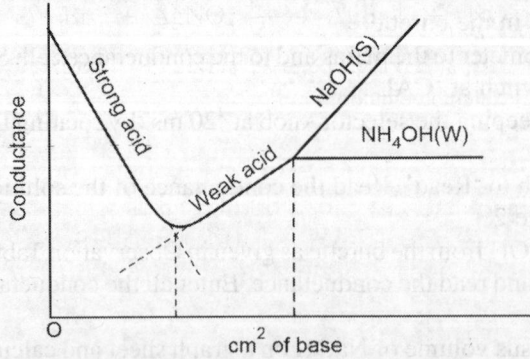

Fig. 4.2: Conductometric titration—a mixture of a strong acid (HCI) and a weak acid (CH₃COOH) vs a strong base (NaOH) or a weak vase (NH₄OH)

Requirements

Apparatus

Same as given in Experiment 4.2.

Chemicals

Sodium hydroxide, hydrochloric acid and acetic acid.

Solutions provided

1. 0.1M sodium hydroxide solution which was standardized with standard oxalic acid.
2. Mixture of ~0.01M HCl (15 ml) and ~0.01M acetic acid (15 ml).

Procedure

1. Take 30 ml of given solution (mixture of ~0.01M HCl (15 ml) and ~0.01M acetic acid (15 ml) in a 50 ml beaker and dip the conductance cell into it.
2. Take NaOH solution in the burette.
3. Connect the conductometer to the mains and to the conductance cell. Switch on the instrument keeping the meter switch at 'CAL'.
4. Calibrate the meter keeping the selector knob at '20 mS' by rotating the sensitivity knob till the meter reads 1.0.
5. Shift the meter switch to 'READ'. Read the conductance of the solution. Record this value in Observation Table 3.
6. Make additions of NaOH from the burette as given in Observation Table 3. After each addition, stir the solution well and read the conductance. Enter all the conductance values in Observation Table 3.
7. Plot conductance versus volume of NaOH on a graph sheet and calculate the volume of NaOH used for the neutralization of HCl and acetic acid respectively.

Observations

Observation Table 3: Conductometric titration of a mixture of a strong acid and a weak acid vs a strong base

Volume of NaOH added (ml)	Conductance (mS)
0.00	
0.30	
0.60 and so on	

Calculations

Volume of the acid mixture taken = 30 ml (mixture of ~0.01M HCl (15 ml) and ~0.01M acetic acid (15 ml).

Molarity of standardized NaOH solution = M_1

1. From the graph, the first change in slope of the conductometric curve gives the first equivalence point (obtained after complete neutralisation of HCl present in the acid mixture). From which volume of NaOH corresponding to this first equivalence point V_1 ml can be determined.

2. Similarly, the volume of NaOH, corresponding to the second equivalence point V_2 cm^3 (total volume of NaOH used for the complete neutralization of both the acids can be determined from the graph. Volume NaOH used for the neutralisation of weak acid = $(V_2 - V_1)$ ml.

3. The molarity of strong acid (HCl) = M_2

Volume of the strong acid taken = 15 ml
Molarity of the weak acid (CH$_3$COOH) = M_3
Volume of the weak acid taken = 15 ml
Molarity of HCl = $M_1 V_1$/15 ml
Molarity of CH$_3$COOH = M_1 $(V_2 - V_1)$/15 ml

Result

Molarity of HCl = …… M
Molarity of CH$_3$COOH = …… M

POTENTIOMETRIC TITRATIONS

Potentiometric titration is a volumetric method in which indicator is not used; instead, the potential between two electrodes is measured (referent and indicator electrode) as a function of the added reagent volume. The part of the curve that has the maximum change marks the equivalence point of the titration.

The main advantage of using potentiometric titration method is that it is an inexpensive method. It uses small quantities of substances. These kinds of titrations are more sharp and accurate as the equivalence point is not determined by using coloured indicators.

General Principle

A typical cell for potentiometric analysis consists of a reference electrode, an indicator electrode and a salt bridge. This cell can be represented as

$$\underbrace{\text{Reference electrode}}_{E_{\text{ref}}} \mid \underbrace{\text{Salt bridge}}_{E_j} \mid \text{Analyte solution} \mid \underbrace{\text{Indicator electrode}}_{E_{\text{ind}}}$$

A reference electrode, E$_{\text{ref}}$, is a half-cell having a known potential that remains constant at constant temperature and independent of the composition of the analyte solution. The reference electrode is always treated as the left-hand electrode in potentiometric measurements. Calomel electrodes and silver/silver chloride electrodes are types of reference electrodes. An indicator electrode has a potential that varies with variations in the concentration of an analyte. Most indicator electrodes used in potentiometry are selective in their responses. Metallic indicator electrode and membrane electrodes are types of indicator electrodes. The third component of a potentiometric cell is a salt bridge that prevents the components of the analyte solution from mixing with those reference electrode. A potential develops across the liquid junctions at each end of the salt bridge. The junctions potential across the salt bridge, E_j, is small enough to be neglected. The potential of the cell is given by the equation

$$E_{\text{cell}} = E_{\text{ind}} - E_{\text{ref}} + E_j$$

A typical set up for potentiometric titrations is given in Fig. 4.3. Titration involves measuring and recording the cell potential (in units of millivolts or pH) after each addition of titrant. The titrant is added in large increments at the outset and in smaller and smaller increments as the end point is approached (as indicated by larger changes in response per unit volume). Sufficient time must be allowed for the attainment of equilibrium after each addition of the reagent by continuous stirring. For this, a magnetic stirrer with a stirring magnet bar is used.

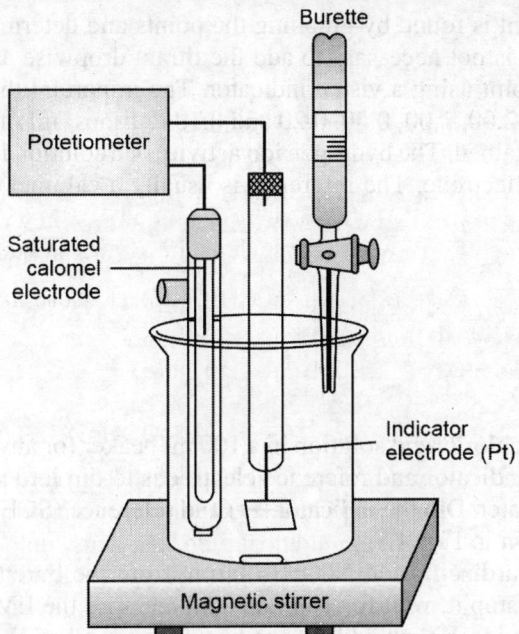

Fig. 4.3: Apparatus setup for potentiometric titrations

End-Point Detection with Potentiometric Titrations

Several methods can be used to determine the end point of a potentiometric titration. The most straightforward one involves a direct plot of potential as a function of reagent volume, as in Fig. 4.4.

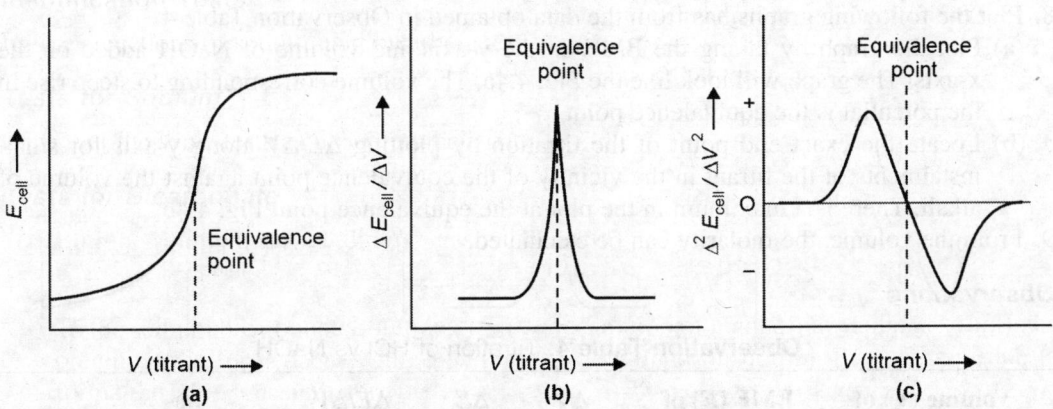

Fig. 4.4: Titration curve. (a) Typical plot of EMF vs volume; (b) Typical first derivative titration curve; (c) Typical second derivative titration curve

Experiment 4.4: Potentiometric titration of strong acid with strong base

Principle

The potentiometric titration is a useful means of characterizing an acid. The pH of a solution is measured as a fraction of the amount of titrant added. The change in pH is small until the end point where there is a sharp change. The strength of an acid or base determines the sharpness of the change. The end point is found by graphing the points and determining the location of the sudden change in pH. It is not necessary to add the titrant dropwise as was required to obtain the exact equivalence point using a visual indicator. The important thing is that a good graph with increments such as 2.00, 1.00, 0.50, 0.20 and 0.10 (2 drops) ml of titrant be added and the resulting pH readings obtained. The hydrogen ion activity of a solution is conveniently measured using a glass indicator electrode. The reference is usually a calomel or silver–silver chloride electrode.

Requirements
- Hydrochloric acid
- Sodium hydroxide

Procedure
1. Take 20 ml the hydrochloric acid solution in a 100 ml beaker (or any other measured volume enough to allow the indicator and reference electrodes to dip into solution).
2. Add some distilled water. Dip the indicator (Pt) and reference (SCE) electrodes in the above acid solution as shown in Fig. 4.3.
3. Add 1–2 ml of standardized 0.1M NaOH solution from the burette, operate the magnetic stirrer for 2 minutes, stop it, wait for 1 minute and measure the EMF.
4. Repeat the above step, each time adding one or two more ml of NaOH at a time and go on noting the EMF after each addition.
5. When the volume reached near about 1 ml of the expected equivalence point (approximate), add the solution from the burette in 0.5 ml instalments and note the potential each time.
6. Continue adding these instalments even after the equivalence point (this can be easily observed from the change in the measured potentials). The change becomes very small. Continue for another 3–4 additions and note the potential readings.
7. Record the observations in the Observation Table 4.
8. Plot the following graphs has from the data obtained in Observation Table 4.
   (a) Plot the graph by taking the EMF on the y-axis and volume of NaOH added on the x-axis. The graph will look like the Fig. 4.4a. The volume corresponding to steep rise in the potential is the equivalence point.
   (b) Locate the exact end point of the titration by plotting $\Delta E/\Delta V$ along y-axis for small instalments of the titrant in the vicinity of the equivalence point against the volume of alkali. There is a maximum in the plot at the equivalence point Fig. 4.4b.
9. From the volume, the molarity can be calculated.

Observations

Observation Table 4: Titration of HCl vs NaOH

Volume (V) of NaOH (ml)	EMF (E) of the cell (mV)	ΔV	ΔE	$\Delta E/\Delta V$	
1.					
2.					
3.					
4.					
...					

Note:

How to determine the endpoint from the following data by the first derivative method.

	Volume (mL)	mV	First derivative	
1.	19.0	235	$(19.5 - 19)/2 = 19.25$	$(240 - 235)/(19.5 - 19) = 10$
2.	19. 5	240	$19.75 = 12$	
3.	20	246		
And so on				

Qualitative Inorganic Analysis

PART I: IDENTIFICATION TESTS FOR INORGANIC DRUGS

Identification tests are performed to determine the quality of a drug for its safe use. These identifications tests for inorganic drugs are based generally on reactions of an anion or a cation or both present in a molecule.

Identification tests of some inorganic substances, feasible in the laboratory, are presented in this chapter.

Ammonium chloride	Iodine
Barium sulphate	Magnesium sulphate
Boric acid	Mercuric oxide
Borax	Potassium permanganate
Bentonite	Potassium iodide
Calcium gluconate	Sodium benzoate
Chlorinated lime	Sodium bicarbonate
Copper sulphate	Sodium chloride
Ferrous gluconate	Sodium thiosulphate
Ferric ammonium citrate	Zinc sulphate
Ferrous sulphate	Zinc oxide
Hydrogen peroxide	

AMMONIUM CHLORIDE (NH_4Cl)

Ammonium chloride is an expectorant, diuretic and systemic acidifier.

It is available as odourless, colourless or white crystalline powder with saline taste. The salt is freely soluble in water but slightly soluble in ethanol.

Identification Tests

Identification tests are based on characteristics of ammonium and chloride ions.

Tests for ammonium ion

(i) Heat a small amount of ammonium chloride with solution of sodium hydroxide, ammonia gas is evolved. The evolved NH_3 is identified by the following tests:

$$NH_4Cl + NaOH \longrightarrow NH_3\uparrow + H_2O + NaCl$$

(a) It has a characteristic smell.

(b) Bring a glass rod dipped in concentrated hydrochloric acid at the mouth of the test tube. Ammonia gas forms dense white fumes of ammonium chloride.

(c) Bring a wet red litmus paper at the mouth of the test tube. It turns red litmus blue.

(ii) Add a few drops of sodium cobaltinitrite to ammonium chloride solution. Yellow precipitate of ammonium cobaltinitrite is formed.

$$3NH_4Cl + Na_3[Co(NO_2)_6] \longrightarrow (NH_4)_3[Co (NO_2)_6] + 3NaCl$$

Sodium cobaltinitrite   Ammonium cobaltinitrite

Test for Chloride Ion

Add dilute nitric acid (1 ml) to ammonium chloride solution (3 ml). Add a few drops of silver nitrate solution, a white precipitate of silver chloride, is formed. On addition of dilute ammonia solution, the precipitate dissolves due to formation of a complex.

$$NH_4Cl + AgNO_3 \longrightarrow AgCl \downarrow + NH_4NO_3$$

Silver chloride

$$AgCl + 2NH_3 \longrightarrow [Ag(NH_3)_2]^+Cl^-$$

Soluble complex

BARIUM SULPHATE (BaSO₄)

It is used as a diagnostic aid. It is used for making the intestinal tract opaque to X-rays. It is heavy, odourless, tasteless, white fine powder. Barium sulphate is insoluble in water, organic solvents and in dilute solution of acids and of alkalies.

Identification Tests

Identification tests are based on the presence of barium and sulphate ions.

Boil barium sulphate (0.2 g) with 50% solution of sodium carbonate (5 ml) for five minutes. The salt is insoluble. It is converted into more soluble salt by fusion with anhydrous sodium/ potassium carbonate. Treat the resulting mass with hot water and filter. Perform the test for sulphate in filtrate and for barium in the residue.

$$BaSO_4 + Na_2CO_3 \longrightarrow Na_2SO_4 + BaCO_3\downarrow$$

Tests for Sulphate

(i) Add barium chloride solution (1 ml) to a part of the filtrate. A white precipitate due to formation of barium sulphate is formed.

$$Na_2SO_4 + BaCl_2 \longrightarrow BaSO_4\downarrow + 2NaCl$$

Barium sulphate
(White precipitate)

(ii) Add lead acetate solution (1 ml) to the filtrate (1 ml). A white precipitate of lead sulphate is formed.

$$Na_2SO_4 + (CH_3COO)_2Pb \longrightarrow PbSO_4 \downarrow + 2CH_3COONa$$

Lead acetate   Lead sulphate
(white precipitates)

The precipitate is soluble in ammonium acetate solution and sodium hydroxide solution.

Tests for Barium

(i) Dissolve a portion of residue in hydrochloric acid and perform flame test. Yellowish green colour indicates the presence of barium.

(ii) Wash the above residue with successive small quantities of water. To the residue, add dilute hydrochloric acid (5 ml), filter and to the filtrate, add dilute sulphuric acid (0.3 ml). A white precipitate of barium sulphate is formed.

$$BaCO_3 + 2HCl \longrightarrow BaCl_2 + CO_2 + H_2O$$
$$BaCl_2 + H_2SO_4 - \longrightarrow BaSO_4\downarrow + 2HCl$$
$$\text{Barium sulphate}$$
$$\text{(white precipitate)}$$

BORIC ACID (H$_3$BO$_3$)

Boric acid is a local anti-infective agent. It is mainly used in eyedrops and in dusting powders. Boric acid is a colourless or white crystalline powder. It is odourless and taste is slightly acidic and bitter with a sweetish after taste. Boric acid is sparingly soluble in water and ethanol, freely soluble in boiling water, boiling ethanol and glycerine.

Identification Tests

(i) Dissolve boric acid (0.1 g) with gentle warming in methyl alcohol (5 ml) containing a few drops of sulphuric acid. Ignite the solution, the flame has green border (flame test). The green colour is due to formation of methyl borate

$$\underset{\text{Boric acid}}{H_3BO_3} + 3CH_3OH \longrightarrow \underset{\text{Methyl borate}}{B(OCH_3)_3\uparrow} + 3H_2O$$

(ii) Dissolve boric acid (3 g) in boiling water (90 ml) and cool. The solution is faintly acidic.

BORAX (Na$_2$B$_4$O$_7$.10H$_2$O)

It is available as transparent, colourless crystals, odourless, with saline and alkaline taste. It is slightly soluble in boiling water, but insoluble in alcohol. It is used as bacteriostatic and pharmaceutical aid.

Identification Tests

(i) Acidify a 5% w/v solution with hydrochloric acid, moisten a piece of turmeric paper with this solution and dry; the colour of the paper becomes pink or brownish red. Pour dilute ammonia solution or solution of NaOH on the paper, the colour changes to blue or greenish black.

(ii) Ignite in a porcelain dish a mixture of borax with sulphuric acid and alcohol, the flame is tinged green.

(iii) It gives the following characteristic reactions of sodium.

(a) To the substance (0.1 g) dissolved in water (2 ml), add 15% potassium carbonate solution (2 ml) and heat to boiling. Then add freshly prepared potassium antimonate solution (4 ml) and heat to boiling. Cool the solution in ice water and if necessary, rub the inside of the test tube with glass rod, a white precipitate forms:

$$NaCl + KH_2SbO_4 \longrightarrow NaH_2SbO_4\downarrow + KCl$$
$$\text{Sodium dihydrogen antimonate}$$
$$\text{(white precipitate)}$$

(b) Acidify the solution of the substance with acetic acid and then add excess of magnesium uranyl acetate solution, a yellow crystalline precipitate is formed:

$$Na^+ + Mg^{2+} + 3UO_2^{2+} + 8C_2H_2O_2^- + 9H_2O \longrightarrow \underset{\text{Magnesium uranyl acetate}}{NaMg(UO_2)_3(C_2H_3O_2)_9.9H_2O} + H^+$$

BENTONITE

Bentonite, a colloidal hydrated aluminium silicate, is used as a suspending agent. It is odourless, pale buff or cream coloured powder with slightly earthy test. It is insoluble in water but swells to approximately twelve times its volume on addition of water. It is insoluble in organic solvents in which it does not swell.

Identification Tests

Identification tests are performed mainly on the basis of the presence of aluminium ion.

Fuse the sample (1 g) with anhydrous sodium carbonate (2 g). Warm the residue with distilled water (10 ml). Filter and wash the residue with water (5 ml). Combine the filtrate and washings. Perform the test with residue for the presence of aluminium and filtrate for silica.

Tests for Aluminium

Dissolve the residue in dilute hydrochloric acid (10 ml) and perform the following tests:

(i) Take the above solution (2 ml), add thioacetamide reagent (0.5 ml), no precipitate is formed. Add dropwise 2N sodium hydroxide solution, a gelatinous white precipitate of aluminium hydroxide is obtained.

$$AlCl_3 + 3NaOH \longrightarrow Al(OH)_3\downarrow + 3NaCl$$
$$\text{(White precipitate)}$$

Add excess of sodium hydroxide solution, the precipitate is redissolved due to formation of tetrahydroxy aluminate but reappears on addition of ammonium chloride solution.

$$Al(OH)_3 + NaOH \longrightarrow [Al(OH)_4]^- Na^+$$
$$\text{Sodium tetrahydroxy aluminate}$$

$$[Al(OH)_4]^- Na^+ + NH_4Cl \longrightarrow Al(OH)_3\downarrow + NH_3 + NaCl + H_2O.$$

(ii) To the above solution (2 ml), add a few drops of freshly prepared 0.05% w/v solution of quinalizarin in 1% w/v solution of sodium hydroxide, boil, cool and acidify with excess of acetic acid; a reddish-violet colour is produced.

Aluminium is precipitated into aluminium hydroxide in the presence of the dye, quinalizarin. The hydroxide forms a coloured lake with the dye. The aluminium complex is reddish violet in dilute acetic acid. Quinalizarin is a 1,2,5,8-tetrahydroxy anthraquinone.

Test for Silica

To the above filtrate and washings, add dilute hydrochloric acid (3 ml), a gelatinous precipitate of metasilicic acid, H_2SiO_3 is formed.

CALCIUM GLUCONATE ($C_{12}H_{22}CaO_{14}.H_2O$)

It is used as an electrolyte replenisher. It is an odourless, tasteless, white crystalline powder. Calcium gluconate is slightly soluble in water, freely soluble in boiling water and insoluble in ethanol.

Identification Tests

Identification tests are performed on the basis of presence of calcium and D-gluconic acid.

Tests for Gluconic Acid

(i) To a solution of 3% w/v calcium gluconate (1 ml), add a few drops of ferric chloride solution, a yellow colour appears.

Gluconic acid is an α–hydroxy acid. It reacts with ferric chloride to form a yellow coloured complex.

(ii) To the sample (0.75 g) in warm water (7.5 ml), add glacial acetic acid (1 ml) and freshly distilled phenylhydrazine (1.5 ml). Heat the mixture on a water bath for half an hour and allow to cool. Scratch the inner surface of the tube with a glass rod until crystals of gluconic acid phenylhydrazine begin to form. Keep the test tube for 10 minutes, filter, dissolve the precipitate in hot water (10 ml), add a small amount of decolourising charcoal and filter. Allow to cool and scratch the test tube to recover the white crystals which melt at about 200°C with decomposition (gluconic acid hydrazide).

Phenylhydrazine forms gluconic acid. Phenylhydrazine with gluconic acid which is purified by boiling with charcoal and identified on the basis of melting point determination.

$$
\begin{array}{l}
\text{COOH} \\
\text{H—C—OH} \\
\text{HO—C—H} \\
\text{H—C—OH} \\
\text{H—C—OH} \\
\text{CH}_2\text{OH}
\end{array}
+ C_6H_5NHNH_2 \longrightarrow
\begin{array}{l}
\text{CONHNH—C}_6\text{H}_5 \\
\text{H—C—OH} \\
\text{HO—C—H} \\
\text{H—C—OH} \\
\text{H—C—OH} \\
\text{CH}_2\text{OH}
\end{array}
$$

Gluconic acid   Gluconic acid phenylhydrazide

Test for Calcium Ion

(i) To a little quantity of calcium gluconate, add a few drops of a solution of ammonium oxalate. A white precipitate is obtained which is slightly soluble in dilute acetic acid but soluble in hydrochloric acid.

$$Ca^{++} \xrightarrow{\text{Ammonium oxalate solution}} Ca(COO)_2\downarrow$$
$$\text{Calcium oxalate (white precipitate)}$$

(ii) Dissolve the calcium gluconate solution (20 ml) in minimum quantity of dilute hydrochloric acid and neutralize with dilute sodium hydroxide solution. Add ammonium carbonate solution (5 ml), a white precipitate is formed which after boiling and cooling the mixture is only sparingly soluble in ammonium chloride solution.

Calcium ion reacts with ammonium carbonate to form a white precipitate of calcium carbonate.

$$Ca^{++} \xrightarrow{\text{Ammonium carbonate}} CaCO_3\downarrow$$
$$\text{White precipitate}$$

(iii) Dissolve the calcium gluconate solution (20 ml) in glacial acetic acid (1 ml). Add potassium ferrocyanide (0.5 ml), the solution remains clear. Add ammonium chloride (50 ml), a white precipitate, due to formation of ammonium calcium ferrocyanide, $(NH_4)_2Ca[Fe(CN)_6]$, is produced.

$$Ca^{2+} + 2NH_4Cl + K_4Fe(CN)_6 \longrightarrow Ca(NH_4)_2Fe(CN)_6 + 4K^+$$
$$\text{Ammonium calcium}$$
$$\text{ferrocyanide}$$

CHLORINATED LIME [Ca(OCl)₂]

It contains not less than 30.0% of available chlorine.

It occurs as white powder and has chlorine like odour. It is partially soluble in water. The solution changes red litmus paper to blue. It is widely used for water treatment and as bleaching agent.

Identification Tests

(i) To chlorinated lime, add dilute hydrochloric acid, chlorine gas is evolved. The gas changes moistened starch potassium iodide paper to blue.

$$Cl_2 + 2I^- \longrightarrow I_2 + 2Cl^-$$

$$I_2 + \text{Starch mucilage} \longrightarrow \text{Blue colour}$$

(ii) Shake chlorinated lime (1 g) with water (10 ml) and filter. Perform the quantitative test for calcium salt as in calcium gluconate.

COPPER SULPHATE (CuSO$_4$.5H$_2$O)

Copper (II) sulphate, also known as cupric sulphate, is the inorganic compound with the chemical formula $CuSO_4(H_2O)_x$, where x can range from 0 to 5. The pentahydrate ($x = 5$) is the most common form. Older names for this compound include blue vitriol, blue stone, vitriol of copper, and Roman vitriol.

The pentahydrate (CuSO$_4$.5H$_2$O), the most commonly encountered salt, is bright blue. It exothermically dissolves in water to give the aqua complex $[Cu(H_2O)_6]^{2+}$, which has octahedral molecular geometry.

Copper sulphate pentahydrate is a fungicide. Several chemical tests utilize copper sulphate. It is used in Fehling's solution and Benedict's solution to test for reducing sugars, which reduce the soluble blue copper (II) sulphate in insoluble red copper (I) oxide. Copper (II) sulphate is also used in the Biuret reagent to test for proteins.

Copper sulphate is used to test blood for anaemia. The blood is tested by dropping it into a solution of copper sulphate of known specific gravity—blood which contains sufficient hemoglobin sinks rapidly due to its density, whereas blood which does not sink or sinks slowly has insufficient amount of hemoglobin.

Identification tests

Identification of copper sulphate is based on presence of copper and sulphate ions.

Test for copper ion

Add a few drops of 2M NH$_4$OH to 1 ml of CuSO$_4$ solution. The precipitate is white-bluish basic salt (CuOH)$_2$SO$_4$ that stabilizes in an excess of ammonia, giving the dark-blue colour product—a tetra ammonium (II) copper sulphate–[Cu(NH$_3$)$_4$]SO$_4$.

$$2CuSO_4 + 2NH_3.H_2O \rightarrow (CuOH)_2SO_4\downarrow + (NH_4)_2SO_4$$

$$(CuOH)_2SO_4 + 6NH_3.H_2O + (NH_4)_2SO_4 \rightarrow 2[Cu(NH_3)_4]SO_4 + 8H_2O$$

Test for sulphate ion

Barium chloride precipitates a barium sulphate sediment from sulphate ions solution. Barium sulphate is sparingly soluble in acids and bases.

Add a few drops of barium chloride to 1 ml of copper sulphate ions solution and observe formation of abundant white barium sulphate sediment.

FERROUS GLUCONATE

Ferrous gluconate is haematinic in action. It is yellowish-grey or pale greenish yellow fine powder. Its odour slightly resembles with burnt sugars. Ferrous gluconate is soluble in water but insoluble in ethanol.

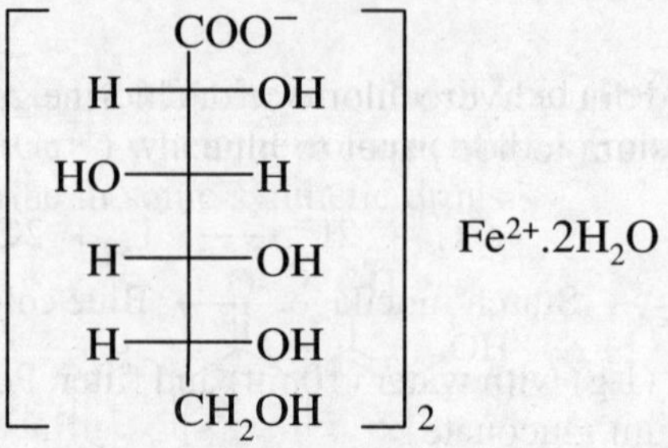

$$
\begin{bmatrix}
\text{COO}^- \\
\text{H} \!-\!\!-\! \text{OH} \\
\text{HO} \!-\!\!-\! \text{H} \\
\text{H} \!-\!\!-\! \text{OH} \\
\text{H} \!-\!\!-\! \text{OH} \\
\text{CH}_2\text{OH}
\end{bmatrix}_2 \text{Fe}^{2+}.2\text{H}_2\text{O}
$$

Ferrous gluconate

Identification Tests

Identification tests are based on reaction of ferrous ion and D-gluconic acid.

Tests for D-Gluconic Acid

Carry out the same tests as in case of calcium gluconate for gluconic acid.

Tests for Ferrous Ion

A solution (1 in 20) gives the reactions of ferrous salt.

(i) Take solution of ferrous gluconate (2 ml), add dilute sulphuric acid (2 ml) and 0.1% w/v solution of ortho-phenanthroline (1 ml). An intense red colour is produced; the colour is discharged by addition of slight excess of 0.1N ceric ammonium sulphate.
   Ferrous ion forms red coloured complex with ortho-phenanthróline (see Chapter 3). The colour disappears on addition of ceric ammonium sulphate due to oxidation of ferrous ion into ferric ion.

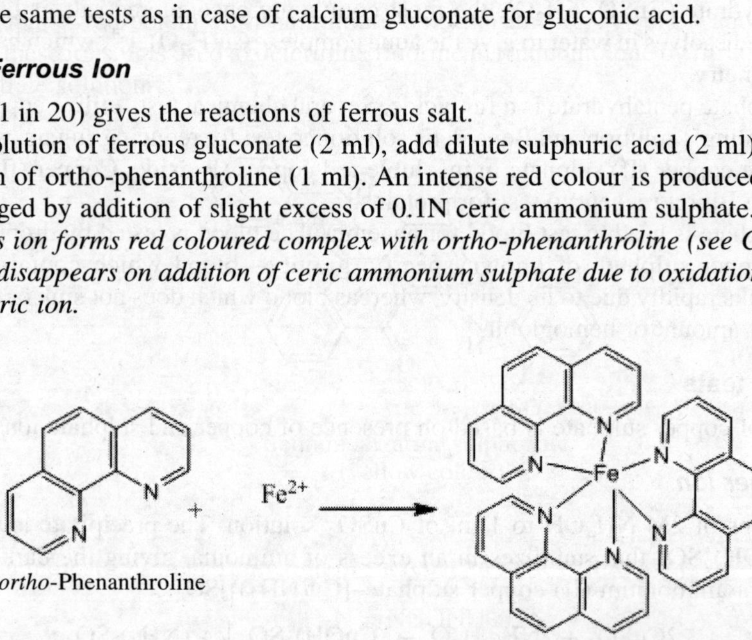

*ortho-*Phenanthroline $+$ Fe^{2+} $\longrightarrow$

Ferrous-tris-*o*-phenanthroline
(red colour)

(ii) Take solution of ferrous gluconate (1 ml), add potassium ferricyanide solution (1 ml), a dark blue precipitate is formed which is insoluble in dilute hydrochloric acid and is decomposed by sodium hydroxide solution. *Ferricyanide oxidizes ferrous into ferric, themselves reduces into ferrocyanide [Fe (CN)$_6$]$^{4-}$.*

$$\text{Fe}^{2+} + 2\text{K}_3\text{Fe (CN)}_6 \longrightarrow \text{Fe}_3 \, [\text{Fe (CN)}_6]_2 + 6\text{K}^+$$

Ferrocyanide ion reacts with ferric ions to form dark blue colour due to formation of ferriferricyanide.

$$4\text{Fe}^{+++} + [\text{Fe (CN)}_6]^{4-} \longrightarrow \text{Fe}_4[\text{Fe (CN)}_6]_3$$

Blue white

(iii) Take solution of ferrous gluconate (1 ml), add potassium ferrocyanide solution (1 ml), a white precipitate is formed due to formation of potassium ferroferrocyanide which rapidly becomes blue in colour in presence of oxygen.

$$Fe^{2+} + K_4Fe(CN)_6 \longrightarrow K_2Fe[Fe(CN)_6] + 4K^+$$

$$K_2Fe[Fe(CN)_6] + O_2 + 2H_2SO_4 \longrightarrow Fe_4[Fe_4(CN)_6]_3 + K_4Fe(CN)_6 + 2K_2SO_4 + 2H_2O$$

The precipitate is insoluble in dilute hydrochloric acid solution.

FERRIC AMMONIUM CITRATE

Synonym: Scale Preparation

It is haematinic, used in iron deficiency. It occurs as thin, transparent, dark red scales or granules or a brownish-red granular powder; odourless with astringent taste. It is very soluble in water but insoluble in ethanol.

Identification Tests

These are performed for ferric, ammonium and citrate ion.

Test for Ammonium (NH$_4$$^+$) Ion

Heat ferric ammonium citrate solution (2 ml) with dilute solution of sodium hydroxide (1 ml). Ammonia gas is evolved. Evolution of ammonia indicates the presence of ammonium ion (see the ammonium chloride).

Test for Citrate Ion

To the solution (5 ml) of ferric ammonium citrate, add calcium chloride solution (1 ml) and boil. A white precipitate of calcium citrate is formed. This white precipitate is soluble in acetic acid solution.

CH$_2$COOH   CH$_2$—COOCa
| |
C(OH)COOH + CaCl$_2$ $\longrightarrow$ C(OH)COOCa
| |
CH$_2$COOH   CH$_2$—COOCa

Citric acid   Calcium citrate
                                          (white precipitate)

To the solution (5 ml) of ferric ammonium citrate, add sulphuric acid (0.5 ml), potassium permanganate solution (3 ml) and warm until the colour of the permanganate is discharged. Add 10% w/v solution of sodium nitroprusside (0.5 ml) in 2N sulphuric acid and sulphamic acid (4 g). Make alkaline with addition of strong ammonia solution until all the sulphamic acid has dissolved. Add more of strong ammonia solution, a violet colour is produced which changes into violet-blue odour.

Citrate decolourizes acidified potassium permanganate due to oxidation into carbon monoxide and acetone dicarboxylic acid.

$$\text{Citrate salt} \xrightarrow{\text{KMnO}_4} CO + \underset{\text{Acetone dicarboxylic acid}}{HOOCCH_2CCH_2COOH} \longrightarrow CH_3 - \overset{\overset{\displaystyle O}{\|}}{C} - CH_3 + CO_2$$

Sodium nitroprusside
NH$_3$ solution

Violet colour $\longrightarrow$ Violet-blue colour

Acetone dicarboxylic acid is converted into acetone. It also reacts with sodium nitroprusside, $Na_2[Fe(CN)_5NO]2H_2O$ in the presence of sulphamic acid, NH_2SO_3H to give a violet colour which changes into violet-blue colour.

Tests for Ferric Salt

(i) Gently ignite the sample in a China dish. Dissolve the residue in hydrochloric acid. Carry out the following tests with the solution:

(ii) To the solution (1 ml), add 5% w/v solution of potassium ferrocyanide (1 ml). An intense blue precipitate is formed due to formation of ferricyanide, $Fe_4[Fe(CN)_6]_3$.

$$Fe^{+++} \xrightarrow{\text{HCl}} FeCl_3$$

$$\underset{\text{Potassium ferrocyanide}}{4FeCl_3 + 3K_4[Fe(CN)_6]M} \longrightarrow \underset{\text{Ferriferrocyanide}}{Fe_4[Fe(CN)_6]_3 + 12KCl}$$

(iii) To the above solution (4 ml), add ammonium thiocyanate solution (1 ml). Red colour is produced due to formation of ferric thiocyanate.

$$FeCl_3 + NH_4SCN \longrightarrow \underset{\text{Ferric thiocyanate}}{Fe(SCN)_3 + 3NH_4Cl}$$

Divide this solution into two portions. To one portion add ether (5 ml), shake and allow to stand. The ether layer becomes pink due to solubility of ferric thiocyanate in ether. To another portion add 0.2M mercuric chloride (3 ml). The red colour disappears due to formation of non-dissociated mercuric thiocyanate Hg (SCN)$_2$.

$$2Fe(SCN)_3 + 3HgCl_2 \longrightarrow \underset{\text{Mercuric thiocyanate}}{3Hg(SCN)_2 + 2FeCl_3}$$

(iv) To the above solution (3 ml), add acetic acid followed by addition of 0.2% w/v solution of 8-hydroxy-7-iodoquinoline-5-sulphonic acid (2 ml). A stable green colour is produced. The reagent 8-hydroxy-7-iodiquinoline-5-sulphonic acid (also called ferron reagent), forms green-coloured complex in acidic medium (Part III).

This reagent forms complex with ferric cation to impart green colour.

8-Hydroxy-7-iodiquinoline-5-sulphonic acid

FERROUS SULPHATE (FeSO$_4$.7H$_2$O)

Synonym: Green vitrol

It is a haematinic compound, available as transparent, green crystals or as a pale bluish green, crystalline powder. It occurs as heptahydrate. It is efflorescent in dry air and on exposure to moist air, the crystals rapidly oxidize and become coated with brownish yellow basic ferrous sulphate.

It is soluble in water but insoluble in ethanol. It is used in the treatment of anaemia.

Identification Tests

Identification tests are performed for the ferrous salts and sulphates.

Tests for Ferrous Salts

Carry out the same tests for ferrous salts as in ferrous gluconate.

Tests for Sulphate

(i) Take the solution of ferrous sulphate (1 g in 20 ml) (5 ml) in a test tube, and dilute hydrochloric acid (1 ml) and barium chloride solution (1 ml), white precipitate or turbidity appears due to formation of barium sulphate.

$$FeSO_4 + BaCl_2 \longrightarrow BaSO_4\downarrow + FeCl_2$$
$$\text{Barium sulphate}$$

(ii) Add lead acetate solution (2 ml) to ferrous sulphate solution (5 ml); a white precipitate of lead sulphate is formed.

HYDROGEN PEROXIDE (H$_2$O$_2$)

It is an antiseptic and topical anti-infective agent. It occurs as a colourless, odourless liquid with slightly acidic taste. It contains not less than 5% v/v and not more than 7% v/v of H$_2$O$_2$ corresponding to about 20 times its volume of available oxygen.

Identification Tests

(i) Add dilute sodium hydroxide solution (1 ml) to hydrogen peroxide and heat. Oxygen is evolved due to decomposition.

$$2H_2O_2 \longrightarrow 2H_2O + O_2$$

(ii) Acidify hydrogen peroxide solution with dilute sulphuric acid (2 ml) and shake well. Add 1 drop of potassium chromate solution and solvent ether (2 ml), the ethereal layer is coloured blue due to formation of chromium pentaoxide, CrO$_5$, which is more soluble in diethyl ether.

$$K_2CrO_4 + H_2SO_4 + 2H_2O_2 \longrightarrow CrO_5 + K_2SO_4 + 3H_2O$$
$$\text{Chromium}$$
$$\text{pentaoxide}$$

IODINE (I$_2$)

Iodine is a topical anti-infective agent. It occurs as heavy, bluish-black, rhombic prism or plates with a metallic lustre and characteristic odour. It is volatile at room temperature. It is slightly soluble in water, soluble in ethanol, freely soluble in carbon disulphide, chloroform, solvent ether, carbon tetrachloride and concentrated aqueous solution of iodides.

Identification Tests

(i) On gentle heating, it gives violet coloured vapours which condense forming a bluish-black crystalline sublimate.

(ii) Dissolve a few crystals of iodine in potassium iodide solution and add a few drops of starch mucilage. A deep blue colour is produced which disappears on boiling but reappears on cooling.

MAGNESIUM SULPHATE ($MgSO_4.7H_2O$)

Synonym: Epsom Salts

It occurs as odourless, colourless crystals with cool, saline and bitter taste. It effloresces in warm dry air. Its 1 part is soluble in 1 part of water but slightly soluble in ethanol and dissolves slowly in 1 part of glycerin.

Identification Tests

It gives reactions characteristic of magnesium and sulphate.

Tests for Magnesium

Prepare a solution (1 in 20) of the given sample and perform the following tests.

(i) To the above solution (2 ml), add dilute ammonia solution (1 ml). A white precipitate of magnesium hydroxide is formed. The precipitate dissolves on addition of 2M ammonium chloride solution (1 ml).

$$MgSO_4 + 2NH_4OH \longrightarrow \underset{\substack{\text{Magnesium hydroxide} \\ \text{(white precipitate)}}}{Mg(OH)_2\downarrow} + [(NH_4)_2]_2SO_4$$

(ii) To the above solution (1 ml), add 0.025M disodium hydrogen phosphate solution (1 ml), white precipitate of magnesium ammonium phosphate, $Mg(NH_4)PO_4$ appears.

$$Mg^{2+} + NH_3 + HPO_4^{2-} \longrightarrow \underset{\substack{\text{Magnesium ammonium phosphate} \\ \text{(white precipitate)}}}{Mg(NH_4)PO_4\downarrow}$$

Test for Sulphate

Carry out the same test as in barium sulphate.

MERCURIC OXIDE Yellow (HgO)

It contains not less than 99% w/w of HgO, calculated with reference to the substance, and dired at 105°C for 1 hour.

It is an orange yellow, heavy, amorphous powder. It is odourless, stable in air but becomes discoloured on exposure to light. It is antibacterial in action.

Identification tests

(i) Heat gently, it produces red colour but on strong heating, it decomposes into oxygen and mercury.

(ii) Add sodium hydroxide solution to acidified solution of mercuric oxide, white precipitate appears.

(iii) Add potassium iodide solution to a neutral solution. Scarlet precipitate is produced due to formation of HgI_2, soluble in excess of potassium iodide solution.

$$Hg^{2+} + 2KI \longrightarrow HgI_2 + 2KCl$$

$$\underset{\text{Potassium mercuric iodide}}{HgI_2 + 2KI \longrightarrow K_2HgI_4 \text{ (soluble)}}$$

POTASSIUM PERMANGANATE (KMnO$_4$)

It is a topical anti-infective agent. It occurs as dark purple, prismatic crystals with metallic lustre. It is odourless with sweet astringent taste. Potassium permanganate is soluble in water and freely soluble in boiling water.

Identification Tests

It gives reactions characteristic of permanganate and potassium ions.

Test for Permanganate

To the aqueous potassium permanganate solution (2 ml), add dilute sulphuric acid (1 ml) and warm to 50°C temperature. Add hydrogen peroxide solution. Permanganate solution is decolourized, due to oxidation of hydrogen peroxide and conversion of permanganate ion into colourless manganese ions.

$$2KMnO_4 + 5H_2O_2 + 3H_2SO_4 \longrightarrow 5O_2\uparrow + 2MnSO_4 + K_2SO_4 + 8H_2O$$

Tests for Potassium

Heat the compound to redness, it decrepitates, evolves oxygen and leaves a black residue which forms potassium hydroxide on addition of a few ml of water. Neutralize the solution with dilute hydrochloric acid solution and perform the following tests with the resulting solution.

(i) Take the above solution (1 ml), add dilute acetic acid (1 ml) and freshly prepared 10% w/v solution of sodium cobaltinitrite (1 ml). A yellow or orange precipitate of potassium cobaltinitrite, $K_3[Co(NO_2)_6]$, is formed.

$$3CH_3COOK + Na_3[Co(NO_2)_6] \longrightarrow K_3[Co(NO_2)_6]\downarrow + 3CH_3COONa$$
$$\text{Potassium cobaltinitrite}$$

(ii) Take the above solution (2 ml), add sodium carbonate solution (1 ml) and heat. No precipitation appears. Add sodium sulphide solution (0.5 ml) ; no precipitate forms. Cool in ice bath. Add 15% w/v solution of tartaric acid (2 ml), a white precipitate is formed due to formation of potassium hydrogen tartarate.

$$CH_3COOK + \begin{matrix} CH(OH)COOH \\ | \\ CH(OH)COOH \end{matrix} \longrightarrow \begin{matrix} CH(OH)COOK \\ | \\ CH(OH)COOH \end{matrix} + CH_3COOH$$

$$\qquad\qquad\quad \text{Tartaric acid} \qquad\qquad \text{Potassium hydrogen tartarate}$$

POTASSIUM IODIDE (KI)

Potassium iodide is used as an antifungal, expectorant and source of iodine. It occurs as colourless crystals or white powder. It is odourless with saline and slightly bitter taste. Potassium iodide is soluble in water, glycerin and ethanol.

Identification Tests

It gives reactions characteristic of potassium and iodide ions.

Test for Potassium

Carry out the same test as for potassium permanganate.

Tests for Iodide

(i) Take potassium iodide solution (2 ml), acidify with dilute nitric acid, add silver nitrate solution (0.5 ml) and shake. A pale yellow precipitate appears due to formation of silver iodide.

$$KI + AgNO_3 \xrightarrow{\text{HNO}_3} AgI \downarrow + KNO_3$$

Silver iodide
(Yellow precipitate)

The precipitate is insoluble in ammonia solution.

(ii) Take a solution of potassium iodide (2 ml), add 2N sulphuric acid (0.5 ml), potassium dichromate solution (0.15 ml), water (2 ml), and chloroform (2 ml). Shake for a few seconds and allow to stand. The chloroform layer becomes violet or violet-red in colour. *Potassium iodide is oxidized by potassium dichromate and liberates iodine gas which imparts violet colour due to its more solubility in chloroform.*

$$6I^- + 14H^+ + Cr_2O_7^{2-} \longrightarrow 2Cr^{3+} + 7H_2O + 3I_2 \uparrow$$

(iii) To a solution containing equivalent of about 5 mg of iodide ion, add mercuric chloride solution (0.5 ml). A dark red precipitate is formed which is slightly soluble in an excess of this reagent and very soluble in an excess of potassium iodide solution forming potassium mercuric iodide.

$$2I^- + HgCl_2 \longrightarrow HgI_2 + 2Cl^-$$
$$HgI_2 + 2I^- \longrightarrow [HgI_4]^{2-}$$

Complex salt (soluble)

SODIUM BENZOATE (C_6H_5COONa)

Sodium benzoate is a pharmaceutical aid, most commonly used as antifungal preservative. It is white, amorphous, granular or crystalline powder. It is odourless or possess faint odour, and its taste is unpleasant, sweetish and saline. It is freely soluble in water and slightly soluble in ethanol.

Identification Tests

Sodium benzoate gives reactions for benzoic acid and for sodium ions.

Tests for Benzoic Acid

(i) To a 10% w/v solution, add ferric chloride solution. A buff coloured precipitate is produced due to formation of basic ferric benzoate. The precipitate is soluble in dilute hydrochloric acid.

$$3C_6H_5COONa + 2FeCl_3 + 3H_2O \longrightarrow (C_6H_5COO)_3Fe.Fe(OH)_3 + 3NaCl + 3HCl$$

Sodium benzoate   Ferric benzoate

(ii) Dissolve the substance (0.5 g) in water (5 ml). Add hydrochloric acid (0.5 ml). A precipitate of benzoic acid appears. Filter the precipitate, wash and dry and take its melting point which should be 120°C.

$$C_6H_5COONa + HCl \longrightarrow C_6H_5COOH \downarrow + NaCl$$

Benzoic acid

Tests for Sodium

Prepare a solution (1 in 20) of the substance and carry out the following tests:

(i) Take the above solution (2 ml), add 15% w/v solution of potassium carbonate (2 ml) and heat to boiling; no precipitate forms. Add freshly prepared potassium antimonate solution (4 ml) and heat to boiling. Cool in an ice bath. Rub, if necessary, the inside layer of the test tube with a glass rod. A dense white precipitate is formed due to formation of sodium antimonate.

$$KH_2SbO_4 + Na^+ \longrightarrow NaH_2SbO_4\downarrow + K^+$$

Potassium   Sodium
antimonate   antimonate

(ii) Acidify the above solution (1 ml) with acetic acid. Add an excess of magnesium uranyl acetate solution. A yellow crystalline precipitate is formed.

Magnesium uranyl acetate solution is of uranyl acetate, $UO_2 (CH_3COO)_2$ and magnesium acetate, $Mg (CH_3COO)_2$, in dilute acetic acid. Sodium ions on reaction with this reagent form white precipitate of sodium magnesium uranyl acetate.

$$Na^+ + Mg^{2+} + 3UO_2^{2+} + 8C_2H_3O_2^- + 9H_2O \longrightarrow NaMg(UO_2)_3 C_2H_3O_2^-.9H_2O + H^+$$

Sodium magnesium uranyl acetate
(Precipitate)

SODIUM BICARBONATE (NaHCO₃)

It, also known as sodium hydrogen carbonate, is used as an electrolyte replenisher and systemic alkalinizer. Sodium bicarbonate is a white crystalline powder. It is odourless with saline taste. Sodium bicarbonate is soluble in water but insoluble in ethanol.

Sodium bicarbonate, referred to as **baking soda**, is primarily used in baking, as a leavening agent. Sodium bicarbonate mixed with water can be used as an antacid to treat acid indigestion and heartburn. Its reaction with stomach acid produces salt, water, and carbon dioxide:

$$NaHCO_3 + HCl \rightarrow NaCl + H_2O + CO_2(g)$$

It is used for treatment of hyperkalemia, as it will drive K^+ back into cells during periods of acidosis. Since sodium bicarbonate can cause alkalosis, it is sometimes used to treat aspirin overdoses. Aspirin requires an acidic environment for proper absorption, and the basic environment diminishes aspirin absorption in the case of an overdose.

Identification Tests

It gives reactions of sodium and bicarbonates.

Tests for Sodium

Carry out the same tests as in sodium benzoate.

Tests for Bicarbonate

(i) Boil the solution; carbon dioxide gas is liberated.

$$2NaHCO_3 \longrightarrow Na_2CO_3 + H_2O + CO_2\uparrow$$

(ii) To the sodium bicarbonate solution (1 ml), add solution of magnesium sulphate (1 ml) ; no precipitate is formed but white precipitate is obtained on boiling the solution, due to formation of magnesium carbonate.

$$Mg^{++} + 2HCO_3^- \longrightarrow MgCO_3\downarrow + H_2O + CO_2$$

Magnesium carbonate

(iii) Add 2N acetic acid solution (2 ml) to a solution of the substance (0.1 g in 2 ml of water). Close the tube immediately using a stopper fitted with a glass tube bent at two right angles. Heat gently and pass the generated carbon dioxide gas into barium hydroxide solution (5 ml); a white precipitate of barium carbonate appears which is soluble in dilute hydrochloric acid.

$$NaHCO_3 + CH_3COOH \longrightarrow CH_3COONa + H_2O + CO_2\uparrow$$

$$CO_2 + Ba(OH)_2 \longrightarrow BaCO_3\downarrow + H_2O$$
$$\text{Barium carbonate}$$
$$\text{(white precipitate)}$$

$$BaCO_3 + 2HCl \longrightarrow BaCl_2 + CO_2 + H_2O$$

SODIUM CHLORIDE (NaCl)

Sodium chloride is used as a pharmaceutical aid. It is an odourless, colourless or white crystalline powder with saline taste. It is soluble in water, glycerin and slightly soluble in ethanol.

Identification Tests

It is identified on the basis of presence of sodium ion and chloride ion. Carry out the same tests for sodium as in sodium benzoate and for chloride as in ammonium chloride.

SODIUM THIOSULPHATE ($Na_2S_2O_3.5H_2O$)

It is used as antidote to cyanide poisoning. It occurs as an odourless, colourless crystalline mass or coarsely crystalline powder with saline taste. It is deliquescent in moist air and effloresces in dry air at temperature above 30°C.

Identification Tests

It gives characteristic reactions of sodium ion and thiosulphate. It is also identified on the basis of its reducing properties.

  (i) To a 10% w/v solution, add a few drops of iodine solution; the colour is discharged. *It is an oxidation–reduction reaction. Iodine is an oxidising agent and so reduced into colourless iodide.*

$$2Na_2S_2O_3 + I_2 \longrightarrow 2NaI + Na_2S_4O_6$$

 (ii) Solution of thiosulphate decolourizes bromine solution; the decolourized solution give the reactions of sulphate.

(iii) Dissolve the substance (0.1 g) in water (5 ml), add dilute hydrochloric acid (2 ml). A white precipitate, which soon turns yellow due to separation of sulphur, recognized by its characteristic odour.

$$Na_2S_2O_3 + 2HCl \longrightarrow S\downarrow + SO_2\uparrow + H_2O + 2NaCl$$

(iv) Add ferric chloride solution (2 ml) to its dilute solution. A deep violet colour is produced which quickly disappears.

ZINC SULPHATE ($ZnSO_4.7H_2O$)
Synonym: White vitrol

Zinc sulphate contains not less than 99% and not more than 104% of $ZnSO_4.7H_2O$.

It occurs as colourless, odourless, transparent crystals or white, crystalline powder. It is efflorescent in nature. It is highly soluble in water but practically insoluble in 95% ethanol. It is used as astringent.

Identification Tests

Dissolve zinc sulphate (2.5 g) in sufficient amount of carbon dioxide free water to produce 50 ml. This solution gives the reactions of zinc salt and sulphate.

Tests for Zinc Salt

(i) Take the above solution (5 ml), add sodium hydroxide solution (10.2 ml); white precipitate is produced. Add further sodium hydroxide solution (2 ml), the precipitate dissolves. Add ammonium chloride solution (10 ml), the solution remains clear. Add sodium sulphide solution (0.1 ml), a flocculent white precipitate is produced.

(ii) Acidify the above solution (5 ml) with dilute sulphuric acid, add one drop of 0.1% w/v cupric sulphate solution and ammonium mercurithiocyanate solution (2 ml); a violet precipitate is formed.

This test depends upon the violet crystalline precipitate which is probably a triple thiocyanate of mercury, copper and zinc. The ammonium mercuric-thiocyanate reagent is prepared by dissolving 8 g of mercuric chloride and 9 g of ammonium thiocyanate in 100 ml of water.

(iii) To the above solution (5 ml), add potassium ferrocyanide solution (2 ml), a white precipitate, insoluble in dilute hydrochloric acid, is produced.

$$2Zn^{2+} + K_4Fe(CN)_6 \longrightarrow Zn_2[Fe(CN)_6]\downarrow + 4K^+$$

Zinc ferrocyanide
(white precipitates)

Test for sulphate

Carry out the same tests as for barium sulphate.

ZINC OXIDE (ZnO)

Zinc oxide contains not less than 99% and not more than 100.5% of ZnO, calculated with reference to ignited substance.

It is available as soft, white or faintly yellowish white amorphous powder, free from grittiness. It gradually absorbs carbon dioxide from the air. It is used as mild astringent and topical protective.

Identification Tests

1. It becomes yellow when strongly heated; the yellow colour disappears on cooling.
2. Dissolve zinc oxide (0.1 gm) in 2M hydrochloric acid solution (1.5 ml) and add sufficient water to make up the 5 ml. This solution gives the characteristic reactions of zinc salt as in zinc sulphate.

PART II: TEST FOR PURITY

Test for purity can be done by physical comparison with pure standard, determination of physical constants (mp, bp, refractive index, etc.). It also involves the test for specific property on which use of particular compound is based. Some of the examples are give here as per PCI syllabus.

Bentonite

Bentonite ($Al_2H_4Na_2O_{13}Si_4$) is used as suspending agent. Chemically, it is natural, colloidal hydrated aluminum silicate. It is available as very fine, pale, buff, or cream-coloured to greyish white powder.

Test for purity for bentonite includes determination of its swelling power.

Swelling power: Add 2.0 g in twenty portion at a intervals of 2 minutes to 100 ml of a 1% w/v solution of sodium lauryl sulphate in a 100 ml graduated cylinder about 3 cm in diameter.

Allow each portion before adding the next. Allow to stand for 2 hours. The apparent volume of the sediment at the bottom of the cylinder is not less than 24 ml.

Aluminum hydroxide gel

Aluminum hydroxide gel is white, viscous suspension, translucent in thin layers; small amounts of clear liquid may separate on standing. It is used as antacid.

Test for purity for aluminum hydroxide gel includes determination of its neutralizing capacity.

Neutralizing capacity: Disperse 5.0 g in 100 ml of water, heat to 37°C temperature. Add 100 ml of 0.1M HCl acid previously heated to 37°C. and stir continuously, maintain the temperature at 37°C; determine the pH of the mixture; pH of the solution at 37°C, after 10, 15 and 20 minutes, should not be less than 1.8, 2.3 and 3.0, respectively, and at no time is more than 4.0. Add 10.0 ml of 0.5M HCl previously heated to 37°C, stir continuously for 1 hour and titrate the solution with 0.1M NaOH solution to pH 3.5; not more than 50.0 ml of 0.1M NaOH should be required.

Potassium iodide (KI)

Potassium iodide is colourless or white crystalline odourless powder. It has saline and bitter taste. It is used as antifungal, expectorant and source of iodine.

Determination of potassium iodate and iodine

Dissolve 0.5 g of sample in 10 ml of freshly boiled and cooled water, and add 2 drops of dilute sulphuric acid and a drop of starch solution—no blue colour should be produced within 2 minutes.

Potassium iodate and potassium iodide in acidic media interact to release iodine which imparts blue colouration on reaction with starch solution.

$$KIO_3 + KI \xrightarrow{\hspace{1.5cm}} I_2 \xrightarrow{\text{Starch}} \text{Blue coloration}$$

PART III: QUALITATIVE INORGANIC GROUP ANALYSIS

The inorganic salts are identified on the basis of cation and anion present in it. It is, however, advisable for beginners to proceed with the analysis of simple, inorganic salt, salts first and then try for analysis of difficult mixtures. A clear understanding of the behaviour of individual ions and an acquaintance of the common laboratory processes including those involved in dry tests are, however, prerequisite for anyone to make successful attempts for systematic analysis.

The systematic analysis is divided into three parts:

I. Preliminary examination
II. Systematic examination of cations or basic radicals
III. Systematic examination of anions or acid radicals

I. PRELIMINARY EXAMINATION

The preliminary examination consists largely of dry tests. An examination of the physical appearance of the substance and of the gases evolved on heating or on reaction with sodium hydroxide (for ammonia) or with dilute and concentrated sulphuric acid (for anions) heating or on important clues regarding the nature of the substance.

(i) **Physical characteristics:** The colour, crystalline form, odour, etc., should be examined and in doing so the students must be guided by their own experience and knowledge of the appearance of individual inorganic salts, oxides, etc. A detailed account of physical characteristics of inorganic compounds cannot be given here. The indications obtained from the observation of physical characteristics are frequently negative rather than positive, e.g. a colourless substance is not likely to contain hydrated salts of copper, chromium, cobalt, nickel, etc. Similarly all the cations of the light, colourless powder may not be derived from heavy metals like lead, mercury, silver, etc.

The following preliminary tests must be made with a portion of the powdered substance and not with the whole of it. The remainder should be reserved for tests in solution and also for unforeseen accidents.

(ii) **Heating in a test tube:** Place a little of the substance (nearly 0.2 g) in a dry ignition tube in such a way that none of it remains adhering to the sides. Heat continuously holding the tube in a nearly horizontal position and note the changes taking place carefully. Observe the following changes from which following appropriate inferences can be drawn.

Observation	Inference
A. Steam evolved: The substance changes colour from:	**Hydrated salts of:**
1. Blue or green to white or brown	Copper
2. Violet to green	Chromium
3. Green to white	Iron
4. Green to yellow	Nickel
5. Red or blue to violet or green	Cobalt
B. Substance decomposes with evolution of a gas:	
1. Vapour is alkaline and smells of ammonia	Ammonium salt
2. Vapour is acidic	Readily decomposable salts
3. Brown fumes (nitrous) acidic in reaction	Nitrate or nitrite of heavy metals
4. Carbon dioxide (test by lime water)	Carbonates, bicarbonates and oxalates
5. Sulphur dioxide (odour is characteristic)	Sulphate sulphite or sulphide
6. Oxygen (test by glowing splinter)	Ammonium nitrate
7. Carbon monoxide (combustible)	Oxalate
8. Hydrogen sulphide (distinguished by odour of rotten eggs)	Acid sulphides or hydrated sulphides
9. Chlorine evolved (yellowish green gas)	Unstable chlorides of copper, gold, platinum
10. Bromine vapour (red colour and pungent odour)	Bromides of less basic metals
11. Iodine vapour (violet coloured vapour condenses to blue black crystals on cooler part of tube	Free iodide or iodides of certain metals
C. A sublimate is formed:	
Nature of sublimate:	
1. White, ammonia is also evolved	Ammonium salt
2. White when cold and yellow when hot	Hg_2Cl_2
3. White, formed after solid melts	$HgCl_2$
4. White octahedral crystalline	As_2O_3
5. Yellow melting into reddish drops	Sulphur from sulphide
6. White fusing to yellow liquid	Sb_2O_3 or Sb_2S_3
7. Yellow in cold which becomes dark on heating	Arsenic trisulphide
8. Yellow turns red on rubbing	Mercuric sulphide
9. Black mirror-like deposit and globules	Mercury from its salts
10. Steel grey having garlic odour	Arsenic
11. Blue-black, violet vapour	Iodine

D. A residue remains which gives different colours in hot and cold

Colour	*When hot*	*When cold*
1. Yellow	White	Zinc oxide
2. Yellow	Red (after rubbing)	Mercuric iodide
3. Brown	Yellow	Bismuth trioxide or stannic oxide
4. Dark brown	Reddish brown	Cadmium oxide
5. Brownish	Buff	PbO, lead oxide
6. Black	Brown	Fe_2O_3, ferric oxide
7. Blackening	No change in colour	Copper, manganese and nickel salts (only at high temperature)

E. Substance fuses without decomposition

Certain compounds of alkali or alkaline earth metals

(iii) (a) **Charcoal cavity test:** A block of wood charcoal is employed as a support for substances which are to be strongly heated in blowpipe flame. It possess advantage of being cheap, infusible and of being a very poor conductor of heat. Charcoal is also selected on account of its reducing or deoxidizing power which it can exert at a high temperature. Mix the solid substance with about twice its bulk of anhydrous sodium carbonate. Place it in a small cavity in a charcoal block (Fig. 5.1), and heat in the reducing blowpipe flame. Observe the changes.

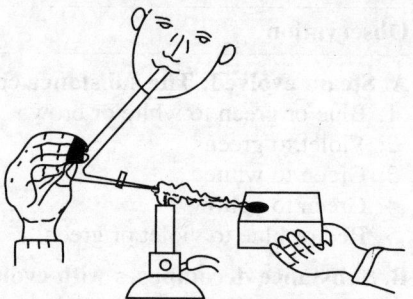

Fig. 5.1: Charcoal cavity test

Observation	Inference
1. The substance decrepitates or crackles	Crystalline salts, e.g. NaCl, KCl
2. The substance causes the charcoal to burn rapidly	Chlorates, nitrates, etc.
3. The substance fuses or forms a liquid bead	Salts of alkalis and certain salts of alkaline earth metals
4. An infusible residue is left on the charcoal:	
(i) The residue is white and very luminous when hot	BaO, CaO, SrO, MgO, Al_2O_3, ZnO
(ii) The residue is metallic with incrustation:	
(a) White incrustation; brittle metallic bead	Antimony
(b) Yellow incrustation; brittle bead	Bismuth
(c) Yellow incrustation; grey and soft metal marking paper	Lead
(iii) The metallic residue without incrustation	
(a) Grey particles attracted by magnet	Fe, Co, Ni
(b) Malleable beads	Ag and Sn (white shining) copper (red flakes)
5. An incrustation without metal:	
(i) White (cold), yellow (hot)	ZnO
(ii) White, garlic odour	As_2O_3
(iii) Brown	CdO

(iii) (b) **Cobalt nitrate tests:** The test is actually an extension of charcoal cavity test and only employed if the residue obtained in (a) is white and infusible. Moisten the residue with a few drops of a solution of cobalt nitrate and reheat the same in the oxidizing flame of the burner strongly. Observe the colour of the residue in cold condition.

Observation	Inference
1. Blue	Aluminium or a phosphate
2. Pink (colour often less distinct)	Magnesium
3. Green	Zinc
4. Dirty bluish green	Tin

Cobalt nitrate decomposes into cobaltous oxide on heating and combines with the oxide present in the cavity to give a double oxide having a characteristic colour, e.g. if Al_2O_3 is present in the cavity, the following reactions take place:

$$2Co(NO_3)_2 \xrightarrow{\Delta} 2CoO + 4NO_2 + O_2$$

$$Al_2O_3 \xrightarrow{CoO} CoO.Al_2O_3$$

(iv) **Borax bead tests:** The test involves the detection of metallic cations by making the use of a bead of borax. Heat the platinum wire in flame and then bring into contact with some borax placed in a watch glass. Thus a little of borax sticks to the loop. Now heat the loop in a flame so that borax loses water of crystallization, swells to a porous mass and finally melts to a transparent glass bead having the composition, $2NaBO_2.B_2O_3$.

$$Na_2B_4O_7.10H_2O \xrightarrow[-10H_2O]{heat} Na_2B_4O_7 \xrightarrow{heat} 2NaBO_2 + B_2O_3$$
$$\quad\quad\quad\quad\quad\quad\quad\quad\quad\quad\quad\quad\quad\quad\quad\quad\quad\quad\quad\quad\quad\text{Sodium}\quad\quad\text{Boric}$$
$$\quad\quad\quad\quad\quad\quad\quad\quad\quad\quad\quad\quad\quad\quad\quad\quad\quad\quad\quad\quad\quad\text{metaborate}\quad\text{anhydride}$$

Touch the glassy bead with a particle of coloured salt and heat again, first in the oxidising flame and then in reducing flame (Fig. 5.2).

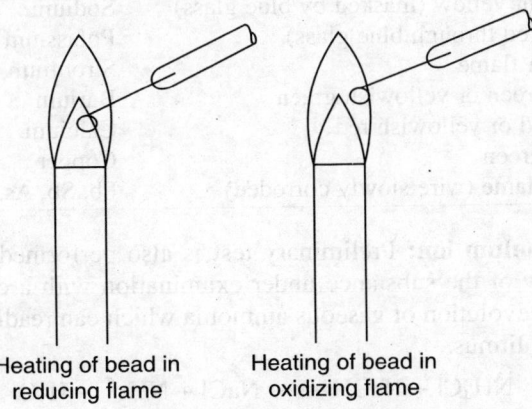

Heating of bead in reducing flame   Heating of bead in oxidizing flame

Fig. 5.2: Borax bead test

Examine the colour in hot and cold in oxidising and reducing flame.

Observation	Observation	Inference
Oxidizing flame	**Reducing flame**	
1. Green (hot), Blue (cold)	Colourless (hot) Red and opaque (cold)	Copper
2. Yellow (hot and cold)	Green (hot and cold)	Iron
3. Bright green (cold), Yellow (hot)	Green (hot and cold)	Chromium
4. Violet (hot and cold)	Colourless (hot and cold)	Manganese
5. Blue (hot and cold)	Bright blue (hot and cold)	Cobalt
6. Reddish brown (hot and cold)	Grey (cold)	Nickel

Borax bead test is based on the fact that when a particular coloured salt, e.g. copper sulphate is heated with a bead of borax, the bead acquires a characteristic bluish-green colour. The formation of cupric metaborate thus gives information about the presence of metallic copper cation in the salt.

$$CuSO_4 + B_2O_3 \xrightarrow{\Delta} Cu(BO_2)_2 + SO_3\uparrow$$
Cupric metaborate
(bluish-green)

(v) **Flame test:** On heating certain metals in the oxidizing (non-luminous) Bunsen flame, they get converted into vapours and impart characteristic colours to the flame.

Since chlorides are amongst the most volatile compounds, the salts under examination are first converted into chlorides before subjecting to flame test.

For performing test, take platinum wire and clean by dipping it in concentrated HCl (Fig. 5.3) and then heating it. Now take a small quantity of powdered mixture under examination on a watch glass, add a little conc. HCl and make a thin paste. Take the paste on a loop of platinum wire, introduce it into outer part of the oxidizing flame. Observe the colour of the flame with nacked eye as well as through blue (cobalt) glass and draw the inference as given below:

Observation	Inference
1. Persistent yellow (masked by blue glass)	Sodium
2. Violet (red through blue glass)	Potassium
3. Crimson flame	Strontium
4. Apple green or yellowish green	Barium
5. Brick red or yellowish red	Calcium
6. Bluish green	Copper
7. Bluish flame (wire slowly corroded)	Pb, Sb, As, Bi or Sn

(vi) **Test for ammonium ion:** Preliminary test is also performed for ammonium ion by boiling a small quantity of the substance under examination with a concentrated solution of sodium hydroxide. The evolution of gaseous ammonia which can readily detected by its odour and alkaline reaction to litmus.

$$NH_4Cl + NaOH \longrightarrow NaCl + NH_3\uparrow + H_2O$$

II. SYSTEMATIC EXAMINATION OF CATIONS OR BASIC RADICALS

It consists of following steps:

(A) **Preparation of a solution of the solid:** Bringing the unknown solid into solution often involves difficulties which may, however, afford valuable information if understood and

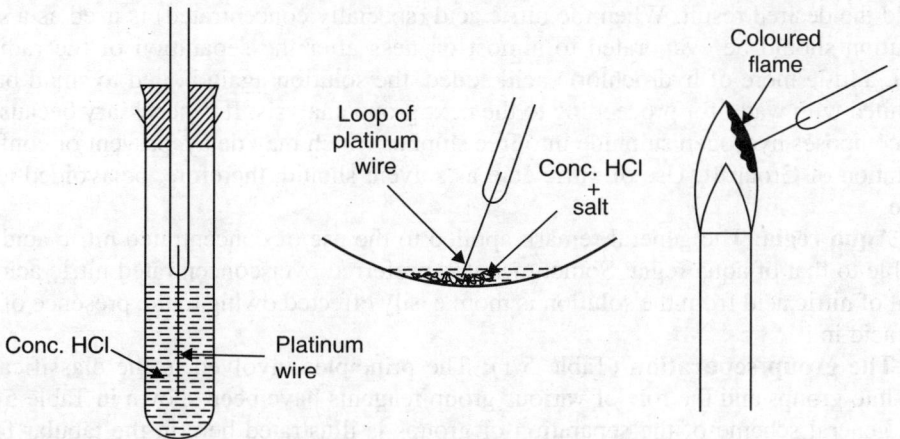

Fig. 5.3: Flame test

overcome properly. The selection of the proper solvent is made by trial on a small quantity (10–15 mg) of the substance. The following solvents may be tried in the order given:

 (i) Distilled water.
 (ii) Hydrochloric acid (dilute and concentrated).
(iii) Nitric acid (dilute and concentrated).
(iv) Aqua regia (3 parts conc. HCl + 1 part HNO_3)

The solvent action of the reagents should be tested first in cold and then on warming and the solvent dissolving total or maximum part of the substance should be used for the preparation of the solution.

After deciding upon the solvent treat nearly 0.5–1 g of the substance and note the changes occurring and remarks thereon as follows:

(i) **Distilled water:** If the substance is completely soluble in water proceed immediately for the analysis of metal ions after cooling the solution.

(ii) **Hydrochloric acid:** It should be ascertained by trial whether the substance is soluble in dilute hydrochloric or concentrated hydrochloric acid. Use nearly 15–20 ml of dilute hydrochloric acid for dissolving 0.5–1 g of the substance. If the solution is obtained on warming it should be cooled first and then diluted to twice its bulk with water. The concentrated acid is used only when it is more effective than the dilute. Only 4–5 ml of concentrated hydrochloric acid should be used for dissolving the above amount of the substance and the solution obtained in this case should also be cooled before it is diluted to nearly four times with water.

A white crystalline precipitate which separated out when the hot solution is cooled is **lead chloride**; it should be filtered off and the presence of lead confirmed by test (page 78). Sometimes a granular white precipitate separates on further dilution which is probably due to oxychlorides of bismuth or antimony. It is redissolved by the addition of just sufficient concentrated hydrochloric acid. Silver chloride also dissolves in concentrated hydrochloric acid but is distinguished by being precipitated on slight dilution and also by its curdy appearance from chlorides of bismuth and antimony. Chlorides of sodium, barium, etc. metals appear to be more soluble in water or dilute hydrochloric acid than in concentrated HCl, which is to be borne in mind.

(iii) **Nitric acid:** If the use of the hydrochloric acid (dilute) apparently results into the formation of a precipitate distinguishable from the original substance, use of dilute nitric acid is favoured. Concentrated nitric acid should only be employed when the dilute nitric acid does not yield the desired result. When the nitric acid (specially concentrated) is used as a solvent, the solution should be evaporated to almost dryness after the separation of the radicals of Group I, a little more of hydrochloric acid added, the solution again boiled to small bulk and then diluted with water for proceeding to the next group analysis. It is necessary because nitric acid decomposes hydrogen sulphide into free sulphur which may delay, prevent or confuse the precipitation of Group II. Use of nitric acid as solvent should, therefore, be avoided as far as possible.

(iv) **Aqua regia:** The general remark applied to the use of concentrated nitric acid is also applicable to that of aqua regia. Sometimes it is preferred over concentrated nitric acid as the removal of nitric acid from the solution is more easily effected owing to the presence of hydrochloric acid in it.

(B) **The group separation** (Table 5.1): The principles involved in the classification of cations into groups and the role of various group reagents have been shown in Table 5.1.

The general scheme of the separation of groups is illustrated here in the tabular form. In doing so, it is, however, assumed that the "original solution"* meant for the group separation contains most of the metal ions in question. Following points may be kept in mind before actually applying the scheme for analysis:

 (i) Group reagents should always be employed in succession.
 (ii) A group reagent separates the particular group only from those which follow it and not from those which precede it. It is most important, therefore, that one group, should be completely precipitated before proceeding for the next group.
(iii) All precipitates must be washed to remove adhering liquid in order to avoid contamination by the metals remaining in the filtrate.
(iv) The coordinations for precipitation and for other treatments must be rigidly followed.

Comments on Table 5.1—Group I: Changes taking place on the dilution and cooling of the original solution are important. If the substance dissolves in cold dilute HCl the absence of group I metals may be concluded. Lead chloride is deposited in crystalline form on cooling the solution, when lead is present. If further dilution results into the formation of a precipitate it may be due to the metals of group I or due to the precipitation of oxychlorides of bismuth, antimony and tin. Sodium and barium chlorides crystallise out from a concentrated solution on addition of conc. HCl which dissolve on diluting with water.

Group II: On passing hydrogen sulphide for the precipitation of metals of group II, the following facts may be borne in mind:

(i) Strength of HCl should not be very high. The precipitation of lead, cadmium and tin sulphides will be incomplete unless the concentration of HCl is reduced to nearly 0.3N. It should also not be too low as the sulphides of zinc group may be precipitated at this point. The solution before passing H_2S should, therefore, be suitably diluted either with water or with a solution of ammonia; the latter should be used with a view to avoid the unnecessary increase in the volume of the solution.

(ii) Group II should be precipitated from a hot solution because heating favours coagulation of the sulphides and its subsequent filtration.

(iii) In case large quantity of nitrates has been detected in the original substance (mixture) or the original solution has been prepared in nitric acid or aqua regia, the removal of nitric acid should be effected as described previously (preparation of a solution of the solid).

(iv) If As is detected in preliminary examination, the possibility of the presence of arsenate should be considered. The arsenate is slowly precipitated by H_2S, it should, therefore, be reduced

---

* By "original solution" is meant the solution of the substance to which no group reagent has been added.

Table 5.1: The separation of groups of cations

Add dilute HCl to the original solution of the substance in cold. If any precipitate forms, continue to add HCl until no further precipitation takes place and filter.

Residue: Wash the residue with cold water acidified with hydrochloric acid and examine as outlined in Table 5.2, Group I

Filtrate or solution is evaporated to almost dryness to expel HNO_3, if used, the residue is dissolved in HCl and diluted to adjust the HCl concentration to approx. 0.3 N. Heat it nearly to boiling and then saturate with H_2S and filter.*

Residue: Normally coloured and consists of the sulphides of metals of group II. It may be washed with a solution of H_2S gas in water diluted with HCl. Examine the residue as outlined in Tables 5.4 and 5.5, Group II

Filtrate or solution is boiled in a porcelain dish until the vapour ceases to blacken lead acetate paper and, thus, the removal of H_2S is ensured. Add 3–4 ml of concentrated nitric acid to oxidize any ferrous ion into ferric and boil the liquid further. If any of the interfering radicals has been detected in acid radicals, their removal should be carried out at this stage (see the removal of interfering radicals).

If interfering radical is absent, add nearly 1.5 g of solid NH_4Cl and an excess of ammonium hydroxide, and filter immediately, wash the precipitate with ammoniacal water and reject the washings

Residue: Examine as outlines in Table 5.6, Group III

Filtrate or solution Add about 2 ml of NH_4OH, pass H_2S and heat it to almost boiling for a minute. Filter.

Residue: Examine as outlined in the Table 5.8, Group IV

Filtrate or solution. Boil off H_2S and concentrate the solution by evaporating the liquid. Make it alkaline by adding a little of NH_4OH and then add ammonium carbonate. Warm gently and filter

Residue: Examine as outlined in the Table 5.9, Group V

Filtrate or solution. Examine according to instructions given in Table 5.10, Group VI

* To ensure the complete precipitation the filtrate or solution is diluted and H_2S is passed again into it. The process is repeated if necessary.

by passing sulphur dioxide to arsenite; the excess of SO_2 should be boiled off. This operation also helps in reducing oxidising salts, e.g. permanganate, dichromate, ferric salt, etc. The use of sulphur dioxide is objected to owing to the possibility of the formation of sulphuric acid from it which may precipitate lead strontium and barium as their sulphates. The precipitate if any formed in this way, should be examined for these metals (refer to scheme of analysis of insoluble substances).

An alternative method for reducing arsenate into arsenite is to add 4–5 ml of concentrated HCl and 1 ml (not more) of 10% solution of ammonium iodide into the solution and to heat the solution to boil. Pass H_2S for about five minutes to precipitate arsenic completely and to confirm the same treat a small test portion with H_2S.

(v) The complete precipitation should always be ascertained by diluting a little of the final filtrate and heating it with hydrogen sulphide.

Group III: (i) Take the filtrate from group II, boil off the hydrogen sulphide, add a little concentrated nitric acid to oxidize any iron and the last traces of H_2S and boil it again. Treat a little of this solution with NH_4OH, if it forms any precipitate attempt for the removal of interfering anions at this stage. If no interfering anion has been detected, precipitate the metals of Group III by adding excess of NH_4Cl and ammonium hydroxide.

(ii) The use of ammonium chloride is essential to prevent the precipitation of hydroxides of metals of subsequent groups.

(iii) Only a slight excess of ammonium hydroxide should be added as too much of it does not precipitate chromium hydroxide completely.

(iv) The precipitate formed in this group should be filtered off immediately because a delay in the filtration may result into the partial precipitation of hydrated manganese dioxide due to atmospheric oxidation if the substance contains manganese. Reprecipitation is favoured to prevent the precipitation of manganese hydroxide; dissolve the precipitate in dilute HCl and add ammonium hydroxide in slight excess, warm and filter the precipitate without any delay.

Group IV: (i) Filtrate or solution from Group III may be coloured, blue by Ni and pink by Co or otherwise colourless.

(ii) This solution should be made distinctly alkaline by adding a little of NH_4OH. When ammonium sulphide is used as the precipitant the solution need not be necessarily ammonical but neutral only.

(iii) Hydrogen sulphide should not be passed for more than one minute in this group as in the presence of too much of H_2S, NiS partially forms a colloidal solution and escapes in the filtrate.

(iv) The filtrate from Group IV is coloured (brown or dark) may be suspected to contain NiS in colloidal form. Acidifying this solution with acetic acid and boiling subsequently coagulate NiS which should be filtered before the precipitation for Group V is attempted.

(v) If the filtrate from Group IV is allowed to stand in contact with air before further treatment, some of the ammonium sulphide (H_2S is ammoniacal solution) may be oxidized to sulphate which may cause the precipitation of sulphates of barium, strontium. To avoid the oxidation of sulphide into sulphate the filtrate should be acidified immediately.

Group V: (i) The precipitation should be effected by a freshly prepared concentrated solution of $(NH_4)_2CO_3$ as the solution of this reagent slowly gives out ammonia and carbon dioxide due to decomposition of ammonium carbonate and thus becomes very dilute on long-standing.

(ii) The complete precipitation is aided by allowing the solution to stand or better by digesting it on a water bath (50°C) after the addition of ammonium carbonate.

(iii) The solution meant for this group should be ammonical and should contain ammonium chloride solution.

(iv) Owing to the slight solubility of carbonates of metals of Group V, the filtrate from this group may contain traces of these metals when these metals are present. Since these metals may interfere to an extent with tests at the metals of the next group (flame tests for K and Na and phosphate precipitate for Mg), it is recommended that the filtrate of this group may be treated with a little of ammonium sulphate and ammonium oxalate solution and the precipitate, if any, formed is filtered.

Group VI: Follow the instructions for the analysis of alkali group metals including Mg as given in Table 5.10. As they are not precipitated out collectively, nothing is described in the scheme of group separations.

(C) Analysis of Various Groups

(i) Analysis of Group I (Silver Group)

Add dilute HCl to the original solution of the substance in cold until no further precipitation takes place and filter. The precipitate obtained may consist of $PbCl_2$, AgCl and Hg_2Cl_2. Wash the precipitate on the filter once with a little HCl (2N) and two or three times with cold water. Transfer the precipitates to a boiling tube and boil with 10 ml of water. Filter while hot.

Table 5.2: Analysis of group I cations		
Add dilute HCl to the original solution in cold. If precipitates appear, filter.		
Filtrate: The solution may contain $PbCl_2$; brilliant crystals are deposited on cooling. Redissolve the crystals by heating the filtrate and confirm the presence of lead taking a small portion of the solution each time by following tests: (i) K_2CrO_4 solution gives a yellow precipitates insoluble in acetic acid. (ii) A solution of KI forms PbI_2, brilliant yellow precipitates. (iii) A portion of the solution gives white precipitates $PbSO_4$ with dilute H_2SO_4. The precipitates are soluble in ammonium acetate. **Pb⁺⁺**	**Residue:** May contain AgCl and Hg_2Cl_2. It should be washed with hot water free from traces of $PbCl_2$. Take the residue in a boiling tube, warm with 10 ml of NH_4OH and filter	
	Filtrate: May contain silver. Confirm by following tests taking a portion of the solution each time: (i) Acidify with dilute HCl. White precipitates of AgCl becomes curdy on warming. (ii) KI solution gives a pale yellow precipitates of AgI. (iii) K_2CrO_4 solution produces red precipitates of Ag_2CrO_4. **Ag⁺**	**Residue** is black if Hg is present. Scrap the precipitate from the filter and dissolve it in 2 ml of conc. HCl and a few drops of conc. HNO_3. Boil the solution for 1–2 minutes, dilute and filter, if necessary. Confirm Hg by testing a portion of the solution each time as given below: (i) $SnCl_2$ forms a white precipitates which turns grey in presence of excess of $SnCl_2$ solution. (ii) KI solution gives a bright yellow precipitates soluble in excess of potassium iodide solution. **Hg⁺⁺**

Comments on Table 5.2: The separation of the metal of the group is based upon the following facts:

(i) Lead chloride is soluble in hot water and AgCl and Hg_2Cl_2 are not. Boiling the precipitate with water, therefore, dissolves $PbCl_2$ leaving the other two in the residue. The tests for lead ion are applied with this solution.

(ii) Silver chloride is separated from mercurous chloride on the basis of the fact that silver chloride is soluble in ammonia solution forming $Ag(NH_3)_2Cl$ salt.

(iii) The ammonia solution forms a black residue consisting of $Hg(NH_3)Cl$ and free Hg when it reacts with Hg_2Cl_2. This helps the separation of mercurous mercury from silver.

Test for lead: (a) Add potassium chromate solution to the filtrate—yellow precipitates due to formation lead chromate appears. The precipitates are insoluble in acetic acid.

$$PbCl_2 + K_2CrO_4 \longrightarrow PbCrO_4 + 2KCl$$

(b) Add KI solution to the filtrate or salt solution—yellow crystalline precipitate appears due to lead iodide. These precipitates are less soluble than the chloride (0.5% in boiling water.

$$Pb^{2+} + 2KI \longrightarrow PbI_2\downarrow + 2K^+$$

Test for silver: (a) Acidify the filtrate with dilute HCl solution—a white precipitate of silver chloride appears.

(b) Add KI solution to be filtrate or salt solution—yellow precipitates of AgI appear. These are insoluble in ammonia solution but soluble in sodium thiosulphate or KCN solution forming complex compounds.

$$Ag^+ + KI \longrightarrow AgI\downarrow + NO_3^-$$

(c) Add potassium chromate solution to the filtrate or salt solution—red precipitate of silver chromate soluble in nitric acid appears:

$$2Ag^+ + K_2CrO_4 \longrightarrow Ag_2CrO_4 + 2K^+$$
$$\text{Red precipitate}$$

Confirmatory test for mercury, Hg: (a) To the above solution or O.S., add SnCl_2 solution—white precipitates which turn grey in presence of excess of SnCl_2 due to reduction of mercurous chloride to grey metallic mercury.

$$2HgCl_2 + SnCl_2 \longrightarrow SnCl_4 + Hg_2Cl_2$$
$$\text{Mercuric} \qquad\qquad\qquad \text{Mercurous}$$
$$\text{chloride} \qquad\qquad\qquad \text{chloride}$$

$$Hg_2Cl_2 + SnCl_2 \longrightarrow SnCl_4 + 2Hg$$

(b) To the above solution or O.S., add KI chloride solution—red precipitates of mercuric iodide appear which is soluble in excess of KI solution due to formation of complex, K_2HgI_4.

$$HgCl_2 + 2KI \longrightarrow HgI_2 + 2KCl$$
$$\text{Mercuric}$$
$$\text{iodide}$$

$$HgI_2 + 2KI \longrightarrow K_2HgI_4 \text{ (soluble)}$$

Analysis of Group II

Separation into A and B sub-groups: Evaporate the filtrate from Group I or solution to almost dryness to expel HNO_3 if used, dissolve the residue in HCl adjusting the concentration of HCl to approx 0.3N, heat the solution to nearly boiling and pass H_2S till a little of the filtrate on dilution forms no precipitates with H_2S. Group II is divided into two sub-groups. Collect the precipitates produced by H_2S in the HCl solution. Wash with hot water and then heat with yellow ammonium sulphide (5–10 ml) to 50–60°C and maintained at this temperature for about three minutes. Filter it (Table 5.3).

Comments on Table 5.3: Group II is divided into two sub-groups, generally known as the copper and arsenic sub-groups. The sub-group IIA includes the metals (Hb, Pb, Bi, Cu and Cd), whose sulphides are insoluble in yellow ammonium sulphide whilst the metals included in the sub-group IIB give sulphides which are soluble in yellow ammonium sulphide, these are As, Sb and Sn. Yellow ammonium sulphide thus serves as a separating reagent for these two sub-groups. The sulphides of arsenic, antimony and tin dissolve in yellow ammonium sulphide all the members of this group are oxidized into their highest valency states by this treatment. This

Residue: It may consist of HgS, PbS, Bi$_2$S$_2$, CuS and CdS, which constitute group IIA. Wash the residue first with a little of diluted ammonium sulphide solution and then with 10% NH$_4$NO$_3$ solution. Analyse the precipitate as directed in the Table 5.4. **IIA**	**Filtrate:** May contain solutions of the thiosalts of As, Sb and Sn. Acidify the solution by adding drops of concentrated HCl (not excess). A coloured precipitate, yellow, orange or dirty brown settling at the bottom indicates the presence of As, Sb and Sn. This precipitate should be analysed as outlined in the Table 5.5. **IIB**

helps the oxidation of stannous sulphide and antimonous sulphide (Sb$_2$S$_3$) into stanic (SnS$_2$) and antimonic sulphide (Sb$_3$S$_5$) respectively which are easily soluble in this reagent. The stannous and antimonous sulphides are comparatively much less soluble. The following reactions take place in this separation:

(a) As$_2$S$_3$ + 3(NH$_4$)$_2$S$_2$ $\longrightarrow$ S + 2(NH$_4$)$_2$AsS$_4$ (ammonium thioarsenate)

(b) Sb$_2$S$_3$ + 3(NH$_4$)$_2$S$_2$ $\longrightarrow$ S + 2(NH$_4$)$_2$SbS$_4$ (ammonium thioantimonate)

(c) SnS$_2$ + (NH$_4$)$_2$S$_2$ $\longrightarrow$ S + 2(NH$_4$)$_2$SnS$_3$ (ammonium thiostannate)

SnS + (NH$_4$)$_2$S$_2$ $\longrightarrow$ (NH$_4$)$_2$SnS$_3$

The solution containing the thiosalts on acidification, produces the precipitate of sulphides and the excess of ammonium sulphide is also decomposed to produce free sulphur (see below):

(d) 2(NH$_4$)$_2$AsS$_4$ + 6HCl $\longrightarrow$ As$_2$S$_5$ + 6NH$_4$Cl + 3H$_2$S

(e) 2(NH$_4$)$_2$SbS$_4$ + 6HCl $\longrightarrow$ Sb$_2$S$_5$ + 6NH$_4$Cl + 3H$_2$S

(f) (NH$_4$)$_2$SnS$_3$ + 2HCl $\longrightarrow$ SnS$_2$ + 2NH$_4$Cl + H$_2$S

(g) (NH$_4$)$_2$S$_3$ + 2HCl $\longrightarrow$ S$\downarrow$ + 2NH$_4$Cl + H$_2$S

The separation of Group IIA and Group IIB can also be effected by using a solution of 2N KOH solution and saturated H$_2$S water instead of ammonium sulphide. Similar reactions take place in this case too.

Comments on Table 5.4: The separation of the metals of Group IIA is based on the following facts:

(i) Mercuric sulphide (HgS) is insoluble in dilute HNO$_3$(3N) whereas the sulphides of Pb, Bi, Cu and Cd are soluble. The black precipitate of HgS on boiling with moderately concentrated nitric acid becomes whitish owing to the formation of an insoluble compound Hg(NO$_3$)$_2$2HgS. The residue suspected to contain mercury, is dissolved in aqua regia to obtain a solution of mercuric chloride which responds more favourably to confirmatory tests.

(ii) Lead is precipitated from the nitric acid solution as lead sulphate by sulphuric acid. The evaporation of the solution is recommended to expel most of nitric acid which by its solvent action prevents the complete precipitation of lead sulphate. The addition of alcohol also retards the solvent action of the acid.

(iii) Only Bi(OH)$_3$ is precipitated when an excess of ammonium hydroxide is added to the solution containing bismuth copper and cadmium ions. The other two cations (copper and cadmium) form soluble complex ions, [Cu(NH$_3$)$_4$]$^{++}$ and [Cd(NH$_3$)$_4$]$^{++}$ respectively.

Confirmatory test for bismuth, Bi. (a) To a part of precipitates, add a sodium stannite solution when Bi(OH)$_3$, gives a black precipitate that is of metallic bismuth.

$$2Bi(OH)_3 + 3Na_2SnO_2 \longrightarrow 2Bi + 3Na_2SnO_3 + 3H_2O$$

Table 5.4: Analysis of Group IIA (Copper group)

The residue insoluble in yellow ammonium sulphide may contain HgS, PbS, Bi_2S_3, CuS and CdS. Boil it with dilute HNO_3 (3N) and filter

Residue: Black or white may contain HgS. Dissolve the residue in aqua regia, boil off most of the acid and dilute. Test for the presence of mercury as directed in Group I. **Hg^{++}**	**Filtrate:** May contain Pb^{++}, Bi^{+++}, Cu^{++}, Cd^{++}. Test a little of the solution with a dilute sulphuric acid and alcohol, if a precipitate appears, add dilute H_2SO_4 and a little of alcohol to the remainder of the solution, evaporate the solution until white fumes appear, cool, dilute with 10 ml of water, allow to stand for 2–3 minutes, filter and wash with a little water		
	Residue: White precipitates may be $PbSO_4$. Dissolve the precipitate in ammonium acetate. Test for lead as outlined in Group I. **Pb^{++}**	**Filtrate:** May contain Bi^{+++}, Cu^{++}, Cd^{++}. Add a slight excess of ammonium hydroxide to it. If a precipitate is formed, filter	
		Residue: White precipitates may be $Bi(OH)_3$. (i) Treat a part of the precipitate with a solution of sodium stannite. A black precipitate confirms Bi. (ii) Dissolve another part of the precipitate in dilute HCl (1 ml). Add a few drops of this solution to a beaker full of water. A white turbidity confirms Bi. **Bi^{+++}**	**Filtrate:**
			The solution is blue: may contain copper: (i) Add a little of the solution of $K_4[Fe(CN)_6]$ to a part of the solution acidified with acetic acid. A red precipitate confirms Cu^{++}. **Cu^{++}** The solution is colourless: Copper is absent. Test for Cd. Pass H_2S to the solution acidified with acetic acid. Yellow precipitates confirms Cd. When copper is present test for Cd as below: (i) Add a solution of KCN in excess to a part of the solution and then pass H_2S. Yellow precipitates confirm Cd. (ii) To another part add H_2SO_4 and iron powder filter and pass H_2S through the filtrate. A yellow precipitates confirm Cd. **Cd^{++}**

(b) To another part of precipitate, add dilute HCl solution to dissolve. Add a few drops of this solution to a beaker containing water. The white turbidity appears caused by the excessive dilution of bismuth chloride due to BiOCl.

$$BiCl_3 + HOH \longrightarrow BiOCl\downarrow + 2HCl$$
$$\text{Bismuth}$$
$$\text{oxychloride}$$

(iv) The deep blue colouration in ammoniacal solution is a conclusive evidence for copper in this sub-group.

Confirmatory test for copper: (a) To the above filtrate or O.S., add potassium ferrocyanide solution. The reddish brown precipitate appears which dissolves in ammonia solution to give a deep blue colour.

$$2CuSO_4 + K_4Fe(CN)_6 \longrightarrow Cu_2Fe(CN)_6 + 2K_2SO_4$$
$$\text{Copper ferrocyanide}$$

Copper ferrocyanide is decomposed to give blue solution of copper hydroxide.

(b) To the above filtrate, add KI solution—precipitates of cupric iodide appear first which changes readily to white cuprous iodide and free iodine which colours the solution brown. Red coloured precipitate formed with potassium ferrocyanide is due to copper ferrocyanide.

(v) Both copper and cadmium form complex cyanide ions with excess of KCN, $[Cu(CN)_4]^{3-}$ and $[Cd(CN)_4]^{2-}$. The cupro-cyanide complex is much more stable than the cadmium cyanide complex. Thus when H_2S is passed into such a solution, cadmium is precipitated as CdS and copper is not.

(vi) When to an acidic solution, containing copper and cadmium, iron powder is added and solution is warmed, copper is replaced by iron and thrown out as a precipitate from the solution. Cadmium remains in solution in the ionic form and is precipitated when H_2S is passed into it.

Confirmatory test for Cadmium, Cd: (a) Add potassium ferrocyanide to the above filtrate or O.S.—a white precipitates of cadmium ferrocyanide appears (distinction from copper).

$$K_4Fe(CN)_6 + 2CdSO_4 \longrightarrow Cd_2Fe(CN)_6\downarrow + 2K_2SO_4$$
$$\text{Cadmium ferrocyanide}$$
$$\text{(white precipitate)}$$

(b) Moisten a test paper with diphenylcarbazide reagent and dry it. Put a drop of the test above filtrate or O.S. and hold it near the mouth of concentrated ammonia solution—a bluish violet colour develops.

Analysis of Group IIB (arsenic group): To the filtrate obtained after treating the precipitate of Group II with yellow ammonium sulphide, add dilute HCl with stirring until the solution is just acidic to litmus. A fine yellowish white precipitate of sulphur is formed. In addition to that if a yellow or orange flocculent precipitate is also formed the presence of this group may be considered. Filter and wash this precipitate and reject the filtrate. Treat the precipitate with 5–10 ml of concentrated HCl, heat to almost boiling for about 5 minutes, dilute to three times and then filter.

Table 5.5: Analysis of IIB group	
Residue: Yellow, may contain As_2S_3, As_2S_5 and S. Dissolve the ppt. in 2–3 ml of conc. HNO_3, boil to expel most of the acid, dilute and filter, if necessary. Divide it into two parts: (1) Neutralise one part of the solution with NH_4OH and add magnesia mixture solution. White precipitate confirms As. (2) Add to the other part a solution of ammonium molybdate. Yellow precipitate on warming and standing confirms As. $$As^{++}$$	**Filtrate:** May contain Sb and Sn. Boil to expel H_2S completely. Use only a part of the solution every time for the following tests. (a) Add nearly 0.5 g of clean thin iron wire to the solution, warm gently and allow the reaction to proceed for five minutes. A black precipitate confirms—Sb. Filter out the precipitates out and add a solution of $HgCl_2$ to the filtrate. A white precipitate turning to grey confirms Sn. (b) Neutralise the solution with NH_4OH and add 1–2 g of oxalic acid crystals, boil and pass H_2S. An orange coloured precipitate confirms Sb. Filter and utilize the filtrate for testing tin by $HgCl_2$ once again. (c) Add a solution of KOH to another part of the solution till the precipitate that forms is just dissolved. Add a few drops (2–3) of bromine water and solid NH_4Cl. Boil the mixture. A white precipitate confirms Sn. $$Sb^{+++} \text{ and } Sn^{++}$$

Comments on Table 5.5: Yellow ammonium sulphide dissolves the sulphides of As, Sb and Sn forming thio-salts. The precipitate obtained on acidifying this solution contains As_2S_5 (also As_2S_3), Sb_2S_5, SnS_2 and S. When the precipitates is treated with concentrated HCl, Sb_2S_3 and SnS_2 dissolve and As_2S_5 is left unaffected.

Confirmatory test for Arsenic, As: (a) Dissolve the residue of arsenic sulphide treating it with nitric acid. Neutralise a part of this solution or better make alkaline with NH_4OH and then treat with magnesia mixture. The white precipitate of $Mg(NH_4) AsO_4$ thus formed indicates the presence of As.

$$(NH_4)_2AsO_4 + Mg(NO_3)_2 \longrightarrow \underset{\text{White precipitate}}{Mg(NH_4)AsO_4} + 2NH_4NO_3$$

(b) Add ammonium molybdate solution to the other alkaline solution or O.S.—yellow precipitate appears.

$$Na_2HAsO_4 + 12(NH_4)_2MoO_4 + 23\,HNO_3 \rightarrow \underset{\text{Yellow precipitates}}{(NH_4)_3AsO_412MoO_3} + 21NH_4NO_3 + 2NaNO_3 + 12H_2O$$

Confirmatory test for Tin, Sn: (a) Add 0.5 g of clean thin iron wire to the filtrate, warm gently and allow the reaction proceed for 5–10 minutes. A black precipitate appears which confirm the presence of Sb.

The action of iron wire is of two-fold. It replaces antimony from the solution giving a black precipitate of metallic Sb and reduces stannic ion into stannons.

Filter out the precipitates. Add mercuric chloride solution to the filtrate.

The white precipitate appears is due to formation of Hg_2Cl_2. Its darkening is caused owing to the precipitation of metallic Hg.

$$SnCl_2 + 2HgCl_2 \longrightarrow SnCl_4 + Hg_2Cl_2$$
$$SnCl_2 + Hg_2Cl_2 \longrightarrow SnCl_4 + 2Hg$$

(a) Add KOH solution to the above filtrate till precipitates dissolve. Add a few drops of bromine solution and solid NH_4Cl. Boil the mixture. A white precipitate appears.

Stannic chloride forms K_2SnO_3 with a slight excess of alkali. The stannate solution is hydrolysed by the addition of NH_4Cl into stannic hydroxide. Ammonium chloride serves to remove alkali.

$$K_2SnO_3 + 2H_2O \longrightarrow 2KOH + H_2SnO_3$$

Confirmatory test for Antimony, Sb: (a) To the substance (0.1 g), dissolved in water (5 ml), add HCl solution (2 ml) and then pass H_2S gas—orange precipitate of antimonous sulphide (Sb_2S_3) from dilute acid appears. Pentavalent antimony gives a similar precipitate of pentasulphide under similar condition. Both the trisulphide and pentasulphide which are orange, dissolve in concentrated HCl, the former giving antimony trichloride in solution while the latter gives a solution of trichloride with the separation of sulphur.

$$2SbCl_3 + 3H_2S \rightleftharpoons Sb_2S_3 + 6HCl$$
$$2SbCl_5 + 5H_2S \rightleftharpoons Sb_2S_5 + 10HCl$$

Both tri- and pentasulphide dissolve in yellow ammonium sulphide forming thioantimonate from which the pentasulphide is reprecipitated on acidification.

$$Sb_2S_3 + 3(NH_4)_2S_2 \longrightarrow 2(NH_4)_2SbS_4 + S\downarrow$$
$$Sb_2S_5 + 3(NH_4)_2S \longrightarrow 2(NH_4)_2SbS_4$$
$$2(NH_4)_2SbS_4 + 6HCl \longrightarrow Sb_2S_5 + 6NH_4Cl + 2H_2S$$

Analysis of Group III (Iron Group)

(Interfering acids absent)

Boil off H_2S from the filtrate from Group II, add 3–4 ml of conc. HNO_3 and boil the liquid. If any of the interfering radicals has been detected in acid radicals their removal should be affected by the scheme described earlier. If interfering radical is absent, add nearly 1.5 g of solid NH_4Cl and an excess of ammonium hydroxide and filter immediately. The precipitate may consist of

$Fe(OH)_3$, $Cr(OH)_3$ and $Al(OH)_3$. Traces of $MnO_2.XH_2O$ may also be present. Wash the precipitate with very dilute hot solution of NH_4Cl; reject the washings. Transfer the precipitates in a boiling tube with the aid of 10 ml of water and sprinkle in 0.5–1 g of Na_2O_2 (or add 5 ml of NaOH followed by 5 ml of 3% of H_2O_2). Heat gently and then boil and filter. Then, continue according to Table 5.6.

Table 5.6: Analysis of Group III cations

Residue: May contain $Fe(OH)_3$ and $MnO_2. XH_2O$ (only traces). Dissolve in dilute HCl and divide the filtrates into two parts:	Filtrate: May contain chromium (if yellow) and aluminium. If the solution is colourless, tests for chromium need not be done. Divide the solution in three parts and perform following tests:
A. Solution: (i) To one part of the solution add NH_4CNS solution. A deep blood red colouration confirms Fe. (ii) To the other part of the solution add a solution $K_4[Fe(CN)_6]$, a deep blue colour or ppt, confirms Fe. **B. Residue:** To the residue add concentrated HNO_3, and 1 g of PbO_2. Boil the mixture for 3 minutes, cool and dilute with water. A permanganate colour in the supernatant liquid confirms Mn. $\mathbf{Fe^{3+}}$ **and** $\mathbf{Mn^{2+}}$	(i) Acidify one part with acetic acid and add a solution of lead acetate. Formation of yellow precipitates confirm Cr. (ii) Acidify another part with dilute HNO_3 and add 1 ml of amyl alcohol or ether and 3 drops of H_2O_2 to it. Shake the mixture well and allow to settle. Blue colouration in the upper layer (due to the perchromic acid) confirms—Cr. (iii) Acidify the other part with dilute HCl (first acidic, test with litmus paper) and add NH_4OH until just alkaline. A white gelatinous ppt on warming confirms Al. (Alternatively Al may be tested by adding 2–3 g of solid NH_4Cl to a part of the filtrate from Na_2O_2 treatment and boiling. A white gelatinous ppt. confirms Al.). $\mathbf{Cr^{3+}}$ **and** $\mathbf{Al^{3+}}$

Comments on Table 5.6: (i) When the precipitate of hydroxides of iron (ic) chromium and aluminium is treated with Na_2O_2 and water or NaOH and H_2O_2, ferric hydroxide remains unaffected. Aluminium hydroxide dissolves forming aluminate ion AlO_2^- and chromium hydroxide is oxidized to give yellow solution of sodium chromate. Traces of $MnO_3.XH_2O$ remain unchanged.

$$Al(OH)_3 + NaOH \longrightarrow NaAlO_3 + 2H_2O$$

$$2Cr(OH)_3 + 3H_2O_3 + 4NaOH \longrightarrow 2Na_2CrO_4 + 8H_2O$$

(ii) Ferric hydroxide present in the residue dissolves in dilute HCl giving a solution of $FeCl_3$. The solution is tested with $K_4[Fe(CN)_6]$ or KSCN solution to confirm the presence of iron.

Confirmatory test for iron, Fe: (a) To one part of the above solution or O.S., add NH_4CNS solution—a deep red colouration confirms the iron (herein ferric form):

$$FeCl_3 + 3NH_4CNS \longrightarrow Fe(CNS)_3 + 3NH_4Cl$$
$$\text{Ferric}$$
$$\text{triocyanate}$$

(b) To another part of above solution, add a solution of $K_4Fe(CN)_6$—a deep blue colour confirm the presence of iron (herein ferric form):

$$4FeCl_3 + 3K_4Fe(CN_6) \longrightarrow Fe_4[Fe(CN_6)_3 + 12KCl$$

Note: Iron is always detected as ferric ion. To ascertain the oxidation state of iron in original substance, boil a little of the mixture with conc. HCl and filter. Dilute and divide into parts. To one part, add $K_3[Fe(CN)_6]$, if a dark blue precipitate is formed, iron is present as ferrous. To another part, add KCNS solution, a blood red colouration shows ferric ion.

Confirmatory test for Chromium: (a) To one part of the above filtrate or O.S., add lead acetate solution—yellow precipitates appear.

(b) Acidify another part of filtrate, and add 1.0 ml of amyl alcohol or ether and 3 drops of H_2O_2 to it. Shake well the mixture and allow to settle. The colouration (due to the formation of perchromic acid) confirms the Cr^{3+}.

(c) Yellow solution containing CrO_3^{2-} forms yellow precipitate of $PbCrO_4$ on treatment with a soluble lead salt.

$$Na_2CrO_4 + (CH_3COO)_2Pb \longrightarrow PbCrO_4\downarrow + 2CH_3COONa$$
Yellow precipitates

Confirmatory test for Aluminium: (a) Acidify the other part of filtrate with dilute HCl (first acidic, test with litmus paper) and add NH_4OH until just alkaline—a white gelatinous precipitate develop. (Alternatively Al^{3+} may be tested by adding solid NH_4Cl (2 g) to a part of filtrate from Na_2O_2 treatment and boiling. A white gelatinous precipitates confirms Al).

The solution of sodium aluminate is hydrolysed when boiled with excess of NH_4Cl. The white precipitate of $Al(OH)_3$ appears.

$$NaAlO_2 + NH_4Cl + H_2O \longrightarrow Al(OH)_3 + NaCl + NH_3$$

REMOVAL OF INTERFERING ACID RADICALS

(i) Interfering Acid Radicals and Special Treatments for their Removal

Certain acid radicals cause precipitation of subsequent group metals or prevent the precipitation of metals of group III by ammonium hydroxide. Thus, the presence of oxalate, borate, fluoride or phosphate will precipitate the metals of subsequent groups excluding alkali metals when the solution is made alkaline after Group II. Similarly, the presence of oxalate, citrate and tartrate ions might prevent the precipitation of hydroxides of Fe, Cr and Al by the group reagent, NH_4OH. It is, therefore, essential to remove or destroy such anions before precipitation of Group III. This is effected by applying the following methods:

(a) **Organic acids:** The filtrate from the Group II is evaporated to dryness and the residue is ignited before the precipitation of Group III. Salts like oxalates, citrates, tartrates are decomposed in this way and then the normal course of analysis is not disturbed. It should be noted that when the residue is heated, Cr_2O_3 and Al_2O_3 may be rendered insoluble or difficultly soluble in HCl and these should be tested in the portion remaining insoluble in hydrochloric acid.

(b) **Fluorides and borates:** The residue obtained after evaporation of the filtrate from Group II is boiled repeatedly with concentrated HCl. The volatilisation of H_2F_3 with HCl and H_3BO_3 in the steam causes their removal from the solution.

(c) **Silicates:** The repeated boiling of the residue with HCl after Group II makes H_2SiO_3 insoluble which is filtered off.

(d) **Phosphates:** The presence of phosphate should be ascertained once more in the filtrate from Group II from which H_2S has been expelled off completely. Take 1 ml of this solution and add 1 ml of conc. HNO_3 and 5 ml of ammonium molybdate solution. Warm the mixed solution. A bright yellow crystalline precipitate confirms PO_4^{3-}.

The removal of phosphate, even if it is present, is not necessary if the Group II filtrate after due treatment does not form any precipitate with NH_4Cl and NH_4OH. It is also not necessary if phosphate radical has not been detected in the original substance. Removal of phosphate is nevertheless essential if it is present and precipitate is caused in Group III by the group reagent. There are several methods for the removal of phosphate but the one more commonly employed is described here. This method which is known as "Acetate Buffer–$FeCl_3$ Method" is based on the two important principles.

(i) The phosphates of Fe, Cr and Al are insoluble in the solution buffered by acetic acid and alkali acetate. The other phosphates being soluble.

(ii) The complete precipitation of phosphate takes place as $FePO_4$ by the addition of an excess of neutral $FeCl_3$ solution to a solution buffered with acetic acid and alkali acetate.

Removal of Phosphate by the Acetate Buffer—$FeCl_3$ Method

If a precipitate appears in Group III and phosphate has been detected, proceed as follows. Dissolve the precipitate by adding the minimum quantity of dilute HCl with stirring. Take a few drops of this solution and test for iron by ammonium thiocyanate or by potassium ferrocyanide. To the main part of the solution add dilute NH_4OH drop wise until a faint precipitate remains after stirring. Add 4.5 ml of dilute acetic acid and 10–12 ml of 3N ammonium acetate solution. A precipitate if formed at this stage is due to phosphates of iron, chromium or aluminium. Add neutral $FeCl_3$ solution drop by drop until the liquid has a deep brown colour. Dilute to nearly 150 ml with hot water, boil first gently and then briskly for 1–2 minutes and filter.

Table 5.7: Removal of phosphate		
Residue (A): May contain phosphates of Al, Cr and Fe in addition to the basic ferric acetate and also $Fe(OH)_3$. Treat the residue as Group III precipitate (Table 5.6) except that the residue obtained after Na_2O_2 or Br_2 water (or H_2O_2) and NaOH treatment consisting chiefly of $FePO_4$ and $(FeOH)_3$ should not be further tested as the presence of iron is ascertained earlier.	**Filtrate:** It should be free from phosphate which is indicated by its red colour due to ferric acetate. Evaporate the solution to small bulk and add 1 g of NH_4Cl and then slight excess of NH_4OH. Filter.	
	Residue (B): Examine the residue for Al and Cr if not tested for in the residue (A).	**Filtrate:** Examine the filtrate for remaining groups in the usual way.

Comments on Table 5.7: (i) Before proceeding for the removal of phosphate, the filtrate from Group II should have been given all the necessary treatments which are normally given when phosphate is not present.

(ii) The addition of buffer solution is aimed to restrict the pH (4.8) which is necessary to keep the cations of further Groups in solution, it is therefore, important to add buffering materials only in amounts prescribed. If too much of acetic acid is added, ferric phosphate will not precipitate on addition of $FeCl_3$.

(iii) The ferric chloride solution provided on the shelf usually contains some free hydrochloric acid. The solution should be neutralized so that it may not lead to incomplete precipitation by disturbing the pH. The solution is made neutral by adding dilute ammonia solution dropwise until a slight permanent precipitate appears. After shaking, this precipitate may either be filtered off or dissolved by addition of a few drops of original ferric chloride solution.

(iv) Ferric chloride solution should always be added in slight excess to ensure the complete removal of phosphate. The excess of iron forms insoluble basic ferric acetate on boiling. But Ferric chloride should not be added in large excess as it exerts a solvent action on ferric phosphate.

(v) The possibility of Al and Cr being in Residue (B) is very little as they go mostly in Residue (A).

Analysis of Group IV (Zinc Group)

Add about 2 ml of NH_4OH to the filtrate from Group III, pass H_2S, heat it to almost boiling for a minute and filter. The precipitate may contain ZnS, MnS, NiS and CoS. Wash the precipitate with a solution containing 1% solid NH_4Cl and reject the washing. Transfer the precipitate to a small beaker, add 10–15 ml of water and nearly equal volume of dilute HCl. Stir it occasionally and filter after 2–3 minutes.

Table 5.8: Analysis of Group IV cations		
Filtrate: May contain $ZnCl_2$ and $MnCl_2$, boil the solution for 2–3 minutes to expel H_2S completely and then add 10–15 ml of a dilute solution of NaOH. Filter.		**Residue:** Black, may contain NiS and CoS. Dissolve the residue in 2–3 ml of concentrated HCl, add a few drops of conc. HNO_3, warm if necessary, and evaporate the solution just to dryness. Dissolve the residue in 10–20 ml of water. Reserve this solution for the following tests:
Filtrate: May contain sodium zincate, Na_2ZnO_2. Divide it in three parts. (i) Pass H_2S in one portion. A white precipitate (ZnS) confirms Zn. (ii) Acidify another portion with concentrated HNO_3, add a few drops of $Co(NO_3)_3$ solution. Soak a folded filter paper in it and ignite it in flame. Greenish ash confirms Zn. (iii) Acidify third portion with dilute HCl and add $K_4[Fe(CN)_4]$. A white or bluish-white ppt confirms Zn. <center>**Zn⁺⁺**</center>	**Residue:** Whitish first but readily darkens in the air, may be hydrated oxide of manganese. (i) Boil a little of the precipitate with PbO_2 and concentrated HNO_3 for 3–4 minutes, dilute and allow it to stand. Pink colouration (MnO_4^-) confirms Mn. (ii) Fuse a part of the residue in a borax bead. Amethyst bead confirms Mn. <center>**Mn⁺⁺**</center>	(i) Take a little of the solution, add 3–5 ml of dimethylglyoxime and then add NH_4OH drop by drop. A pink coloured precipitate in just alkaline solutions confirms Ni. (ii) Add KCN solution to a part of the solution till the precipitate formed just dissolves; and then add NaOH and bromine water and warm. A black precipitate confirms Ni. (iii) Add NH_4Cl and NH_4OH to about 2 ml of the solution and then add $K_3[Fe(CN)_6]$. A red colour or reddish brown ppt. on warming confirms Co. (iv) Take a little of the solution, add a slight excess of ammonia and then acidify it with acetic acid. Add a solution of KNO_2 to it. A yellow precipitate on standing confirms Co. <center>**Ni^{2+} and Co^{2+}**</center>

Comments on Table 5.8: (i) The precipitate produced in this group may contain ZnS, MnS, NiS and CoS. The colour of the precipitate usually shows whether it contains any NiS or CoS which are black or consists of one MnS (buff) or ZnS (white).

(ii) The presence of Ni and Co is also indicated by the change in colour of the solution at different stages. Nickel salts are green while those of cobalt are pink in dilute HCl and deep blue in conc. HCl medium.

(iii) The sulphides of nickel and cobalt are not appreciably soluble in very dilute HCl whereas those of zinc and manganese dissolve readily. The solution containing chlorides of zinc and manganese on treatment with an excess of NaOH solution, precipitates $Zn(OH)_2$ which passes into solution in excess of NaOH whereas manganese remains with residue as manganese hydroxide which is not soluble in NaOH.

(iv) The sulphides of nickel and cobalt dissolve in concentrated HCl in presence of an oxidizing reagent giving a solution of chlorides of these metals. The tests for these cations are, however, specific and usually there is no interference by the other cation present.

Confirmatory test for Zinc, Zn: (a) Acidify the above filtrate with dilute acetic acid and then pass H_2S gas—a white precipitate appears.

$$Zn^{2+} \xrightarrow{H_2S} ZnS\downarrow$$
Zinc oxide
(white precipitate)

(b) Acidify another portion of the filtrate or O.S. with nitric acid and then add a few drops of cobalt nitrate. Moisten the folded paper with it and ignite it in flame. Greenish flame confirms the zinc.

(c) Acidify the third portion of the filtrate or O.S. with dilute HCl solution and add $K_4[Fe(CN)_6]$. A white or bluish white precipitates appear due to zinc ferrocyanide.

$$2Zn^{2+} + K_4Fe(CN)_6 \longrightarrow \underset{\text{Zinc ferrocyanide}}{Zn_2[Fe(CN)_6]} + 4K^+$$

Confirmatory test for Manganese, Mn: (a) Boil a little of precipitates with PbO_2 and concentrated HNO_3 for 3–4 minutes, dilute it and allow to stand for 2 minutes. Pink colour develops owing to formation of permanganic acid (MnO_4^-).

$$5PbO_2 + 2MnCl_2 + 6HNO_3 \longrightarrow \underset{\text{Permanganic acid}}{2HMnO_4} + 3Pb(NO_3)_2 + 2PbCl_2 + 2H_2O$$

Confirmatory test for Nickel, Ni: (a) Add dimethylglyoxime to the above solution or O.S. and then add NH_4OH drop by drop to make alkaline—a pink-coloured precipitate appears due to formation of complex (distinction from cobalt).

Complex
(pink colour)

Confirmatory test for Cobalt, Co: (a) Take the little of above solution or O.S., acidify with acetic acid, and then add potassium nitrite solution—yellow crystalline precipitate of potassium cobaltinitrate appears.

$$Co(NO_3)_2 + 7KNO_2 + 2HC_2H_3O_3 \longrightarrow \underset{\text{Pot. cobalt nitrite}}{K_2[Co(NO_2)_6]} + 2KNO_3 + 2KC_2H_3O_3 + NO + H_2O$$

(b) Add NH_4Cl and NH_4OH to the above solution or O.S. till alkaline. Add potassium ferrocyanide solution and warm—reddish precipitates or colour appear.

Analysis of Group V (Calcium Group)

Boil off H_2S from the solution of filtrate of Group IV and concentrate the solution by evaporating the liquid. Make it alkaline by adding a little of NH_4OH, then add ammonium carbonate and filter. Wash the precipitate with warm water. The precipitate may contain carbonates of Ba, Sr and Ca. Dissolve it in 4–5 ml of dilute acetic acid. Take 0.5–1 ml of this solution and to it add K_2CrO_4 solution dropwise, if a precipitate appears, mix the test solution with the main bulk and add K_2CrO_4 solution to it until the supernatant liquid is yellow. Warm and filter. (In case no precipitate is formed reject the test portion and proceed for Sr and Ca in the rest of the solution).

Comments on Table 5.9: The separation and detection of Ba, Sr and Ca are based upon following facts:
  (i) Barium chromate is insoluble in acetic acid medium whereas strontium and calcium chromates are soluble.
 (ii) Strontium sulphate is much less soluble than calcium sulphate.
(iii) These ions impart characteristic colours individually to Bunsen's flame.

Table 5.9: Analysis of Group V cations

Residue: Yellow, may contain $BaCrO_4$. Wash the precipitates with hot water and apply flame test. Green or yellowish green flame confirms Ba. **Ba^{++}**	**Filtrate:** May contain Sr and Ca acetates. Render it ammonical by adding ammonia solution. Then, add 2–3 ml of saturated solution of $(NH_4)_2SO_4$. Boil and filter.	
	Residue: White, may contain $SrSO_4$. Apply flame test. Crimson flame confirms Sr. **Sr^{++}**	**Filtrate:** (i) If Sr is present boil it with a little of dilute H_2SO_4 to remove Sr completely. Reject the precipitates To the filtrate, add $(NH_4)_2C_2O_4$ solution and NH_4OH—a white crystalline precipitate shows Ca. (ii) If Sr is not present, add ammonium oxalate and ammonia solution to the filtrate from Ba. White crystalline precipitates confirms Ca. Confirm further by flame test (brick red for Ca). **Ca^{++}**

Confirmatory test for Barium, Ba: (a) Addition of potassium chromate solution gives yellow coloured precipitates of barium chromate.

$$Ba^{2+} + K_2CrO_4 \longrightarrow \underset{\substack{\text{Barium chromate} \\ \text{(yellow precipitate)}}}{BaCrO_4} + 2K^+$$

(b) To the O.S., add dilute sulphuric acid (2 ml)—a white precipitates appear due to formation of insoluble barium sulphate.

$$Ba^{2+} + SO_4^{2-} \xrightarrow{\text{HCl}} \underset{\text{Barium sulphate}}{BaSO_4 \downarrow}$$

Confirmatory test for Calcium, Ca: (a) To the above filtrate or O.S., add ammonium oxalate solution above and ammonia solution—white precipitates owing to formation of insoluble calcium oxalate appear.

$$\underset{\substack{\text{Ammonium} \\ \text{oxalate}}}{(NH_4)_2C_2O_4} + Ca^{2+} \longrightarrow \underset{\substack{\text{Calcium oxalate} \\ \text{(White precipitate)}}}{CaC_2O_4} + 2NH_4^+$$

The precipitate is only slightly soluble in dilute acetic acid but soluble in HCl solution.

$$CaC_2O_4 + 2HCl \longrightarrow \underset{\substack{\text{Calcium chloride} \\ \text{(soluble)}}}{CaCl_2} + (COOH)_2$$

(b) To a solution of solid salt (20 mg) if simple salt in acetic acid (5 ml). Add potassium ferrocyanide solution (5 ml), the solution remains clear. Add ammonium chloride (50 mg)—a white precipitate appears.

$$CaCl_2 + 2NH_4Cl + K_4[Fe(CN)_6] \longrightarrow Ca(NH_4)_2[Fe(CN)_6] \downarrow + 4KCl$$

Analysis of Group VI (Alkali Group)

Add a few drops of $(NH_4)_2C_2O_4$ and $(NH_4)_2SO_4$ solution to the filtrate from calcium group, boil and filter. Reject the precipitate. Divide the filtrate into two unequal parts.

Tests for ammonium ion, NH$_4^+$: Ammonium radical should always be tested in the original substance. Following two tests will suffice:

(a) Heat a little of the substance with concentrated solution of NaOH. The gaseous smells of ammonia of alkaline nature confirms ammonium.

(b) Boil nearly 0.5 g of the substance in 2–3 ml of water for three minutes and filter add two drops of Nessler's reagent to the filtrate. A reddish brown precipitate confirms ammonium ion.

The reddish brown precipitate caused by Nessler's reagent with an ammonium salt solution is due to the compound, $HgO.Hg(NH_2)I$.

$$NH_4^+ + 2(HgI_4)^{2-} + 4OH^- \longrightarrow HgO.Hg(NH_2)I \downarrow + 7I^- + 3H_2O$$

Table 5.10: Analysis of Group VI cations	
(i) Add to the smaller part an equal volume of Na_2HPO_4 solution and a few drops of concentrated NH_3 solution. Shake well and scratch the wall of the test tube with a glass rod. A white crystalline precipitate—on standing confirms Mg. (Apply magneson test for magnesium which is very sensitive and is suitable for detecting smaller amounts of Mg.) $\mathbf{Mg^{++}}$	(ii) Evaporate the larger portion to complete dryness and ignite the residue gently in a porcelain dish till fumes of ammonia no longer evolve. Cool and extract the residue in water and divide it into two or three parts as the case may be. (a) To one part add zinc uranyl acetate, shake and allow it to stand. A yellow crystalline precipitates confirms Na. Perform flame test. Persistent yellow colour shows the presence of Na. (b) To another part add 1 ml of a freshly prepared concentrated solution of sodium cobaltinitrite. A bright yellow precipitate on standing confirms K. Flame test—Crimson flame, lilac through cobalt glass shows K. $\mathbf{Na^+, K^+}$

Comments on Table 5.10: (i) **Confirmatory test for magnesium:** Magnesium forms insoluble magnesium ammonium phosphate, $Mg(NH_4)PO_4$ when sodium hydrogen phosphate is added to the solution containing Mg in ammoniacal solution.

(ii) The ignition of the residue meant for sodium and potassium tests is done to decompose ammonium salts which interfere with the sodium cobaltinitrite test for K, as ammonium also forms similar type of complex which is indistinguishable. The flame tests may be performed with the precipitate produced to ascertain that K is present.

Confirmatory test for potassium, K^+:

(a) To the another part (Table 5.10) or O.S., add concentrated solution of sodium cobaltinitrite, a yellow orange precipitate due to potassium cobaltinitrite appears.

$$2K^+ + Na_3Co(CN)_6 \longrightarrow K_2[NaCo(CN)_6] \downarrow + 2NaCl$$
$$\text{Potassium cobaltinitrite}$$

(b) Tartaric acid produces, in a moderately concentrated neutral solution of potassium salt, a white crystalline precipitates of potassium acid tartrate.

$$K^+ + H_2C_4H_4O_6 \longrightarrow KHC_4H_4O_6 + H^+$$
$$\text{Potassium tartrate}$$
$$\text{(white precipitates)}$$

Confirmatory test for Sodium, Na^+: (a) To a concentrated solution of sodium salt, add zinc uranyl acetate reagent—a yellow crystalline precipitate of sodium zinc uranyl acetate appears.

$$NaCl + 3UO_2(C_2H_3O_2)_2 + Zn(C_3H_3O_2)_2 + CH_3COOH + 6H_2O \longrightarrow$$
$$NaZn(UO_2)_3(C_2H_3O_2)_9.6H_2O \downarrow + HCl$$
$$\text{Sodium zinc uranyl acetate}$$

(b) A white crystalline precipitate of sodium hydrogen antimonate is formed when a concentrated solution of sodium salt is treated with potassium hydrogen antimonate.

$$Na^+ + KH_2SbO_4 \longrightarrow NaH_2SbO_4\downarrow + K^+$$

Sodium dihydrogen
antimonate (white precipitates)

III. SYSTEMATIC EXAMINATION OF ANIONS OR ACID RADICALS

There is no generalised scheme for the separation of anions into groups from which members of each group can be separated and identified as is the case of cations. Most of them are usually detected in the course of analysis by special test.

However, anions are classified on the basis of test to make the easy detection of anions. This consists of two broad divisions, A and B.

Class A: The anions in this category are indicated by evolution of characteristic volatile products on treatment with acids. These are further classified as:

(i) Gases evolved with dilute sulphuric or hydrochloric acid: *Carbonate, bicarbonate, sulphite, thiosulphate, sulphide and nitrite.*

(ii) Gases evolved with concentrated sulphuric acid: *Fluoride, chloride, bromide, iodide, nitrate, chlorate, borate, oxalate, acetate, tartrate, citrate in addition to those given under (i).*

Class B:

(i) Precipitation reaction: These are identified with the formation of precipitates on adding some reagent: *Sulphate, phosphate, arsenate, arsenite and chromate.*

(ii) Oxidation or reduction in solution. The anions of this category possess either oxidizing or reducing properties: *Chromate, dichromate, etc.*

The above classification is, however, not the exact one and has no theoretical basis. Because, sometimes one anion belongs to more than one of the above classes, an iodide, e.g. is tested sometimes by the evolution of iodine A(ii) and also by the precipitation of silver iodide, B(i). Similarly, a chromate is indicated by the precipitation of lead chromate, B(i) and also by its reduction in solution B(ii).

Class A(i) Anions

Carbonates, CO_3^{2-}

(i) Place about 0.5 g of the substance in a boiling test tube, add 1–2 ml of dil H_2SO_4 or HCl and apply the cork with delivery tube immediately. Pass the gas evolved through lime water. The formation of white turbidity or precipitate indicates the carbonate.

All normal carbonates except those of alkali metals and ammonium are insoluble in water. Dilute acid reacts with carbonates with effervescence due to evolution of CO_2 which may be recognized by its property of rendering lime water turbide.

$$-CO_3^{2-} + 2HCl \longrightarrow 2Cl^- + H_2O + CO_2\uparrow$$
$$Ca(OH)_2 + CO_2 \longrightarrow CaCO_3\downarrow + H_2O$$

(ii) To the solution of carbonate salt, add barium chloride—white voluminous precipitates of barium carbonate appear. The precipitates dissolve on adding dilute HCl solution.

$$CO_3^{2-} + BaCl_2 \xrightarrow{-2Cl^-} BaCO_3\downarrow \xrightarrow{HCl} BaCl_2$$

Barium
carbonate

Bicarbonate, HCO_3^-

(i) Place the bicarbonate salt (0.5 g) in boiling test tube. Add dilute sulphuric or hydrochloric acid like carbonate, it also gives effervescence of CO_2, may be on slight warming the solution.

Distinguishing test for carbonate and bicarbonate: Add a solution of magnesium sulphate (1 ml) to a solution of bicarbonate salt (1 ml). No precipitation takes place in cold but on boiling, white precipitates are formed.

The carbonate salt reacts with magnesium salt to give the precipitates of magnesium carbonate in cold.

$$CO_3^{2-} + MgSO_4 \longrightarrow MgCO_3\downarrow$$

In contrast, bicarbonate salt react with magnesium sulphate to give the soluble magnesium bicarbonate. This is converted into insoluble, magnesium carbonate on boiling.

$$HCO_3^{2-} + MgSO_4 \longrightarrow Mg(HCO_3)_2$$
$$\text{Magnesium bicarbonate}$$

$$Mg(HCO_3)_2 \longrightarrow MgCO_3\downarrow + CO_2 + H_2O$$
$$\text{Magnesium carbonate}$$

Test of bicarbonate in presence of a carbonate: Add an excess of calcium chloride solution (1 ml) to the solution (1 ml) containing carbonate and bicarbonate. Filter off the precipitates of calcium carbonate and add a little of ammonia solution to the filtrate—a precipitates formed indicates bicarbonate.

The test is based upon the fact that calcium bicarbonate is soluble in water and is converted into carbonate by the addition of ammonia solution.

Sulphite, SO_3^{2-}

(i) Place the solid salt (0.5 g) in boiling test tube. Add dilute H_2SO_4 or HCl solution (1–2 ml). The evolution of SO_2 indicate the presence of sulphite anion. The evolution becomes more rapid on warming. The gas, SO_2 is identified (a) by its suffocating odour which is that of burning sulphur, (b) by green colouration produced on a piece of filter paper moistened with acidified dichromate solution and held over the mouth of the test tube. The green colour is produced by the reaction of dichromate and SO_2 gas. (c) by forming a precipitate of calcium sulphite when passed through lime water.

$$K_2Cr_2O_7 + 3SO_2 + H_2SO_4 \longrightarrow K_2SO_4 + Cr_2(SO_4)_3 + H_2O$$
$$\text{(green colour)}$$

(ii) To 3–4 drops of soda extract, add 0.5 ml of $BaCl_2$ solution. Separate the white precipitates and to the precipitate, add 1–2 drops of $KMnO_4$ and 2–3 drops of H_2SO_4. The disappearance of pink colour indicates the presence of sulphite.

$$SO_3^{2-} + Ba^{2+} \longrightarrow BaSO_3\uparrow$$
$$\text{White precipitate}$$

$$BaSO_3 + 2H^+ \longrightarrow Ba^{2+} + H_2O + SO_2$$

$$MnO_4^- + 8H^+ + 5e \longrightarrow Mn^{2+} + H_2O$$

$$2H_2O + SO_2 \longrightarrow SO_4^{2-} + 4H^+ + 2e^-$$

Preparation of soda extract: Boil 100 mg of salt mixture with 200 mg of pure anhydrous sodium carbonate and 5 ml of distilled water for 5 minutes. Decant solution and add 1–2 ml of distilled water to it. Label it sodium carbonate or soda extract.

Thiosulphates, $S_2O_3^{2-}$

(i) Dissolve the solid salt (0.1 g) in water (5 ml) and add HCl solution (2 ml)—a white precipitates is produced which soon turns yellow; sulphur dioxide is liberated simultaneously. It may be recognised as in the sulphite ion.

The solid salt containing thiosulphate gives the $H_2S_2O_3$ and sulphur (responsible for white turbidity or precipitation). The $H_2S_2O_3$ gives the evolution of sulphur dioxide.

$$S_2O_3^{2-} + H^+ \longrightarrow H_2S_2O_3 + S\downarrow$$
$$\text{Thiosulphuric}$$
$$\text{acid}$$

$$H_2S_2O_3 \longrightarrow SO_2\uparrow + H_2O + S\downarrow$$

(ii) **Ferric chloride test:** Dissolve the solid salt (0.1 g) in water (5 ml) and add ferric chloride solution (2 ml)—a dark violet colour is produced which quickly disappears.

(iii) The solution of thiosulphate salt decolourizes the iodine solution.

(iv) **Silver nitrate test:** Add the silver nitrate solution to a solid compound in a test tube—a white precipitate appears which becomes black on standing for short time or immediately, if the liquid is heated owing to the formation of silver sulphide, Ag_2S.

The silver nitrate on reaction with thiosulphate gives silver thiosulphate which is converted into black coloured, silver sulphide.

$$S_2O_3^{2-} \xrightarrow{\text{AgNO}_3} Ag_2S_2O_3\downarrow \xrightarrow{H_2O} Ag_2S\downarrow + H_2SO_4$$
$$\qquad\quad \text{Silver thiosulphate} \qquad \text{Silver sulphide}$$
$$\qquad\quad \text{(white precipitate)} \qquad \text{(black precipitate)}$$

Sulphide, S^{2-}

(i) Place the solid salt (0.5 g) in a test tube, and add dilute H_2SO_4 or HCl solution (2 ml)—H_2S gas is evolved. The gas is recognised (i) by its characteristic odour resembling that of rotten eggs, (ii) by its property of darkening a piece of filter paper moistened with lead acetate solution and (iii) by turning a filter paper moistened with cadmium acetate solution yellow.

$$S^- + 2HCl \longrightarrow 2Cl^- + H_2S$$

$$Pb(CH_3COO)_2 + H_2S \longrightarrow PbS\downarrow + 2CH_3COOH$$
$$\text{Lead acetate} \qquad\qquad \text{Lead sulphide}$$
$$\qquad\qquad\qquad \text{(black precipitate)}$$

The black precipitates is formed due to formation of lead sulphide.

(ii) Add solution nitroprusside solution to an alkaline solution—purple colour is produced. *Free H_2S produces no such colour with nitroprusside but the colour is produced if a filter paper is alkaline with NaOH and then brought in contact with the free H_2S.*

$$Na_2S + Na_2[Fe(CN)_5NO] \longrightarrow Na_4[Fe(CN)_5NOS]$$
$$\text{Sodium nitroprusside}$$

Note: The reagent must be freshly prepared.

Nitrites, NO_2^-

(i) Add dilute sulphuric acid solution to the solid salt—brown fumes appear.

Dilute sulphuric acid readily decomposes nitrite with the formation of nitric oxide which gives brown fumes of the dioxide when allowed to mix with acid.

$$NO_2^- + H_2SO_4 \longrightarrow NaHSO_4 + HNO_2$$

$$3HNO_2 \longrightarrow HNO_3 + 2NO\uparrow + H_2O$$

$$2NO + O_2 \text{ (air)} \longrightarrow 2NO_2\uparrow$$
$$\text{Nitrogen dioxide}$$

(ii) Add cold ferrous sulphate solution (1 ml) to nitrite salt solution—dark colour appears. Add a few drops of dilute H_2SO_4 solution—colour becomes more dark.

The dark colour is due to $FeSO_4.NO$ which decomposes on boiling.

$$NO_2^- + H_2SO_4 \longrightarrow NaHSO_4 + HNO_2$$

$$3HNO_2 \longrightarrow HNO_3 + 2NO + H_2O$$

$$FeSO_4 + NO \longrightarrow FeSO_4.NO$$

If the nitrite solution is added carefully to the solution of ferrous sulphate acidified with dilute H_2SO_4, a brown ring is formed at the contact zone.

(iii) Add 2 drops of $KMnO_4$ solution to the salt solution. The disappearance of pink colour indicates the presence of nitrite.

The colour disappears due to redox reaction.

$$2KMnO_4 + 3H_2SO_4 + 5HNO_2 \longrightarrow K_2SO_4 + 2MnSO_4 + 5HNO_3 + 3H_2O$$

Class A(ii)

Fluoride, F^-

(i) Add concentrated H_2SO_4 solution (2 ml) to the solid salt (0.5 g)—H_2F_2 is evolved.

Keep the moistened rod over the mouth of the test tube—a white gelatinous film of silicic acid is formed.

$$Na_2F_2 + H_2SO_4 \longrightarrow Na_2SO_4 + H_2F_2$$

$$2H_2F_2 + SiO_2 \longrightarrow SiF_4 + 2H_2O$$

$$3SiF_4 + 4H_2O \longrightarrow 2H_2[SiF_6] + H_4SiO_4$$
$$\text{Silicic acid}$$

H_2F_2 reacts with glass of rod to form SiF_4. The SiF_4 reacts with water to form a film of silicic acid.

(ii) Add calcium chloride solution (1 ml) to a solution of solid salt—white precipitate appears.

A white precipitates appears due to formation of calcium fluoride. The precipitates is soluble in dilute hydrochloric acid solution but insoluble in acetic acid.

$$Na_2F_2 + CaCl_2 \longrightarrow CaF_2 + 2NaCl$$
$$\text{Calcium fluoride}$$

Chlorides, Cl^-

(i) Add conc. sulphuric acid (1 ml) to the solid salt (0.5 g)—HCl gas is evolved. The gas can be recognized by its odour, by the white fumes which it forms with ammonia or in moist air and by its turning blue litmus paper red.

$$2NaCl + H_2SO_4 \longrightarrow Na_2SO_4 + 2HCl\uparrow$$

White fumes appears due to formation of ammonium chloride.

$$HCl + NH_4OH \longrightarrow NH_4Cl + H_2O$$

(ii) Add silver nitrate solution (1 ml) to a salt solution—a white precipitate appears which is soluble in ammonia solution.

Silver nitrate reacts with chloride salt to give white precipitate of silver chloride. The precipitate of AgCl is soluble in ammonia solution due to formation of soluble complex.

$$Cl^- + AgNO_3 \longrightarrow AgCl\downarrow + NO_3^{2-}$$

$$AgCl + 2NH_3 \longrightarrow Ag(NH_3)_2^+ Cl^-$$
$$\text{Soluble complex}$$

(iii) Place a solid salt (0.1 g) and potassium dichromate (0.3 g) in a test tube. Add sulphuric acid (1 ml). Place a filter paper moistened with diphenyl carbazide solution (0.1 ml) over the mouth of the test tube—the paper turns violet-red.

The chloride ions react with acidified potassium dichromate solution to give chromyl chloride gas.

$$K_2Cr_2O_7 + 4Cl^- + 6H_2SO_4 \longrightarrow 2CrO_2Cl_2 \uparrow + 2KHSO_4 + 4HSO_4^- + 3H_2O$$
$$\text{Chromyl chloride}$$

$$CrO_2Cl + \text{Diphenyl carbazide} \longrightarrow \text{Violet red colour}$$

Bromide, Br⁻

(i) Add concentrated sulphuric acid solution (1 ml) to the solid salt—a pungent acid fumes are evolved. The solution is brown initially but becomes yellow after the brown vapours are given off.

The bromide salt on reaction with sulphuric acid gives hydrobromic acid. Bromine is liberated by the oxidation of hydrogen bromide by sulphuric acid.

$$Br^- + H_2SO_4 \longrightarrow KHSO_4 + HBr\uparrow$$

$$2HBr + H_2SO_4 \longrightarrow Br_2\uparrow + SO_2 + 2H_2O$$

(ii) Add silver nitrate solution (1.0 ml) to a solution of bromide salt—a curdy cream-coloured precipitates appear. Add excess of ammonia solution—precipitates are solubilized.

Silver nitrate reacts with bromide ion to give precipitate of silver bromide which is soluble in excess of ammonia solution.

$$Br^- + AgNO_3 \longrightarrow AgBr\downarrow + NO_3^{2-}$$

$$AgBr\downarrow + 2NH_3 \longrightarrow [Ag(NH_3)_2^+]Br^-$$
$$\text{Soluble complex}$$

Iodide, I⁻

(i) Add concentrated sulphuric acid (1 ml) to a solid salt (0.5 g)—a violet-coloured vapour is evolved.

The hydrogen iodide first formed, is largely oxidized by concentrated sulphuric acid to form iodine gas.

$$I^+ + H_2SO_4 \longrightarrow HI + HSO_4^{2-}$$

$$H_2SO_4 + 2HI \longrightarrow SO_2 + I_2\uparrow + 2H_2O$$

(ii) Add silver nitrate solution (1 ml) to an iodide salt solution—yellow curdy precipitates appear. The precipitates are insoluble in ammonia solution but soluble in potassium cyanide and sodium thiosulphate solutions.

$$I^- + AgNO_3 \longrightarrow AgI\downarrow + NO_3^-$$
$$\text{Yellow precipitate}$$

Nitrate, NO_3^-

(i) Add concentrated sulphuric acid (1 ml) to a solid salt—yellow brown vapours of NO_2 accompanied by the pungent acid vapours of nitric acid.

Nitric acid, initially formed, is converted into NO_2 by heating.

$$NaNO_3 + H_2SO_4 \longrightarrow NaHSO_4 + HNO_3$$
$$4HNO_3 \longrightarrow 4NO_2 + O_2 + 2H_2O$$

(ii) **Brown ring test:** Dissolve the solid salt (0.05 g) in water (1.0 ml); add cautiously concentrated sulphuric acid (1.0 ml), mix and cool. Carefully add ferrous sulphate (0.5 ml)—a brown colour is produced at the interface of the two liquids. Alternatively, the sulphuric acid may be added in the last sequence.

$$3Fe^{2+} + 4H^+ + NO_3^- \longrightarrow NO + 3Fe^{3+} + 2H_2O$$

At the junction, a brown ring $FeSO_4.NO$ is formed.

$$FeSO_4 + NO \longrightarrow FeSO_4.NO$$

Nitrites, bromide, iodides, chromates, thiosulphates and cyanide interfere. Nitrite is removed by adding ammonium chloride. Other interfering substances may be removed by adding a solution of silver sulphate which precipitates most of them.

Oxalate, $C_2O_4^{2-}$

(i) Add concentrated sulphuric acid (1.0 ml) to solid salt (0.5 g)—carbon dioxide and carbon monoxide gases are evolved. The former is detected by passing the gas through lime and later is detected by its blue flame on burning.

$$H_2C_2O_4 \longrightarrow H_2 + CO_2 + CO$$
$$\text{Oxalic acid}$$

(ii) To the solution of oxalate, add calcium chloride solution—white precipitate appears. These are insoluble in acetic acid but soluble in dilute mineral acids.

$$CaCl_2 + H_2C_2O_4 \longrightarrow Ca(COO)_2 \downarrow + 2HCl$$
$$\text{Calcium oxalate}$$
$$\text{(white precipitates)}$$

Calcium chloride on reaction with oxalate (oxalic acid) form calcium oxalate which is insoluble in acetic acid.

(iii) Add oxalate solution to the dilute solution of potassium permanganate solution and warm it—decolourization of $KMnO_4$ solution takes place.

$$2KMnO_4 + 3H_2SO_4 + 5C_2O_4H_2 \longrightarrow 2MnSO_4 + K_2SO_4 + 10CO_2$$

Manganese is reduced to manganous state with the evolution of carbon dioxide.

Tartrates, $C_4H_4O_6^{2-}$

(i) Warm the solid salt (0.5 g) with concentrated sulphuric acid (1 ml)—charring occurs with the evolution of carbon monoxide which burns with blue flame.

$$H_2C_4H_4O_6 \longrightarrow CO_2\uparrow + CO\uparrow + 2C + 3H_2O$$

(ii) Dissolve the solid salt (0.5 g) in water (5 ml) or use the prescribed solution (5 ml). Add 1% w/v ferrous sulphate solution (0.05 ml) and hydrogen peroxide solution (10 vol) (0.05 ml)—a transient yellow colour is produced. After the colour has disappeared, add 2M NaOH solution dropwise—an intense blue colour is produced.

Tartaric acid is oxidised into dihydroxymaleic acid.

$$\begin{array}{ccc}
\text{COOH} & & \text{COOH} \\
| & & | \\
\text{H—C—OH} + \text{H}_2\text{O}_2 & \longrightarrow & \text{C—OH} + 2\text{H}_2\text{O} \\
| & & || \\
\text{H—C—OH} & & \text{C—OH} \\
| & & | \\
\text{COOH} & & \text{COOH}
\end{array}$$

Dihydroxymaleic acid

Note: The solution of H_2O_2 and ferrous sulphate is designated as Fenton reagent.

(iii) Heat the solution of tartarate (1 ml) on a water bath for 5 to 10 minutes with 10% KBr solution (0.1 ml), 2% w/v resorcinol solution (0.1 ml) and sulphuric acid (2 ml)—a dark blue appears that changes to red when the solution is cooled and poured into water.

Citrates, $C_6H_5O_7^{3-}$

(i) Concentrated sulphuric acid when heated with a citrates evolves CO, CO_2, acetone vapour and sulphur dioxide. The solution darkens slowly owing to carbonization of part of citric acid.

(ii) To a neutral solution of the citrate salt, add calcium chloride solution—no precipitate is produced. Boil the solution—a white precipitate soluble in 6M acetic acid is produced.

On boiling, the precipitates of calcium citrate, $Ca_3(C_6H_5O_7)_2.4H_2O$ are formed.

(iii) Dissolve a quantity of the substance (0.01 g) in water (5 ml) or use the prescribed solution (5 ml). Add sulphuric acid (0.5 ml) and potassium permanganate solution (3 ml). Warm until the colour of the permanganate is discharged and add 10% w/v sodium nitroprusside solution (0.5 ml) in 1M sulphuric acid and sulphamic acid (4 g). Make alkaline with strong ammonia solution, added dropwise until all the sulphamic acid has been dissolved. Add excess of strong ammonia solution, a violet colour which turns violet-blue is produced.

$$\text{Citric acid} + \text{KMnO}_4 \longrightarrow \text{CO(CH}_2\text{COOH)}_2$$
Acetone dicarboxylic acid

$$\text{Acetone dicarboxylic acid} + \text{NH}_3 \longrightarrow \text{Violet colour}$$

Acetate, CH_3COO^-

All normal acetates except that of silver and mercurous are readily soluble in water. Basic acetates of iron, aluminium, chromium are insoluble in water.

(i) Add dilute sulphuric acid solution to the solid salt (0.5 g)—vapours of acetic acid, recognized by its odour is produced.

$$\text{CH}_3\text{COO}^- + \text{H}_2\text{SO}_4 \longrightarrow \text{CH}_3\text{COOH} + \text{HSO}_4^-$$

(ii) Add concentrated sulphuric acid to the O.S. and then add alcohol. Warm the content— fruity smell of ethyl acetate is produced.

Borates, BO_3^{3-}, $B_4O_7^{3-}$, BO_2^{2-}

Borates of alkalies dissolve in water giving an alkaline solution. Other borates are difficultly soluble in water but readily in acids and ammonium chloride solutions.

(i) Add concentrated acid to the inorganic salt and then warm. Fumes of boric acid liberated. It is capable of imparting green tinge to the non-luminous flame.

$$Na_2B_4O_7 + H_2SO_4 + 5H_2O \longrightarrow 4H_3BO_3 + Na_2SO_4$$

(ii) Add little of borate salt to methyl or ethyl alcohol containing a few drops of conc. H_2SO_4 in a small dish. Stir the mixture and spray the solution in flame. *Green bordered flame appears as a result of the formation of methyl or ethyl borate.*

$$H_3BO_3 + 3CH_3OH \longrightarrow B(OCH_3)_3 + 3H_2O$$
$$\text{Methyl borate}$$

$$H_3BO_3 + 3C_2H_5OH \longrightarrow B(OC_2H_5)_3 + 3H_2O$$
$$\text{Ethyl borate}$$

Class B(i)

Sulphates, SO_4^{2-}

Sulphates of lead, barium and strontium are insoluble. Calcium sulphate is sparingly soluble while all other sulphates are soluble in water.

(i) Add barium chloride solution to O.S.—a white precipitate owing to formation of barium sulphate confirms the presence of sulphate.

$$SO_4^{2-} + BaCl_2 \longrightarrow BaSO_4 + 2Cl^-$$

(ii) Silver nitrate causes no precipitation in dilute solution but in concentrated solution a white crystalline precipitate is produced due to formation of silver sulphate.

$$SO_4^{2-} + 2AgNO_3 \longrightarrow Ag_2SO_4\downarrow + NO_3^{2-}$$

Phosphates, PO_4^{3-}, PO_3^-, $P_2O_7^{4-}$

There are three phosphoric acids known. Their ions are orthophosphate, PO_4^{3-}, meta-phosphate, PO_3^-, and pyrophosphate, $P_2O_7^{4-}$. The last two change into PO_4^{3-} on boiling so that PO_4^{3-} alone may be considered.

(i) Add silver nitrate to the O.S.—a yellow precipitate of silver phosphate appears (different from meta- and pyrophosphate).

$$2HPO_4^{2-} + 3Ag^+ \longrightarrow H_2PO_4^- + Ag_3PO_4$$

The precipitates are readily soluble in nitric acid and ammonia solution.

(ii) Acidify the O.S. with nitric acid. Add ammonium molybdate solution. The yellow crystalline precipitate of ammonium phosphomolybdate appears.

$$12MoO_4 + HPO_4^{2-} + 3NH_4^+ + 23H^+ \longrightarrow (NH_4)_3[P(Mo_{12}O_{40})] + 12H_2O$$
$$\text{Ammonium phosphomolybdate}$$
$$\text{(yellow precipitate)}$$

Note: Ammonium molybdate is the most valuable reagent for the detection of phosphate ions. Heating aids the precipitation.

(iii) Add magnesia mixture (an aqueous solution of $MgCl_2$, NH_4Cl and ammonia, prepared by mixing 100 g each of $MgCl_2$ and NH_4Cl and 40 ml of concentrated ammonia solution and diluting to 1 litre) to O.S.

A white precipitate of magnesium ammonium phosphate is produced. The precipitate is soluble in dilute acids but practically insoluble in ammonia solution.

$$MgCl_2 + HPO_4^{2-} + NH_3 \longrightarrow Mg\,NH_4PO_4 + 2Cl^-$$

Chromates, CrO_4^{2-} and dichromates, $Cr_2O_7^{2-}$

A solution of chromate salt is yellow in neutral or alkaline solution. It turns orange when the solution is acidified owing to the formation of dichromate ion, $C_2O_7^{2-}$.

(i) Add silver nitrate solution to O.S.—a brownish red precipitate of silver chromate is produced.

$$CrO_4^{2-} + 2Ag^+ \longrightarrow Ag_2CrO_4$$

The precipitate is soluble in ammonia and mineral acids and insoluble in acetic acid. In a concentrated solution of a dichromate reddish brown precipitate of silver dichromate is obtained. This precipitate passes onto silver chromate on boiling.

$$Cr_2O_7^{2-} + 2Ag^+ \longrightarrow Ag_2Cr_2O_7\downarrow$$
$$\text{Silver dichromate}$$

$$2Ag_2Cr_2O_7 + H_2O \longrightarrow 2Ag_2CrO_4 + H_2Cr_2O_7$$
$$\text{Silver chromate}$$

(ii) Add barium chloride to the O.S.—yellow precipitate of barium chromate appears. The precipitates are insoluble in acetic acid.

$$CrO_4^{2-} + Ba^{2+} \longrightarrow BaCrO_4\downarrow$$

Class B(ii)

Chromate, CrO_4^{2-}, and dichromates, $Cr_2O_7^{2-}$, are strong oxidizing agents in acidic solution.

(i) Acidify the O.S. with sulphuric acid. Pass H_2S gas—green colour appears.

H_2S gas reduces chromate or dichromate solution to green solution of chromic salt.

$$2CrO_4^{2-} + H_2SO_4 \longrightarrow Cr_2O_7^{2-} + 2H_2O + SO_4^{2-}$$
$$Cr_2O_7^{2-} + 3H_2S + 8H^+ \longrightarrow 2Cr^{3+} + 7H_2O + 3S\downarrow$$

(ii) Diphenyl carbazide forms a deep red colouration when treated with acidified solution of chromate or dichromate (may be used as a spot test).

Special Tests for Certain Anions in the Presence of Another Interfering Anion

Carbonate in the presence of sulphite or thiosulphate: The lime water test is given by all the three CO_3^{2-}, SO_3^{2-} and $S_2O_3^{2-}$. In such cases mix 20 mg of the dry mixture with an equal amount of powdered $K_2Cr_2O_7$ and 0.5 ml of dil. H_2SO_4. Warm the tube and allow the evolved gas to bubble through lime-water. A white milkiness now confirms carbonate.

$$K_2Cr_2O_7 + 2H^+ + 3SO_2 \longrightarrow 2K^+ + 2Cr^{3+} + H_2O + 3SO_4^{2-}$$
$$\underbrace{Ca^{2+} + 2OH^-}_{\text{Lime-water}} + CO_2 \longrightarrow \underset{\substack{\text{White} \\ \text{precipitate}}}{CaCO_3\downarrow} + H_2O$$

Nitrate in the presence of nitrite. First remove interfering nitrite and then carry out ring test for nitrate. Boil 0.5 ml of water extract with 0.2 g of solid NH_4Cl until effervescence (due to N_2) ceases. Then apply brown ring test in the solution for nitrate.

$$NO_2^- + NH_4^+ \xrightarrow{\text{Heat}} N_2\uparrow + 2H_2O$$

Chloride, bromide and iodide in presence of each other. Acidify 0.5 ml of 'soda extract' with dil. H_2SO_4 in a crucible. Add about 0.2 gm of solid potassium persulphate and boil gently (adding distilled water, if necessary, to prevent dryness). If iodide is present, violet fumes of iodine are evolved. If the solution after the elimination of iodine is brown then bromine is indicated. The boiling continue till the solution becomes colourless. Then cool and add 2–3 drops of $AgNO_3$ solution and a few drops of dil. HNO_3 solution. A white precipitate soluble in ammonia indicates chloride also.

$$2I^- + S_2O_8^{2-} \longrightarrow 2SO_4^{2-} + I_2\uparrow \text{ (Violet)}$$

$$2Br^- + S_2O_8^{2-} \longrightarrow 2SO_4^{2-} + Br_2\uparrow \text{ (Violet)}$$
$$\text{(Brown solution)} \qquad\qquad \text{(Reddish-brown)}$$

$$Cl^- + Ag^+ \longrightarrow AgCl\downarrow \text{ (White)}$$

$$AgCl^- + 2NH_3 \longrightarrow [Ag(NH_3)_2]^+Cl^-$$
$$\text{(Soluble complex)}$$

Bromide in presence of iodide: Acidify 5 drops of 'soda extract' with dil. HCl. Add 0.5 ml of CS_2 and then add Cl_2 water dropwise with shaking. A violet colour in the CS_2 layer indicates the presence of iodide. Continue adding Cl_2-water and shake till the violet colour disappears and if CS_2 layer assumes an orange-brown colour, bromide is also present.

$$2I^+ + Cl_2 \longrightarrow 2Cl^-I_2\uparrow \text{ (Violet)}$$

$$I_2 + 5Cl_2 + 6H_2O \longrightarrow 12H^+ + 10Cl^- + 2IO_3^-$$
$$\text{(Excess)} \qquad \text{(Colourless)}$$

$$2Br^- + Cl_2 \longrightarrow 2Cl^- + Br_2\uparrow$$
$$\text{(Orange solution in } CS_2)$$

Sulphate in the presence of fluoride: Acidify 4–5 drops of 'soda extract' with excess of acetic acid. Boil off CO_2. Add a few drops of lead acetate solution. A white precipitate confirms *sulphate*.

$$SO_4^{2-} + Pb^{2+} \longrightarrow PbSO_4 \text{ (White)}$$

Oxalate in the presence of carbonate: Heat 20 mg of the dry mixture with 0.5 ml of dil. H_2SO_4 until effervescence ceases. Then, add a pinch of MnO_2 and warm. If effervescence starts again, oxalate is present.

$$CO_3^{2-} + 2H^+ \longrightarrow H_2O + CO_2\uparrow$$

$$C_2O_4^{2-} + MnO_2 + 4H^+ \longrightarrow Mn^{2+} + 2H_2O + 2CO_2\uparrow$$

Sulphide, sulphite, thiosulphate and sulphate in presence of one another. To 10 drops of 'soda extract' add 5–10 mg of $CdCO_3$ and centrifuge.

Yellow precipitates of CdS confirms sulphide.	**Centrifugate:** Acidify with dil. HNO_3 and add a slight excess of ammonia, boil off excess of ammonia. To neutral solution thus obtained, add 0.5 ml $BaCl_2$ solution and centrifuge.		
	White precipitates (may contain $BaSO_2$, and $BaSO_4$). Add cold dil. HCl and centrifuge.		**Centrifugate:** (May contain thiosulphate). Add a few drops of $AgNO_3$ solution. A white precipitate turning yellow orange, brown and finally black confirms thiosulphate.
	White precipitates of $BaSO_4$ identifies sulphate.	**Centrifuge** (may contain $H_2SO_3 + BaCl_2$). Add a few drops of conc. HNO_3 in bromine water. Warm—formation of white precipitate confirms SO_3^{2-}.	

Analysis of Insoluble Compounds

The systemic analysis of cations in the soluble salt is very simple but the identification of cations in insoluble salt requires a different technique.

All those substances, which remain insoluble in conc. HCl, conc. HNO_3 or aqua regia are practically regarded as insoluble salts. The use of aqua regia is not recommended as it creates many complications in analysis.

The insoluble salt which are under the scope of simple analysis are limited in number. Some of these are identified by their characteristic colours. The list of such insolubles is given below with their colours.

 (i) White: $BaSO_4$, $SrSO_4$, $PbSO_4$, AgCl, SnO_2, Sb_2O_4 and Al_2O_3
 (ii) Yellow: AgBr and AgI
 (iii) Green: Cr_2O_3, $Cr_2(SO_4)_3$ (anhydrous)
 (iv) Black: HgS
 (v) Violet: $CrCl_3$ (mineral)
 (vi) Dark red: Fe_2O_3
 (vii) Brown: SnS_2 of mixture (soluble in aqua regia)

Systemic analysis: That part of mixture which is not dissolve in conc. HCl and conc. HNO_3 is taken out and washed with water. Now observe the colour carefully and proceed accordingly.

Option I: When residue is white: Mix the residue with six times of Na_2CO_3. Add distilled water to it, heat for sufficient time and filter.

Take filtrate for acid radicals (SO_4^{2-}, Cl^- and F^-) analysis in the usual way. Further analysis rests on the presence of acid radical.

 (a) **Sulphate:** If the sulphate ion is present, the salt may be $BaSO_4$, $SrSO_4$ and $PbSO_4$. Take the residue to flame test.
 (i) **$PbSO_4$:** This gives characteristic lemon blue flame. In such a case, dissolve the residue in ammonium acetate by boiling. Add CH_3COOH and K_2CrO_4 solution. A yellow precipitate of lead chromate is obtained.
 (ii) **$BaSO_4$:** This gives the characteristic green flame. Take residue obtained after treatment with Na_2CO_3, put in acetic acid to dissolve. Now add K_2CrO_4 solution. A yellow precipitate of Barium chromate is obtained.
 (iii) **$SrSO_4$:** If in the above treatment, no precipitate is obtained, add ammonium sulphate. A white precipitate of $SrSO_4$ comes.

(b) **Calcium fluoride:** Take the residue obtained by the Na_2CO_3 treatment and dissolve it in acetic acid and add ammonium oxalate – a white precipitate is obtained—CaF_2.

(c) **Silver chloride:** In case of chloride ions, take the insoluble residue and dissolve it in NH_4OH. Add HNO_3 till it becomes acidic. Appearance of white precipitates indicates the presence of AgCl.

(d) **No acidic radical:** If your insoluble white residue fails to give any test as above, the presence of oxides of Sn, Sb or Al is suspected.

(i) **SnO_2 and Sb_2O_4:** Mix a portion of insoluble residue with Na_2CO_3 in almost equal amount and add to it powdered sulphur in excess. Fuse it in a porcelain dish by heating strongly the fused mass with water, add dilute HCl solution and observe.

(a) An orange precipitates indicate Sb_2O_4.

(b) The yellow or grayish yellow precipitates indicate SnO_2.

(ii) Al_2O_3. Test it by charcoal cavity test. A blue mass is obtained.

Option II: When residue is yellow: Boil the residue with Zn and HCl which converts AgI or AgBr to metallic silver. Filter it to get residue. Boil the dissolve metallic residue in HNO_3 and precipitate as AgCl by addition of HCl. Test the filtrate so obtained (after Zn and HCl treatment) for bromide and Iodide ions in the usual way.

Option III: When residue is green (Cr_2O_3) and $Cr_2(SO_4)_3$: Mix the insoluble residue with Na_2CO_3 and KNO_3 in equal amount and fuse by heating it in porcelain dish. Digest the fused mass with water and add CH_3COOH to it. Divide it into two parts.

(i) I part + Lead acetate $\longrightarrow$ yellow precipitate
$\left.\rule{0pt}{2.2em}\right\} \longrightarrow Cr_2(SO_4)_3$
(ii) II part + Barium chloride $\longrightarrow$ white precipitate

If it gives yellow precipitate with lead acetate but not white precipitate with $BaCl_2 \longrightarrow Cr_2O_3$.

Option IV: When residue is black (HgS): This may be tested as follows:

(i) Boil a portion of residue with zinc and sulphuric acid. Pass the evolved gas in lead acetate solution. A black precipitate (PbS) is obtained $\longrightarrow$ HgS is confirmed.

(ii) To another portion of residue, add aqua regia and boil it. Cool, add water to dilute and $SnCl_2$. A white precipitate turning grey on heating with excess of $SnCl_2 \longrightarrow Hg^{2+}$ is confirmed.

Option V: When residue is violet ($CrCl_3$): Proceed as in case III up to acetic acid addition and then divide into two parts.

(i) I part + Lead acetate $\longrightarrow$ yellow precipitate
$\left.\rule{0pt}{2.2em}\right\} \longrightarrow CrCl_3$
(ii) II part + dilute HNO_3 (excess) + $AgNO_3 \longrightarrow$ white precipitate

Option VI: When residue is dark red (Fe_2O_3): This may be confirmed by borax bead test. Brown bead is obtained in oxidizing flame.

Option VII: When residue is brown (SnS_2): Dissolve the residue in yellow ammonium sulphide and then add conc. HCl and iron fillings. Boil for some time and filter. To this, add $HgCl_2$ solution. A white precipitate of mercurous chloride confirms $\longrightarrow SnS_2$.

Preparation of Some Inorganic Pharmaceuticals

PREPARATION OF BORIC ACID FROM BORAX

There are three types of boric acids:

1. Orthoboric acid (H_3BO_3)
2. Metaboric acid (HBO_2)
3. Pyroboric acid ($H_2B_4O_7$)

Orthoboric acid is a white needle like odorless crystalline solid. It is sparingly soluble in cold water and fairly soluble in hot water. It is a weak mono basic acid. It is used as local anti-infective agent.

It is prepared by the reaction of hydrochloric acid with borax. The following equation shows this reaction for hydrochloric acid with borax:

$$Na_2B_4O_7.10H_2O + 2HCl \longrightarrow 4H_3BO_3 + 2NaCl(aq) + 5H_2O$$
$$\text{Borax} \qquad\qquad\qquad\qquad \text{Boric acid}$$

Procedure

1. Dissolve 10 g of sodium tetraborate (borax) in 40 ml of water.
2. Heat the solution.
3. After the heating process was completed, add 5 ml of concentrated hydrochloric acid to the solution.
4. Keep aside the solution in the beaker until the temperature of the solution come down to room temperature.
5. Immerse the beaker in cold water (with ice) to cool down the solution to crystallize out the boric acid.
6. Filter off the boric acid by using suction pump, suction funnel, and filter papers.
7. Record the weight and calculate the yield.

Flame test of the prepared boric acid

1. Transfer a little boric acid (crystal) into the test tube.
2. Add a little methanol and some concentrated sulphuric acid H_2SO_4 to the boric acid in the test tube.
3. Heat the solution.
4. Ignite the vapour produced using a flame splint.
5. Observe the colour of the flame. The flame will have the green-coloured border.

PREPARATION OF FERROUS SULPHATE

Ferrous sulphate ($FeSO_4.7H_2O$), traditionally known as 'green vitriol' or 'copperas', forms beautiful blue-green crystals of the monoclinic system. Ferrous sulphate is useful in chemistry as a reducing agent and a source of ferrous ions. It can also act as a catalyst; an example is Fenton's Reagent, which is used to destroy organic chemical wastes.

It is made by reacting iron with sulphuric acid. This reaction makes hydrogen gas and leaves behind iron (II) sulphate. To follow this method, dip the iron (1 g) in slight excess of dilute sulphuric acid. When evolution of iron ceases, filter the solution, concentrate the filtrate and keep the solution aside for crystallization of ferrous sulphate.

$$Fe + H_2SO_4 \rightarrow FeSO_4 + H_2\uparrow$$

It can also be made by oxidation of pyrite, an iron sulphide material.

$$2FeS_2 + 7O_2 + 2H_2O \rightarrow 2FeSO_4 + 2H_2SO_4$$

It is also prepared from steel wool into following steps:

I. Preparation of $FeSO_4$ solution

For best results the lab temperature should be kept below 25°C. Avoid temperature fluctuations as much as possible, except where indicated in this procedure.

1. Degrease the steel wool by immersing it in acetone for half an hour. Remove it from the acetone and let it dry in a well-ventilated lab where nobody can disturb it.
2. Place the glass beaker in the center of a metal pan or wide glass dish that's reserved just for lab use. The reaction can produce minor spattering as hydrogen bubbles to the surface of the acid.
3. Place the degreased, dry steel wool in the glass beaker and pour in enough 30–40% sulphuric acid to cover it completely. Do not use concentrated acid. If the steel wool is not fully submerged, carefully push it down with a glass rod. The sulphuric acid will begin to dissolve the steel, producing hydrogen gas. Over the course of several hours the steel wool will gradually disappear. Carefully, add more steel wool. Repeat this a few times. Reddish-brown, insoluble ferric compounds will form if you add too much steel wool; just add some dilute sulphuric acid if this happens. The pH of the solution should be acidic at any given time, otherwise the ferrous ions will oxidize to the ferric state.

II. Filtration

Add excess water that's been acidified to a pH between 2 and 4 using sulphuric acid. Add enough of this acidified water to re-dissolve all the green crystals that settled out. If the solution turns brown, add just enough sulphuric acid to make it green again. Filter this solution through filter paper. Discard the solids and the paper. Save the filtrate. It should now be free of steel wool pieces, carbon (from the steel), rust, and other solids. Keep the solution in a covered container to minimize contact with atmospheric oxygen. If the pH is not kept low enough, ferrous sulphate will oxidize to ferric sulphate on standing. Normally, atmospheric oxygen changes Fe^{2+} to Fe^{3+} quite readily. This reaction is reversible, however, by lowering the pH. Below 4 or so, ferrous ion is heavily favored over ferric, with the concentration of Fe^{3+} becoming vanishingly small at pH 1–2. Aqueous $FeSO_4$ in this pH range is stable for days, even with air contact.

III. Evaporation

The filtered solution is put in a shallow, glass container such as a Petri dish or crystallizing dish. Place this on the hot plate and turn it to the lowest setting; even better, use a small, laboratory oven. Slowly heat the solution to about 80 to 90°C; do not boil it. Hold it at this temperature until about half the liquid has evaporated. The colour of the solution may change to yellowish, but do not let this discourage you. On cooling, it becomes green again. Allow the solution to cool to room temperature and place the shallow dish on crushed ice. Leave it there for at least an hour. Remove the dish from the cold and place it on the lab bench in your locked laboratory (remember, the liquid contains sulphuric acid). Let it stand for 24 hours.

Green crystals of ferrous sulphate should form. If not, the cause is probably one of the following:

1. Evaporation of the solution is not proper.
2. The pH was too high.
3. The ambient temperature was too high.
4. Sulphuric acid was contaminated with something that oxidized Fe^{2+}.

IV. Washing

If possible, have a previously-prepared batch of ferrous sulphate crystals which are dissolved to saturation in cold (1 to 4 °C) distilled water. Use this solution, prepared and chilled shortly before use, to wash the crystals you have grown. If you have prepared $FeSO_4$ for the first time and do not have another batch, just use distilled water cooled to just above freezing. There will be some minor losses as some of the crystals go into solution. As the washing removes the strong sulphuric acid from the surface of the crystals, the atmosphere will unfortunately oxidize them more readily. Larger crystals are more desirable; less $FeSO_4$ will oxidize. Conversely, do not crush or powder the crystals, since it will increase the surface area.

V. Drying—Final steps

If no desiccator is available, dry the ferrous sulphate crystals in air at the lowest relative humidity available (e.g. not outside on a foggy day). It is preferable to do the drying in a desiccator having a some calcium chloride drying pellets in the bottom.

Result

The % yield of ferrous sulphate is ....

Note: Ferrous sulphate may be obtained by dissolving 1.0 g of iron in excess of dilute sulphuric acid. After the effervescence ceases, the liquid is filtered, concentrated and cooled. Separate out the ferrous sulphate crystals by filtration at room temperature.

3. PREPARATION OF POTASH ALUM FROM ALUMINUM FOIL

Potash alum is commonly known as "PHITKARI". It is white crystalline solid. It is soluble in water. It is used for the purification of water. It is also used in leather industry and in paper industry. It is used in fire extinguisher. Melting point is 92°C.

Preparation

Method I (from aluminum sulphate)

Potash alum is prepared by mixing equi-molecular masses of potassium sulphate and aluminum sulphate in water followed by evaporation.

$$K_2SO_4 + Al_2(SO_4)_3 + 24H_2O \rightarrow K_2SO_4.Al_2(SO_4)_3.24H_2O$$
$$\text{Alum}$$

Procedure

1. Dissolve 2.5 g of potassium sulphate and 10 g of aluminum sulphate in 40 ml of water in a beaker.
2. Add 2–3 drops of sulphuric acid to make the solution clear. If still the solution has some milkiness, filter.
3. Take the filtrate into a porcelain dish and evaporate to reduce the bulk to half.
4. Cool and allow to remain undisturbed for 3–6 hours.
5. Observe the formation of octahedral crystals of potash alum. Separate it and dry them between filter papers.

Method II (from aluminum foil)

Materials

Aluminum foil, 3M H_2SO_4, 3M KOH, 50%/50% water/ethanol solution.

Procedure

1. Weigh out approximately 1 g of aluminum foil. Tear the foil into small pieces and place into the 250 ml beaker.
2. Slowly, add 25 ml of 3M KOH solution. Gently swirl the beaker while adding the KOH. This reaction will produce some heat and hydrogen gas. Do not directly smell the vapors. The foil should be completely dissolved, leaving only a few small particles of carbon floating in the solution. If the amount of carbon seems excessive, filter the solution with the Buchner funnel.
3. When the solution has cooled to room temperature, slowly add 35 ml of 3M H_2SO_4 with constant stirring. The solution will get hot as the reaction proceeds. The $Al(OH)_3$ precipitate forms, which will then dissolve as more acid is added. If there is still precipitate present after all 35 ml of acid has been added, keep adding acid until all the precipitate is gone.
4. Place the beaker on a ring stand, and boil the solution down until its volume is approximately 50 ml.
5. Gravity filter the hot solution to remove the carbon residue.
6. Cover the beaker with plastic wrap and set it aside to cool for overnight. Make sure to label the beaker with your name.
7. If no crystals have formed the next day, try scraping the bottom of the beaker with a glass stirring rod. If there are still no crystals, try boiling off some more water and cooling again.
8. Pour all of your crystals and remaining liquid from the beaker into the Buchner funnel. Once all the liquid is all drawn through, wash the crystals with 50 ml of the 50/50 water/ethanol mix.
9. Allow the crystals to dry at room temperature. When they are dry, measure the mass of the crystals you produced.

Volumetric Analysis

It is a quite accurate method of quantitative analysis. The quantity of a substance in a solution is determined with accurate measurement of the volume of the reacting solution.

Volumetric analysis may be classified into various categories based on type of reactions involved, e.g.:

- Neutralization titration or acidimetry and alkalimetry
- Precipitation titration
- Oxidation-reduction titration
- Complexometric titration
- Non-aqueous titration
- Diazotization titration

NEUTRALIZATION TITRATIONS

It involves the neutralization of an acid with a base or *vice versa*. End point is determined by means of an indicator or by potentiometric method.

ACIDIMETRY TITRATIONS

It is a direct or residual volumetric analysis of a base with a standard acid.

Direct titration is performed by introducing a standard acid solution gradually from a burette into a solution of base being assayed till the end point is obtained, e.g. assay of sodium bicarbonate.

Residual titration is used when the rate of reaction between a basic compound with an acid is slow. In this, the solution of the base is treated with an excess of accurately measured standard acid and the excess acid is subsequently titrated with standard base, e.g. assay of zinc oxide.

(i) Direct Acidimetric Titrations

Assay of sodium bicarbonate

Sodium bicarbonate I.P. contains not less than 99% and not more than the equivalent of 101.0% w/w of $NaHCO_3$ calculated with reference of the dried substance.

Procedure

Weigh accurately sodium bicarbonate (about 1.5 g), dissolve in water (50 ml) and titrate with 1M hydrochloric acid solution by using methyl orange as an indicator till yellow colour changes into pink colour.

$$2NaHCO_3 + 2HCl \longrightarrow 2NaCl + 2H_2O + 2CO_2$$

Sodium bicarbonate is basic in nature so titrated against standard hydrochloric acid. Methyl orange is used as the indicator because phenolphthalein is affected by carbonic acid, liberated in the reaction which may cause a change of colour before completion of the reaction.

Factor

Each ml of 1M HCl solution = 0.08401 g of $NaHCO_3$.

How to calculate factor

1000 ml of 1.0M HCl contain: 1 mole of HCl
From the equation:
1 mole of $NaHCO_3$ = 1 mole of HCl
1000 ml of 1.0M HCl = 1 mole of HCl = 1 mole of $NaHCO_3$
1000 ml of 1.0M HCl = 84 g of $NaHCO_3$
∴ Mol Wt. of $NaHCO_3$ = 84
1 ml of 1.0M HCl solution = 0.084 g of $NaHCO_3$

How to determine % purity

Weight of sodium bicarbonate sample = W g
Volume 1.0M HCl consumed = V ml
Weight of Sodium bicarbonate sample = W g

$$\% \text{ purity} = \frac{0.08401 \times V \times \text{Molarity (Cal)}}{W \times 1.0 \text{ (Molarity known)}}$$

Assay of Sodium Carbonate

Sodium carbonate contains not less than 99.5% and not more than the equivalent of 100.5% w/w of Na_2CO_3.

Procedure

Weigh accurately sodium carbonate (about 2 g), dissolve in water (20 ml) and titrate with 0.5N sulphuric acid solution by using bromphenol as an indicator till yellow colour appears.

Aqueous solution of sodium carbonate is alkaline in nature. It is assayed by titrating with a standard acid using bromophenol blue as an indicator. At the end point, acidic pH is obtained due to formation of carbonic acid from carbon dioxide.

$$Na_2CO_3 + H_2SO_4 \longrightarrow Na_2SO_4 + H_2O + 2CO_2$$

Hence, bromophenol blue is a choice of indicator as it shows colour change in acidic range. The pH range of bromophenol blue is 2.8 to 4.6.

Factor

Each ml of 0.5N H_2SO_4 solution = 0.0715 g of Na_2CO_3.

Note: Methyl orange indicator may be used in place of bromophenol blue.

How to calculate factor

1000 ml of 1.0N H_2SO_4 contain $= \dfrac{1}{2}$ eq. mole of H_2SO_4

1000 ml of 0.5N H_2SO_4 solution contain $= \dfrac{1}{4}$ eq. mole of H_2SO_4

From the equation:

1 mole of Na_2CO_3 = 1 mole of H_2SO_4

1000 ml of 0.5N H_2SO_4 solution $= \dfrac{1}{4} \times Na_2CO_3.10H_2O$

1000 ml of 0.5N H_2SO_4 solution $= \dfrac{1}{4} \times 286.00$ g of $Na_2CO_3.10H_2O$

Mol Wt. of $Na_2CO_3.10H_2O$ = 286

Each ml of 0.5N H_2SO_4 solution = 0.0715 g of $Na_2CO_3.10H_2O$

Assay of Borax, $Na_2B_4O_7.10H_2O$

Borax was an official in I.P. 1966. It contains not less than 99% and not more than the equivalent of 103% w/w of $Na_2B_4O_7$.

Procedure

Weigh accurately borax (about 3 g), dissolve in water (75 ml) and titrate with 0.5N hydrochloric acid using solution of methyl red as indicator.

On titration with hydrochloric acid, boric acid is formed.

$$2HCl + Na_2B_4O_7 + 5H_2O \longrightarrow 2NaCl + 4H_3BO_3$$

The colour changes when all the boric acid has been set free. Boric acid has a very low ionisation and has no effect on indicators. Methyl red changes its colour in the range 4.2–6.3 and hence is not affected by free boric acid.

Factor

Each ml of 0.5N hydrochloric acid solution = 0.09536 g of $Na_2B_4O_7.10H_2O$.

(ii) Residual Titrations

Assay of Strong Ammonia Solution

Strong ammonia solution contains not less then 24.5% and not more than 25.5% v/v of NH_3.

Procedure

Weigh accurately ammonia solution (3 g) in a flask containing 1N sulphuric acid solution (50 ml) and titrate the excess of acid with 1N sodium hydroxide solution by using methyl red as an indicator till yellow colour changes into red colour.

The ammonia solution is assayed by residual or back titration due to its volatile nature, otherwise some quantity may lost during direct titration with a standard acid.

Ammonia solution is treated with an accurately measured standard acid and the standard acid is back titrated with a standard alkali by using methyl red as an indicator.

$$2NH_3 + H_2SO_4 \longrightarrow (NH_4)_2SO_4$$

Factor

Each ml of 1N H_2SO_4 solution = 0.01703 g of NH_3.

Assay of Zinc Oxide (IP1966 method)

Zinc oxide contains not less than 99% and not more than the equivalent of 100.5% w/w of ZnO, calculated with reference to the ignited substance.

Procedure

Dissolve an accurately weighed quantity of zinc oxide (about 1.5 g) and ammonium chloride (2.5 g) in 1N sulphuric acid solution (50 ml) with the aid of gentle heating. Add a few drops of methyl orange as indicator and the titrate the solution with 1N sodium hydroxide solution till yellow colour appears.

$$ZnO + H_2SO_4 \longrightarrow ZnSO_4 + H_2O$$

It is back titrated due to slow reaction between zinc oxide and sulphuric acid. Ammonium chloride is added to prevent the precipitation of zinc hydroxide both during the titration and also at the end point. The precipitation of zinc hydroxide would give poor end point.

Factor

Each ml of 1N H_2SO_4 solution = 0.04068 g of ZnO.

ALKALIMETRY TITRATIONS

It is an estimation of acid/acidic drugs by titration with standard alkali. It also includes direct titration and residual/back titration methods as in acidimetry.

(i) Direct Alkalimetric Titrations

Assay of Boric Acid (H_3BO_3)

Boric acid I.P. contains not less than 99.5% and not more than the equivalent of 100.5% w/w of H_3BO_3 calculated with reference to the dried substance.

Procedure

Dissolve an accurately weighed quantity of boric acid (about 2 g) in a mixture of water (50 ml) and glycerin (100 ml), previously neutralized to phenolphthalein indicator. Titrate the solution with 1M sodium hydroxide solution by using phenophthalein as indicator till pink colour appears.

Boric acid is a weak acid, hence it cannot be titrated accurately with standard alkali. It can be titrated directly after dissolving in a solution of glycerin (or polyhydroxy compound, e.g. mannitol) in water. In the above method, boric acid reacts with glycerin to form glyceroboric acid which is a strong monobasic acid.

Glycerin is slightly acidic in nature. Therefore, it is neutralized with dilute alkali solution, using phenolphthalein indicator.

Glycerin   Boric acid   Glyceroboric acid

Factor

Each ml of 1N NaOH solution = 0.06183 g of H_3BO_3

Assay of Ammonium Chloride

Ammonium chloride I.P. contains not less than 99.0% and not more than 100.5% w/w of NH_4Cl calculated with reference to the dried substances.

Procedure

Weigh accurately ammonium chloride (about 0.1 g), dissolve in water (20 ml) and add formaldehyde solution (5 ml), previously neutralized to phenolphthalein indicator. After two minutes, titrate slowly with 0.1N sodium hydroxide solution by using phenolphthalein indicator till pink colour appears.

The above method is official in I.P. 2007 while precipitation method is recommended in I.P. 1966. In this method, ammonium chloride is treated with formaldehyde solution to liberate equivalent amount of hydrochloric acid which is subsequently titrated with 0.1N sodium hydroxide solution.

$$4NH_4Cl + H_2O \longrightarrow 4NH_4OH + HCl$$

$$\underset{\text{Urotropine}}{4NH_4OH + 6HCHO \longrightarrow (CH_2)_6N_4 + 10H_2O}$$

$$HCl + NaOH \longrightarrow NaCl + H_2O$$

Factor

Each ml of 0.1N NaOH solution = 0.0053949 g of NH_4Cl.

Assay of Ibuprofen

Procedure

Weigh accurately ibuprofen about 0.4 g, dissolve in 95% ethanol (100 ml) and titrate with 0.1M NaOH using phenolphthalein as indicator. Perform a blank determination.

It is IP official method. *Ibuprofen is acidic in nature so assayed by titration against standard sodium hydroxide solution.*

Factor

Each ml of 0.1M NaOH solution $\equiv$ 0.02063 g of $C_{13}H_{18}O_2$

Ibuprofen   Sodium salt of ibuprofen

Assay of Ibuprofen Tablets

Weigh accurately and powder 20 tablets. Weigh accurately a quantity of the powder equivalent to 0.5 g of Ibuprofen, extract with chloroform (60 ml) and filter. Wash the residue with three quantities of $CHCl_3$ (3 ×10 ml) and gently evaporate the filtrate to dryness. Dissolve the residue in ethanol (100 ml) and do the same as above in the assay of ibuprofen.

(ii) Residual Titrations

In this, acid/acidic drug is treated with excess of accurately measured quantity of base. The unreacted base is then titrated with a standard acid.

Assay of Aspirin

It contains not less than 99.5% and not more than the equivalent of 100.5% w/w of aspirin calculated with reference to the dried substance.

Procedure

Weigh accurately aspirin (1.5 g), dissolve in 95% ethanol (15 ml) add 0.5M sodium hydroxide solution (50 ml) and boil for 10 minutes. Cool the solution and titrate the excess of alkali with 0.5M hydrochloric acid solution using phenol red indicator. Perform a blank titration in the same way.

Aspirin   Sodium salicylate

The reaction of aspirin with NaOH is slow. Hence, aspirin is boiled with excess of standard NaOH solution and then excess of alkali solution is back titrated with standard acid.

On boiling with standard sodium hydroxide solution, aspirin is hydrolysed into salicylic acid and acetic acid. The liberated acid reacts with sodium hydroxide to form sodium salt. At the end point, a slight excess of the base reacts with the indicator to produce colour change.

Factor

Each ml of 0.5M NaOH solution = 0.04504 g of $C_9H_8O_4$.

Furosemide

Furosemide, chemically known as 4-chloro-2-[(2-furanylmethyl) amino]-5-sulphamoyl benzoic acid, is structurally a sulphonamide, an antibacterial agent. However, furosemide is a potent diuretic, widely used in the treatment of edematous states associated with cardiac chronic renal failure hypertension, congestive heart failure and cirrhosis of the liver.

It contains not less than and not more than 101.0% of $C_{12}H_{11}ClN_2O_5S$.

Furosemide

Assay of furosemide tablet

Principle

Furosemide contain acidic group (COOH) so it considered as acid which can be determined by titration against 0.01N NaOH using phenol red as indicator. At the end point the color changes to pink

$$C_{12}H_{11}ClN_2O_5S + NaOH \rightarrow (C_{12}H_{10}ClN_2O_5S) \, Na + H_2O$$

Procedure

1. Weigh 20 tablets and calculate the quantity of powdered tablets equivalent to one tablet and dissolve this amount in 20 ml of hot alcohol then filter it.
2. Titrate the filtrate with 0.01N NaOH solution using phenol red as indicator.

Calculation

$$\text{Furosemide \%} = \frac{\text{Practical content}}{\text{Theoretical content}} = \frac{V_B \times N_B \times \text{Eq. Wt. of furosemide}}{\text{Theoretical content}} \times 100$$

where V_B = Volume of 0.01N NaOH consumed

      N_B = Normality of NaOH

Assay for furosemide powder (IP method)

Wash accurately about 0.5 g, dissolve in 40 ml of dimethylformamide and titrate with 0.1N sodium hydroxide using bromothymol blue solution as indicator. Perform the blank titration.

Factor

Each ml of 0.1N NaOH solution = 0.03308 g of $C_{12}H_{11}ClN_2O_5S$.

PRECIPITATION TITRATIONS

It involves the formation of insoluble substances or precipitate. End point is detected by observing the completion of precipitation or using internal indicator. It is classified into (i) Direct titration method and (ii) Residual or Indirect titration method.

(i) Direct Titration Method

The substance in solution is directly titrated with a titrant (precipitant) and completion of precipitation is detected by the use of an internal indicator.

Assay of Sodium Chloride (IP 1966 method)

It contains not less than 99.5% and not more than the equivalent of 100.5% w/w of sodium chloride calculated with reference to the dried substance.

Procedure

Accurately weigh sodium chloride (about 0.25 g), dissolve in water (50 ml) and titrate with 0.1N silver nitrate solution using a potassium chromate as an indicator.

Sodium chloride is precipitated as silver chloride by adding silver nitrate solution.

$$NaCl + AgNO_3 \longrightarrow AgCl\downarrow + NaNO_3$$
$$\text{White precipitate}$$

On completion of the precipitation, an excess drop of silver nitrate react with the indicator, potassium chromate, to form a red precipitate of silver chromate.

$$2AgNO_3 + K_2CrO_4 \longrightarrow Ag_2CrO_4 \downarrow + 2KNO_3$$
$$\text{Silver chromate}$$
$$\text{(Red precipitates)}$$

This method is also called *Mohr's method* and is applicable in the neutral solution only. In acid solution, potassium chromate cannot be used as the indicator due to solubility of silver chromate in acids.

Factor

1 ml of 0.1N $AgNO_3$ solution = 0.005854 g of NaCl.

(ii) Residual Titration Method

This method is also called *Volhard's* method and is applicable for acidic salts also. In this excess of standard silver nitrate is added to a solution of halide acidified with nitric acid. The unreacted silver nitrate is titrated with standard ammonium thiocyanate solution using ferric ammonium sulphate as an indicator.

At the end point, a permanent red colour is developed due to formation of ferric thiocyanate.

Bromides and iodides can be estimated by Volhard's method without any modification but in the case of chloride, nitrobenzene is added or precipitate of silver chloride is filtered off. Nitrobenzene forms a protective layer on the precipitate of silver chloride (coagulation). The precipitate of silver chloride, if not removed or coagulated, reacts slowly with ammonium thiocyanate (reading will be high).

$$AgCl + NH_4SCN \longrightarrow AgSCN\downarrow + NH_4Cl$$
Silver   Ammonium   Silver
chloride thiocyanate   thiocyanate

Assay of Sodium Chloride

Procedure

This method is official in Indian Pharmacopoeia. Weigh accurately sodium chloride (about 0.2 g), dissolve in distilled water (50 ml), and then add 0.1M silver nitrate solution (50 ml), 2M nitric acid (3 ml) and dibutyl phthalate (5 ml). Shake the solution, add ferric ammonium sulphate indicator and titrate with 0.1M ammonium thiocyanate solution till the colour becomes reddish.

Sodium chloride is precipitated as silver chloride by addition of excess of silver nitrate solution. The precipitate of silver chloride is coagulated by dibutyl phthalate.

$$NaCl + AgNO_3 \longrightarrow AgCl\downarrow + NaNO_3$$

The excess of silver nitrate reacts with ammonium thiocyanate on titration. When whole amount is consumed, a drop of ammonium thiocyanate reacts with ferric ammonium sulphate indicator to give reddish brown colour.

$$AgNO_3 + NH_4SCN \longrightarrow AgSCN + NH_4NO_3$$
$$3NH_4SCN + FeNH_4(SO_4)_2 \longrightarrow Fe(SCN)_3 + 2(NH_4)_2SO_4$$
Ferric thiocyanate
(Red colour)

Factor

Each ml of 0.1M AgNO$_3$ solution = 0.00584 g of NaCl.

Assay of Ammonium Chloride by Volhard's Method

Procedure (Official in I.P. 1966)

Accurately weigh ammonium chloride (0.2 g) dissolve in distilled water (40 ml), add nitric acid (3 ml), nitrobenzene (5 ml) and 0.1N AgNO$_3$ solution (50 ml), shake vigorously for one minute and titrate with 0.1N ammonium thiocyanate using ferric ammonium sulphate as the indicator.

Now the above method is replaced by acid–base titration in I.P. 1996 and 2007 (refer Acidimetry).

Ammonium chloride is precipitated by adding excess of silver nitrate. The unreacted silver nitrate is estimated by titration with standard ammonium thiocyanate solution. At the end point, a drop of NH$_4$SCN solution reacts with ferric ammonium sulphate indicator to give red colour.

$$NH_4Cl + AgNO_3 \longrightarrow AgNO_3 + NH_4NO_3$$
$$FeNH_4(SO_4)_2 + 3NH_4SCN \longrightarrow Fe(SCN)_3 + 2(NH_4)_2SO_4$$
Ferric thiocyanate
(Red colour)

Factor

Each ml of 0.1N AgNO$_3$ solution = 0.005349 g of NH$_4$Cl.

OXIDATION-REDUCTION TITRATIONS

Oxidation and reduction occur simultaneously in oxidation-reduction reaction. The reactant which losses electron is the reducing agent and can be identified as the reactant containing a constituent atom or atoms converted to higher state of oxidation.

$$Fe^{++} \xrightarrow{\hspace{2cm}} Fe^{3+} + e^- \text{ (loss of electron)}$$

Ferrous (ion)   Ferric (ion)

The electrons lost by the reducing agent are gained by the oxidizing agent, the reactant containing a constituent atom or atoms which are converted to a lower state of oxidation, e.g.

$$Fe^{3+} + e^- \xrightarrow{\hspace{2cm}} Fe^{++} \text{ (gain of electron)}$$

Ferric   Ferrous

A combination of oxidizing and reducing agents results in oxidation-reduction reaction which forms the basis for quantitative measurement of one of the reactants. A standard solution of oxidizing agent can be used for estimation of reducing agent, e.g. potassium permanganate is an oxidizing agent and can be used in quantitative estimation of the reducing agent, ferrous sulphate. Similarly sodium thiosulphate, a reducing agent, can be used for iodine which is an oxidizing agent. Oxidation-reduction methods can be classified on the basis of oxidizing agents.

Permanganate Methods

It involves the use of potassium permanganate for estimation of number of reducing substances, e.g. ferrous sulphate.

Potassium permanganate also serves as a self indicator. As a very slight excess of permanganate, it gives a distinct pink colour to the solution due to manganese ion.

Assay of Ferrous Sulphate

Ferrous sulphate contains not less than 98% and not more than equivalent of 105% w/w of $FeSO_4.7H_2O$.

Procedure

Weigh accurately ferrous sulphate (about 1.0 g), dissolve in dilute sulphuric acid (20 ml) and titrate with 0.1N $KMnO_4$ solution till faint pink colour persists for about 30 seconds upon shaking the flask.

This method was official in I.P. 1966. Ferrous sulphate is oxidized by potassium permanganate into ferric sulphate. On complete oxidation of ferrous sulphate, an excess drop of potassium permanganate solution gives pink colour at the end point.

$$10FeSO_4 + 2KMnO_4 \xrightarrow{\hspace{2cm}} 5Fe_2(SO_4)_3 + 2MnSO_4 + K_2SO_4 + 8H_2O$$

Factor

Each ml 0.1N $KMnO_4$ solution = 0.0278 g of $FeSO_4.7H_2O$.

Ferrous Sulphate Tablets

Weigh and powder 20 tablets. Weigh accurately a quantity of the powder equivalent to 0.5 g of dried ferrous sulphate and carry out the assay described under ferrous sulphate.

Assay of Sodium Nitrite

Procedure

Dissolve accurately weighed sodium nitrite (1.0 g) in water to make 100 ml solution in volumetric flask. Accurately measure and add this solution (10 ml) into a mixture of 0.1N potassium permanganate solution (50 ml), sulphuric acid (5 ml) and water (100 ml). (*Precaution*: Immerse the tip of pipette beneath the surface of potassium permanganate solution while adding the sodium nitrite solution.)

Warm the mixture to 40°C, add 0.1N oxalic acid (25 ml). Heat the mixture to 60°C on a water bath and titrate with 0.1N potassium permanganate solution till pink colour persists for 30 seconds after shaking.

Sodium nitrite yields nitrous acid in the presence of sulphuric acid which is volatile in nature; it would be lost if no precaution is taken while adding the sodium nitrite solution by keeping the tip of pipette beneath the surface of the acidified potassium permanganate solution. Nitrous acid is oxidized into nitric acid by KMnO$_4$ solution.

$$10NaNO_2 + 4KMnO_4 + 11H_2SO_4 \longrightarrow 10HNO_3 + 4MnSO_4 + 2K_2SO_4 + 5Na_2SO_4 + 6H_2O$$

Instead of titrating excess of potassium permanganate solution with standard oxalic acid to disappearance of pink colour, the excess of potassium permanganate is reduced by adding an accurately measured excess amount of oxalic acid and subsequently the excess of oxalic acid is titrated with permanganate to the appearance of pink colour. This sequence is followed due to easiness in detecting the appearance of pink colour.

Factor

Each ml 0.1N KMnO$_4$ solution = 0.00345 g of NaNO$_2$.

Assay of Hydrogen Peroxide

Hydrogen peroxide IP is an aqueous solution containing hydrogen peroxide, not less than 5% v/v and not more than 7.0% v/v of H$_2$O$_2$ corresponding to 20 volumes strength. It should not contain more than 0.025% w/v of suitable stabilizing agent. Twenty volumes strength means that it gives 20 times its volume of oxygen on complete decomposition by heat.

Procedure

Dilute hydrogen peroxide (10 to 25 ml) with water to 100 ml. Pipette out 10 ml of this solution, add sulphuric acid solution (20 ml) and titrate with 0.1N potassium permanganate solution to a permanent pink colour.

Hydrogen peroxide has both oxidizing and reducing properties, but if titrated against an acidified potassium permanganate solution (stronger oxidizing agent), it acts as a reducing agent. When hydrogen peroxide is reacted with potassium permanganate, it is oxidized into oxygen. High concentration of the acid is used to prevent the formation of manganese dioxide which may cause decomposition of hydrogen peroxide.

$$5H_2O_2 + 2KMnO_4 + 3H_2SO_4 \longrightarrow 5O_2\uparrow + 2MnSO_4 + K_2SO_4 + 8H_2O$$

Factor

Each ml of 0.1N KMnO$_4$ solution = 0.001701 g of H$_2$O$_2$.

IODIMETRIC AND IODOMETRIC METHODS

It involves the use of iodine as a mild oxidizing agent. Iodine can be used directly for estimation of reducing agents, e.g. sodium thiosulphate. Such direct method is called 'Iodimetry'. In the indirect method, known as Iodometry, the oxidizing agent is reduced with excess of potassium iodide to liberate an equivalent amount of iodine which can be estimated by titrating with standard sodium thiosulphate. Iodometry is used for assays of copper sulphate, available chlorine, etc.

Assay of Iodine

Iodine contains not less than 99.5% and not more than equivalent of 100.5% w/w of I.

Procedure

Weigh accurately iodine (about 0.2 g) and dissolve in a solution of potassium iodide (1 g) in H_2O (5 ml). Dilute it with water to 25 ml, acidify with 2M acetic acid (1 ml) and titrate with 0.1M sodium thiosulphate till light yellow colour appears. At this stage, add starch mucilage and continue the titration till blue colour disappears.

It is iodimetric method, official in I.P. 2007. Iodine is directly estimated by titration with the sodium thiosulphate (reducing agent). Iodine oxidizes the sodium thiosulphate into sodium tetrathionate.

$$I_2 + 2Na_2S_2O_3 \longrightarrow Na_2S_4O_6 + 2NaI$$

Sodium   Sodium

thiosulphate   tetrathionate

Starch is added towards the end of titration (when brown colour changes into yellow colour), when most of iodine is reacted with sodium thiosulphate as starch mucilage forms stable complex with excess of iodine.

Factor

Each ml of 0.1M $Na_2S_2O_3$ solution = 0.01269 g of I.

Assay of Analgin Tablet

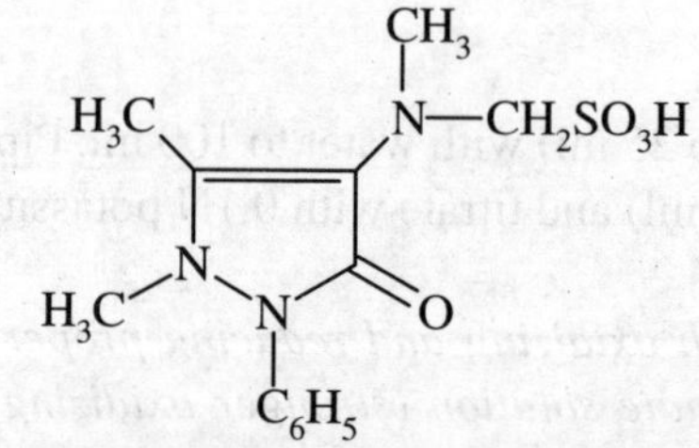

Analgin [(2,3-Dihydro-1,5-dimethyl-3-oxo-2-phenyl-*1H*-pyrazol-1,4-yl)methyl amino] methane sulphonic acid

Procedure

Weigh and powder 20 tablets. Weigh accurately a quantity of the powder equivalent to about 0.5 g of analgin and transfer to 50 ml volumetric flask. Add water (10 ml) and shake for 1 minute. Dilute to volume with ethanol (95%), shake well and filter. Titrate 25.0 ml of the filtrate with 0.05M iodine until yellow colour stable for 30 seconds is produced.

Factor

Each ml of 0.05M iodine solution = 0.01757 g of $C_{13}H_{16}N_3NaO_4S$, H_2O.

The determination of analysis depends upon the oxidation of enolic group present in it with iodine.

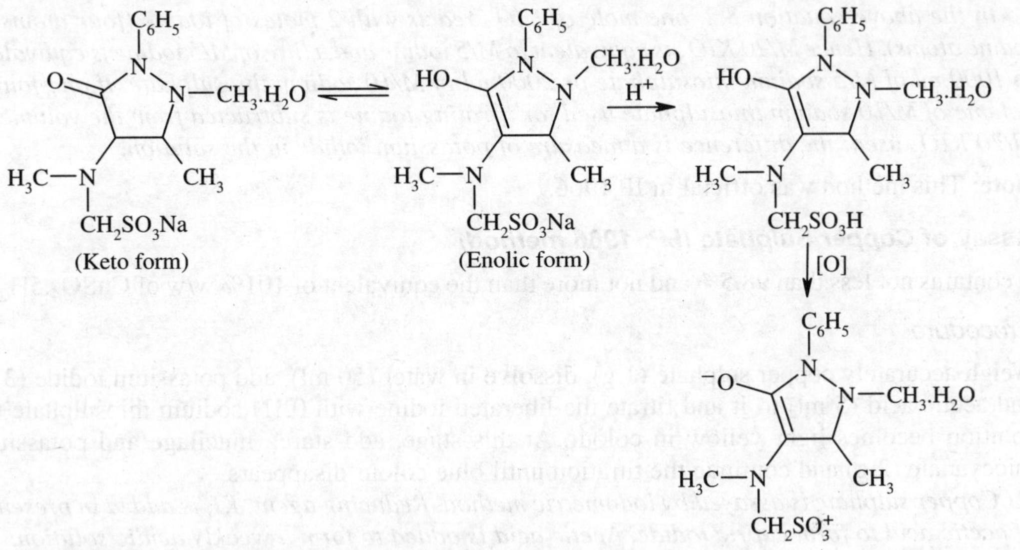

(Keto form) ⇌ (Enolic form)

Assay of Aqueous Iodine Solution (Synonym: Lugol's solution)

It contains 5% w/v of iodine (limits 4.9 to 5.1%) and 10% w/v of potassium iodide (limits 9.8 to 10.2).

Procedure

Estimation is carried for both iodine and potassium iodide. Aqueous iodine solution (25 ml) is diluted to 100 ml with water.

For iodine: To the above solution (20 ml), add water (10 ml) and titrate with 0.1M sodium thiosulphate by using starch mucilage as indicator till blue colour disappears.

Factor

Each ml of 0.1M $Na_2S_2O_3$ solution = 0.01269 g of I.

For potassium iodide: To the above diluted solution (10 ml), add water (20 ml) and conc. HCl (40 ml) and then titrate with 0.05M potassium iodate (KIO_3) solution, with vigorous shaking until brown solution becomes only light yellow in colour. Add chloroform (5 ml) and continue the titration until chloroform becomes colourless and supernatant liquid becomes clear yellow. From the number of ml of 0.05M potassium iodate required substract one-fourth of the number of ml of 0.1M sodium thiosulphate required in the assay for iodine.

Factor

Each ml of 0.05M KIO_3 solution = to 0.0166 g of KI.

Iodides are quantitatively oxidized by iodate to iodine which reacts with more iodate in the presence of strong hydrochloric acid to form iodine monochloride (ICl).

$$5KI + KIO_3 + 6HCl \longrightarrow 3I_2 + 6KCl + 3H_2O \qquad ...(3.1)$$

$$2I_2 + KIO_3 + 6HCl \longrightarrow KCl + 5ICl + 3H_2O \qquad ...(3.2)$$

Starch mucilage cannot be used in this titration due to high concentration of hydrochloric acid (hydrolysis of starch occurs). Iodine monochloride is stable in high concentration of the acid. The end point is detected by disappearance of violet colour of iodine in chloroform.*

---

* Iodine is soluble in chloroform to impart violet colour.

In the above equation 3.2, one mole of KIO_3 reacts with 2 moles of iodine (four atoms of iodine atoms). Hence $M/20$ KIO_3 is equivalent to $M/5$ iodine and a litre of $M/5$ iodine is equivalent to 1000 ml of $M/5$ sodium thiosulphate or 2000 ml of $M/10$ sodium thiosulphate. If one-fourth volume of $M/10$ sodium thiosulphate used for titrating iodine is subtracted from the volume of $M/20$ KIO_3 used; the difference is a measure of potassium iodide in the solution.

Note: This method was official in IP 1966.

Assay of Copper Sulphate (I.P. 1966 method)

It contains not less than 98.5% and not more than the equivalent of 101% w/w of $CuSO_4.5H_2O$.

Procedure

Weigh accurately copper sulphate (1 g), dissolve in water (50 ml), add potassium iodide (3 g) and acetic acid (5 ml) to it and titrate the liberated iodine with 0.1N sodium thiosulphate till solution becomes light yellow in colour. At this stage, add starch mucilage and potassium thiocyanate (2 g) and continue the titration until blue colour disappears.

Copper sulphate is assayed by iodometric method. Reducing agent, KI, is added in presence of acetic acid to form cupric iodide. Acetic acid is added to form a weakly acidic solution.

Cupric iodide is unstable and decomposes into cuprous iodide and iodine. The liberated iodine is titrated with sodium thiosulphate till the solution becomes yellow. Most of the liberated iodine is reacted with sodium thiosulphate, little amount is left (indicated by yellow colour).

Starch mucilage is added towards the end because it forms stable complex with excess of iodine.

$$2CuSO_4 + 4KI \longrightarrow \underset{\text{Cupric iodide}}{2CuI_2} + 2K_2SO_4$$

$$\underset{\text{Cupric iodide}}{2CuI_2} \rightleftharpoons \underset{\text{Cuprous iodide}}{Cu_2I_2} + I_2\uparrow$$

$$I_2 + 2Na_2S_2O_3 \longrightarrow 2Na_2S_4O_6 + 2NaI$$

The decomposition of cupric iodide into cuprous iodide and iodine is reversible, hence to make quantitative, potassium thiocyanate is added which reacts with the reaction product, cuprous iodide, to form cuprous thiocyanate. Potassium thiocyanate is added toward the end of the titration to avoid errors due to adsorption of iodine by cuprous thiocyanate.

$$Cu_2I_2 + KCNS \longrightarrow \underset{\text{Cuprous thiocyanate}}{CuCNS} + 2KI$$

Factor

Each ml of 0.1N $Na_2S_2O_3$ solution is equivalent to 0.02497 gm of $CuSO_4.5H_2O$.

Assay of Chlorinated Lime (Synonyms: Bleaching Powder)

It contains not less than 30% w/w of available chlorine.

Procedure

Triturate accurately weighed bleaching powder (4 g) with little quantity of water in a mortar and transfer to a 1 litre flask. Add sufficient water to make 1000 ml. Take this suspension (100 ml), add 3% potassium iodide solution (100 ml), acidify with acetic acid (5 ml) and titrate the liberated iodine with 0.1N sodium thiosulphate solution, using starch mucilage as indicator.

It is a iodometric method, official in I.P. 1966. On acidification with acetic acid, chlorine is liberated which displaces an equivalent amount of iodine from potassium iodide. The liberated iodine is measured by titration with sodium thiosulphate solution. Starch mucilage is added towards the end of titration. Disappearance of blue colour is an indication of the end point.

$$CaCl\,(OCl) + 2CH_3COOH \longrightarrow Ca\,(CH_3COO)_2 + HCl + HOCl$$

Hypochlorus acid

$$HCl + HOCl + 2KI \longrightarrow 2KCl + I_2 + H_2O$$

$$I_2 + 2Na_2S_2O_3 \longrightarrow Na_2S_4O_6 + 2NaCl$$

Factor

Each ml of 0.1N $Na_2S_2O_3$ solution = 0.003455 g of available chlorine.

Assay of Benzylpenicillin Tablets

Procedure

Weigh and powder tablets. Weigh accurately a quantity of powder equivalent to about 7,50,000 units of penicillin, dissolve in water and dilute to 100 ml with water. Transfer 10.0 ml of this solution to a iodine flask, add 5 ml of 1N NaOH solution and allow to stand for 20 minutes. Add 20 ml of freshly prepared buffer solution containing 5.44% w/v of sodium acetate, 2.40% w/v of glacial acetic acid, and 5 ml of 1N HCl and 25.0 ml of 0.02N iodine solution. Close the flask with a wet stopper and allow to stand in dark place for 20 minutes. Titrate the excess of iodine with 0.02N sodium thiosulphate, using starch mucilage indicator added towards the end of titration. To a further 10.0 ml of initial solution, add 20 ml of buffer solution and 25.0 ml of 0.02N iodine solution, allow to stand for 20 minutes and titrate similarly with 0.02N sodium thiosulphate solution. The difference between the two titrations represents the volume of 0.02N iodine solution equivalent to the total penicillin present.

Note: *Each mg of benzylpenicillin (sodium salt) contain not less than 500 units and not more than 1750 units.*

Each mg of benzylpenicillin (potassium salt) contain not less than 1440 units and not more than 1680 units.

The intact penicillin does not consume iodine while its hydrolytic product, penicilloic acid consumes iodine molecule. NaOH is added to hydrolyze the penicillin molecule. The difference in iodine consumption is analyzed for the estimation of benzylpenicillin.

Benzylpenicillin   Penicilloic acid

Factor

Each ml of 0.02N iodine solution = 0.000764 g of total penicillin calculated as $C_{16}H_{17}O_4N_2SNa$ or 0.000798 of total penicillin calculated as $C_{16}H_{17}O_4N_2SK$.

Assay of Ascorbic Acid

Procedure

Weigh accurately ascorbic acid (about 0.1 g) and dissolve in a mixture of freshly boiled and cooled water (100 ml) and 1M sulphuric acid (25 ml). Immediately titrate with 0.05M iodine solution, using a starch mucilage as indicator.

Ascorbic acid   Dehydroascorbic acid

It is an example of redox titration. Iodine oxidizes the ascorbic acid (reducing agent) into dehydroascorbic acid. At the end point, iodine react with starch mucilage to give blue colour.

Factor

Each ml of 0.05M Iodine solution = 0.008806 g of $C_6H_8O_6$.

Assay of Potassium Permanganate

Procedure

Weigh accurately $KMnO_4$ (about 0.3 g), dissolve in sufficient water to produce 100.0 ml. Add water (20 ml), KI (1 g) and 2M hydrochloric acid (10 ml) and titrate the liberated iodine with 0.1M sodium thiosulphate using starch mucilage added toward the end of titration as indicator.

It is an example of iodometric titration. Potassium permanganate solution react with potassium iodide to liberate an equivalent quantity of iodine. The liberated iodine is titrated with standard sodium thiosulphate solution using starch mucilage as indicator.

$$2KMnO_4 + 10KI + 16HCl \longrightarrow 12KCl + 2MnCl_2 + 5I_2 + 8H_2O$$

Factor

Each ml of 0.1M Sodium thiosulphate solution = 0.003160 g of $KMnO_4$.

CERIC SULPHATE TITRATION METHOD

Solution of ceric sulphate in dilute sulphuric acid is a strong oxidizing agent. It is considered more stable than potassium permanganate solution provided sufficient sulphuric acid is present to prevent its hydrolysis.

Assay of Ferrous Sulphate

Procedure

Dissolve an accurately weighed quantity of ferrous sulphate (about 1.0 g), dissolve in a mixture of water (30 ml) and dilute sulphuric acid (20 ml) and titrate with 0.1M ceric sulphate solution using *o*-phenanthroline-ferrous complex (ferroin) as an indicator.

This method is official in I.P. 1996 and 2007 (permanganate method is official in I.P. 1966). Ferrous sulphate is oxidized into ferric sulphate in acidified solution.

$$2FeSO_4 + 2Ce(SO_4)_2 \xrightarrow{\hspace{3cm}} Fe_2(SO_4)_3 + Ce_2(SO_4)_3$$
$$\text{Ceric sulphate} \qquad\qquad \text{Ferric sulphate} \quad \text{Cerum sulphate}$$

At the end point, when ferrous sulphate is completely oxidized, then ceric sulphate oxidize indicator o-phenanthroline-ferrous complex (ferroin) (red colour) into o-phenanthroline-ferric complex to impart the blue colour (see Chapter 2).

Factor

Each ml of 0.1M ceric ammonium sulphate solution = 0.0278 g of $FeSO_4.7H_2O$.

Assay of Paracetamol

Procedure

Weigh accurately paracetamol (about 0.5 g) and transfer it into mixture of $1MH_2SO_4$ (50 ml) and water (10 ml). Boil the solution on water bath for 1 hour. Cool down, dilute with water to 100 ml. Pipette out 20 ml of this solution and transfer it into water (40 ml) containing 40 g of crushed ice and 2M HCl (15 ml) and ferroin indicator (0.1 ml). Titrate with 0.1M ceric ammonium sulphate solution. Similarly, perform the blank titration.

Factor

Each ml of 0.1M ceric ammonium sulphate solution = 0.00756 g of paracetamol.

Paracetamol on heating with sulphuric acid is hydrolysed into p-aminophenol and acetic acid. The p-aminophenol is oxidized into benzoquinone by ceric sulphate. The difference in two titration indicate the amount required to oxidize the paracetamol.

Paracetamol	*p*-Aminophenol	*p*-Benzoquinone

Assay of Ascorbic Acid Tablets

Procedure

Weigh and powder 20 tablets. Weigh accurately a quantity of powder equivalent to 0.15 g of ascorbic acid and dissolve as completely as possible in a mixture of sulphuric acid and water (30 ml each). Titrate the solution with 0.1M ceric sulphate solution, using ferroin sulphate as indicator as usual.

Ceric sulphate oxidize the ascorbic acid into dehydro ascorbic acid (similar to iodine solution). At the end point, a slight excess of ceric sulphate oxidizes o-phenanthroline–ferrous complex (indicator) into o-phenanthroline-ferric complex to change the colour.

Note: Ascorbic acid injection is assayed by titration against with standard 2,6-dichlorophenol indophenol solution. It acts as titrant as well as indicator. It also oxidises ascorbic acid into dehydro ascorbic acid and changes into reduced form (colourless). The original colour of 2,6-dichlorophenol is blue or pink.

OXIDATION–REDUCTION METHOD WITH 0.1N BROMINE SOLUTION

Bromine is an oxidizing agent used for assay of a number of compounds, e.g. aniline, phenol, etc., as it reacts quantitatively and forms insoluble substitution product, tribromoaniline and tribromophenol, respectively. Standard bromine solution does not contain bromine as such but an equivalent amount of potassium bromide and potassium bromate ($KBrO_3$) which on acidification liberates an equivalent quantity of bromine.

$$5KBr + KBrO_3 + 6HCl \longrightarrow 6KCl + 3Br_2 + 3H_2O$$

Assay of Phenol

Phenol contains not less than 99% and not more than equivalent of 100.5% w/w of C_6H_6O calculated with reference to the anhydrous substance.

Procedure

Weigh accurately phenol (0.5 g) and dissolve in sufficient amount of water to produce 500 ml. Mix this solution (25 ml) with 0.1N potassium bromate solution (25 ml) in 250 ml glass stoppered flask and add potassium bromide (1.0 g) and dilute hydrochloric acid (10 ml) to it. Insert the stopper, previously moistened with a few drops of 10% w/v potassium iodide solution and keep it in dark for 20 minutes with frequent shaking. Add 10% w/v potassium iodide solution (10 ml) to it and keep it in the dark for further 5 minutes with frequent shaking. Wash the stopper and neck of flask with water, add chloroform (10 ml) and titrate the liberated iodine with 0.1N sodium thiosulphate solution using starch mucilage as an indicator. Perform a blank titration in the same way.

When the hydrochloric acid is added, bromine is liberated, which reacts with phenol to form white crystalline precipitate of tribromophenol and hydrobromic acid.

$$5KBr + KBrO_3 + 6HCl \longrightarrow 6KCl + 3Br_2 + 3H_2O$$

$$\underset{\text{Phenol}}{C_6H_5OH} + 3Br_2 \longrightarrow \underset{\substack{\text{Tribromophenol} \\ \text{(white precipitate)}}}{C_6H_2Br_3OH} + 3HBr$$

The flask should be stoppered to prevent the escape of the volatile bromine. Sufficient time should be given to complete oxidation of phenol to tribromophenol.

Potassium iodide liberates an equivalent amount of iodine when reacted with excess of unreacted bromine.

$$2KI + Br_2 \longrightarrow 6KBr + I_2$$

Chloroform is added to dissolve the precipitated tribromophenol otherwise it would interfere in the detection of end point.

The liberated free iodine reacts with sodium thiosulphate. At the end point blue colour disappears as the whole of iodine is consumed by sodium thiosulphate.

$$I_2 + 2Na_2S_2O_3 \longrightarrow 2NaI + Na_2S_4O_6$$

Factor

Each ml of 0.1N bromine solution = 0.01569 g of phenol.

Assay of Isoniazid

Weigh accurately isoniazid (about 0.4 g), dissolve as completely as possible in water, filter and wash the residue with sufficient water to make up 250 ml. Transfer this solution (25 ml) into a glass stoppered flask, add KBr (0.2 g) and hydrochloric acid (20 ml) to it and titrate slowly with continuous shaking with 0.0167M potassium bromate solution using methyl red solution (0.05 ml) until the red colour disappears.

Factor

Each ml of 0.0167M $KBrO_3 \equiv 0.003429$ g of $C_6H_7N_3O$.

Isonicotinic acid

Isoniazid

Bromine (liberated from the reaction of KBr and KBrO$_3$ in acidified solution) oxidizes the isoniazid into isonicotinic acid. At the end point there is a colour change in the indicator after the complete oxidation of isoniazid.

Assay of Isoniazid Tablets

Procedure

Weigh and powder 20 tablets. Weigh accurately a quantity of powder equivalent to 0.4 g of isoniazid and dissolve as completely as possible in water, filter and wash the residue with sufficient water to produce 250 ml. Transfer this solution (25 ml) to a glass stoppered flask, add 0.1N ml bromine solution (25 ml) and hydrochloric acid (5 ml) to it. Shake for one minutes and allow to stand for fifteen minutes in a water bath maintained at about 15°C temperature. Add 10% w/v potassium iodide solution (10 ml) and titrate with 0.1N sodium thiosulphate, using starch mucilage as indicator. Carry out the blank determination with the same quantities of the same reagent but omitting the substance being examined.

Factor

Each ml of 0.1N bromine solution = 0.003429 g of isoniazid.

Bromine oxidizes the isoniazid into isonicotinic acid. Excess of bromine solution react with iodide to liberate an equivalent quantity of iodine. The liberated iodine is titrated with standard sodium thiosulphate solution.With the determination of amount of bromine solution actually required for oxidation of isoniazid, percentage purity is calculated.

Note: According to IP 2007, Isoniazid is assayed by chromatographic method.

OXIDATION-REDUCTION METHOD WITH POTASSIUM IODATE SOLUTION

In this method, potassium iodate is used as oxidizing agent. It involves the formation of iodine monochloride. A number of reducing agents, e.g. potassium iodide, can be estimated by potassium iodate method.

Assay of Potassium Iodide

Potassium iodide contains not less than 99% and not more than 100.5% w/w of KI calculated with reference to the dried substance.

Procedure

Weigh accurately potassium iodide (0.5 g), dissolve in water (10 ml) and add hydrochloric acid (25 ml) and chloroform (5 ml). Titrate it with 0.05M potassium iodate until purple colour disappears from the chloroform layer.

Factor

Each ml of 0.05M Potassium iodate solution = 0.0166 g of KI.

Potassium iodate oxidizes quantitatively iodides into iodine.

$$5KI + KIO_3 + 6HCl \longrightarrow 6KCl + 3I_2 + 3H_2O$$

The liberated iodine reacts with excess of iodate in the presence of strong hydrochloric acid to form iodine monochloride (ICl).

$$2I_2 + KIO_3 + 6HCl \longrightarrow KCl + 5ICl + 3H_2O$$
Iodine
monochloride

In the titration, starch mucilage cannot be used as an indicator due to presence of strong hydrochloric acid which may be hydrolyzed, hence, chloroform is used. Iodine is more soluble in chloroform. The solution becomes colourless when whole iodine reacts with iodate.

COMPLEXOMETRIC TITRATIONS

Earlier aluminium and magnesium salts were assayed by a time consuming gravimetric method but with the introduction of chelate forming agents, mainly disodium salt of ethylenediamine tetra-acetic acid (EDTA), a new volumetric method is developed. The method referred as complexometric titrations which involves the formation of complex of which stability depends on pH of the solution.

Assay of Calcium Carbonate

Calcium carbonate I.P. contains not less than 98% and not more than the equivalent of 100.5% w/w of $CaCO_3$ calculated with reference to the dried substance.

Procedure

Weigh accurately of calcium carbonate (0.1 g) and dissolve in dilute hydrochloric acid (3 ml) in water (10 ml). Boil for 10 minutes, cool, dilute to 50 ml with water. Titrate with 0.05M disodium ethylenediamine tetra-acetate solution (to within a few ml of expected end point), then add sodium hydroxide (8 ml) and calcon mixture (0.1 g) and continue the titration until the colour of the solution changes from pink to full blue colour.

Calcium carbonate forms complex with 0.05M disodium salt of EDTA ethylenediamine tetra-acetate.

Calcon mixture is added as an indicator. It is pink in colour in the presence of calcium salt (calcium-indicator complex) but blue in colour in the absence of calcium carbonate. Hence, at the end point, whole amount of calcium carbonate is reacted to form the Ca-EDTA complex and blue colour appears due to presence of free indicator. Indicator is added towards the end of titration. Sodium hydroxide is added to maintain the alkaline pH to avoid the interference of other metallic salts (like aluminium salt) which also form complex with EDTA salt in a similar manner.

Calcium EDTA complex

Factor

Each ml of 0.05M disodium EDTA solution = 0.0050048 g of $CaCO_3$.

Assay of Magnesium Sulphate

Magnesium sulphate IP contains not less than 99% and not more than equivalent of 100.5% w/w of $MgSO_4$, calculated with reference to ignited substance.

Procedure

Weigh accurately the substance (0.3 g) and dissolve in water (50 ml). Add strong ammonia-ammonium chloride solution (10 ml) and titrate with 0.05M disodium ethylenediamine tetra-acetate solution using mordant black II mixture (0.1 g) as an indicator until pink colour changes into blue colour.

Magnesium forms complex with disodium salt of EDTA at pH 10 maintained by adding ammonia buffer. Mordant black II mixture is used as an indicator. The colour change at the end point is from pink to blue due to release of free indicator.

Factor

Each ml of 0.05M disodium EDTA solution = 0.00602 g of $MgSO_4$.

Assay of Zinc Oxide

Procedure

Dissolve 0.15 g in 1M acetic acid (10 ml) and dilute to 50 ml with water. To the resulting solution, add xylenol orange triturate (50 mg) and sufficient hexamine to produce violet pink colour. Add a further 2 g of hexamine and titrate with 0.1M disodium edetate until the solution becomes yellow.

Factor

Each ml of 0.1M disodium edetate solution = 0.008138 g of ZnO.

NON-AQUEOUS TITRATIONS

This method is used when the analyte is insoluble in water or it is weak acid or weak base in comparison to water. It is again classified into (i) acidimetry and (ii) alkalimetry.

(i) Acidimetry

The estimation of weak base can be performed in glacial acetic acid using perchloric acid as a titrant. End point is detected by using an indicator or by potentiometric method.

Assay of Ephedrine Hydrochloride Tablets

Procedure

Weigh accurately 20 tablets and grind to fine powder. Weigh accurately a quantity of powder equivalent to about 0.15 g of ephedrine hydrochloride, add glacial acetic acid (30 ml), mercuric acetate solution (10 ml) and crystal violet solution (0.1 ml) to it. Warm gently the solution, cool and titrate with 0.1M perchloric acid until the violet colour changes to green blue. Perform a blank titration in the same way.

It is difficult to titrate halogen salt directly with acetous perchloric acid because there is not sufficient difference in the proton attracting capabilities of halide and perchlorate anions in glacial acetic acid. Therefore, reaction does not proceed toward completion. Addition of mercuric acetate (which is undissociated in acetic acid solution) to halide salt replaces ion by an equivalent quantity of acetate ion which is a strong base in acetic acid and can react quantitatively with perchloric acid.

$$2HClO_4 + 2CH_3COOH \longrightarrow 2CH_3COOH_2^+ + 2ClO_4^-$$
$$\text{Onion ion}$$

$$\underset{\text{Ephedrine HCl}}{2C_{10}H_{15}N^+HOCl^-} + \underset{\text{Mercuric acetate}}{(Ac)_2Hg} \longrightarrow 2C_{10}H_{15}N^+HO.Ac + HgCl_2$$

$$CH_3COO^- + CH_3COOH_2^+ \longrightarrow 2CH_3COOH$$

$$2C_{10}H_{15}N^+HO.Ac + 2CH_3COOH_2^+ \longrightarrow 2C_{10}H_{15}N^+HO + 4CH_3COOH$$

The overall reaction

$$2C_{10}H_{15}N^+HOCl^- + (Ac)_2Hg + 2HClO_4 \longrightarrow 2C_{10}H_{15}N^+H + AcOH + 2ClO_4^- + HgCl_2$$

Factor

Each ml of 0.1M perchloric acid solution = 0.02017 g of $C_{10}H_{15}NO.HCl$.

Assay of Bisacodyl tablets

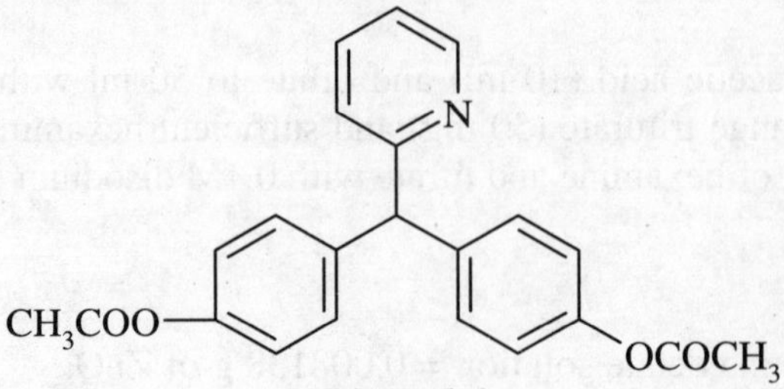

Bisacodyl

Procedure

1. Weigh accurately about 20 tablets and powder them.
2. Weigh accurately the powder equivalent to 0.5 g of bisacodyl and extract with chloroform thrice each of 25 ml.
3. Evaporate off the chloroform to get residue and dissolve in glacial acetic acid.
4. Titrate with 0.1N $HClO_4$ solution by using 1-naphthol benzein solution as indicator.
5. Similarly carry out the blank titration.

Factor

Each ml of 0.1N $HClO_4$ = 0.0314 g of $C_{22}H_{19}NO_4$.

Assay of Chloroquine tablets

Chloroquine is an aminoquinoline used for the prevention and therapy of malaria. It is also effective in extraintestinal amoebiasis and as an anti-inflammatory. It is used as phosphate and sulphate salt.

It contains not less than 98.0% and not more than 102.0% of $C_{18}H_{26}ClN_3.2H_3PO_4$. It contains not less than 98.0% of $C_{18}H_{26}ClN_3.H_2SO_4$.

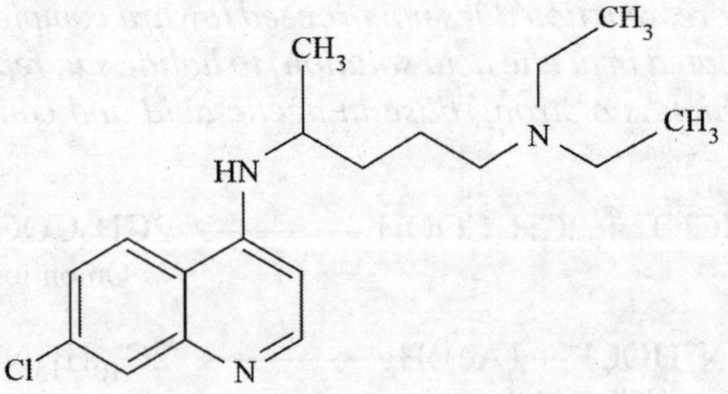

Chloroquine

Principle

Chloroquine is a weekly basic drug, so estimation is done by non-aqueous titration. When weakly basic chloroquine is dissolved in acetic acid, the acetic acid exerts its levelling effect and enhances the basic properties of chloroquine. Hence, chloroquine can be titrated to get sharp end point.

Procedure

Weigh accurately 20 tablets and powder them. Find out average weight of tablet. Weight the powder accurately, equivalent to 0.5 g of chloroquine sulphate/phosphate. Transfer this powder in dry 100 ml flask and add 10 ml of glacial acetic acid. Add 2–3 drops of crystal violet indicator and titrate with 0.1N perchloric acid solution until violet colour changes to green.

Factor

Each ml of 0.1N perchloric acid solution = 0.0418 g chloroquine sulphate
Each ml of 0.1N perchloric acid = 0.0 257 g of chloroquine phosphate

Assay of Metronidazole

Metronidazole is a chemotherapeutic agent that is used to treat a wide variety of infections. It works by stopping the growth of certain bacteria and parasites.

It contains not less than 99.0% and not more than 101.0% of $C_6H_9N_3O_3$.

Metronidazole

Principle

It is weak basic drug, so estimated by non-aqueous titration with perchloric acid. Drug is dissolve in glacial acetic acid to enhance it acidity.

Procedure

Metronidazole: Weigh accurately about 0.45 g powdered metronidazole and dissolve in glacial acetic acid. Add few drops of 1-naphtholbenzein solution and titrate with 0.1N perchloric acid solution until a pale-green colour is produced. Perform a blank determination and make necessary correction.

Metronidazole tablets: Weigh and powder 20 tablets. Weigh accurately a quantity of powder equivalent to about 0.2 g of metronidazole and transfer to a sintered glass crucible. Extract with six quantities of, each of 10 ml of hot acetone. Cool, add to the combined extract 50 ml of acetic anhydride, 0.1 ml of 1% w/v solution of brilliant green in glacial acetic acid and titrate with 0.1N perchloric acid solution until a yellowish-green colour is produced. Perform a blank determination and make necessary correction.

Factor

Each ml of 0.1N perchloric acid = 0.01712 g of metronidazole.

Assay of Phenobarbitone

Phenobarbitone is used for the treatment of certain types of epilepsy in developing countries. Phenobarbital is occasionally used to treat trouble sleeping, anxiety, and drug withdrawal and to help with surgery.

It contains not less than 98.0% and not more than 101.0% of $C_{12}H_{12}N_2O_3$.

Principle

Assay is based on the acidic nature of the imido hydrogen in pheno-barbitone. The titration in water is hindered by their insolubility and weakly acidic nature so titration is carried out in alcoholic or hydro-alcoholic medium.

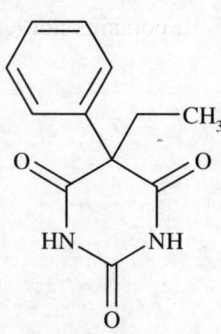

Phenobarbitone

Procedure

Phenobarbitone powder: Weigh accurately about 0.1 g of phenobarbitone, dissolve in 5 ml of pyridine, add 0.25 ml of thymolphthalein solution, 10 ml of silver nitrate–pyridine reagent and titrate with 0.1N alcoholic sodium hydroxide until a full blue colour is obtained.

Factor

Each ml of 0.1N alcoholic NaOH solution = 0.0116 g of phenobarbitone.

Phenobarbitone sodium tablet: Weigh and powder 20 tablets. Weigh accurately a quantity of powder equivalent to 0.3 g of phenobarbitone sodium and dissolve in 30 ml of glacial acetic acid. Add 10 ml of mercuric acetate and few drops of 1-naphtholbenzein solution. Titrate with 0.1N perchloric acid solution to a green end point.

Factor

Each ml of 0.1N perchloric acid solution = 0.0254 g of phenobarbitone sodium.

Assay of Atropine sulphate

Atropine is an enantiomeric mixture of d-hyoscyamine and l-hyoscyamine, with most of its physiological effects due to l-hyoscyamine. Its pharmacological effects are due to binding to muscarinic acetylcholine receptors. The most common atropine compound used in medicine is atropine sulphate.

It contains not less than 98.5% and not more than 101.5% of $C_{34}H_{48}N_2O_{10}S$.

Principle

It is a alkaloid, weak basic in nature and so estimated by non-aqueous titration.

Procedure

Weigh accurately about 1.0 g and dissolve in 50 ml of glacial acetic acid. Titrate with 0.1N perchloric acid, determining the end-point potentiometrically. Perform a blank titration and make any necessary correction.

Factor

Each ml of 0.1N perchloric acid = 0.0677 g of atropine sulphate.

Assay of Chlorpheniramine maleate

Chlorphenamine (also known as CPM) is a first-generation antihistamine used in the prevention of the symptoms of allergic conditions such as rhinitis and urticaria. It is used as maleate salt.

It contains not less than 98.0% of $C_{16}H_{19}ClN_2.C_4H_5O_4$.

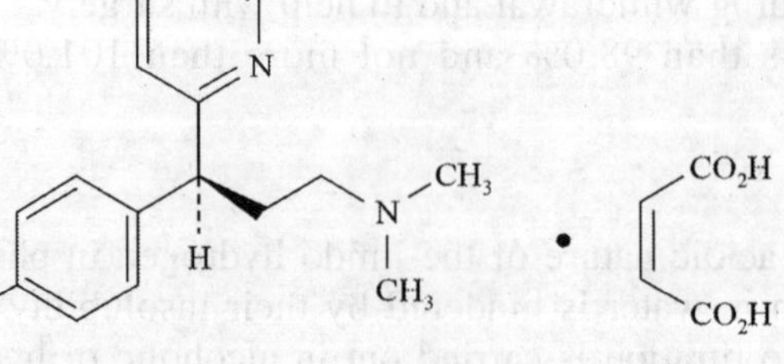

Principle

It is weak basic in nature and estimated by titration with standard perchloric acid. Acidity is enhanced by dissolving it in glacial acetic acid.

Procedure

Chlorpheniramine maleate powder. Dissolve about 0.5 g of chlorpheniramine maleate powder in 20 ml of glacial acetic acid. Add 2–3 dops of crystal violet indicator. Titrate with 0.1N perchloric acid solution until colour changes from purple though blue-green to green. Perform a blank titration and make necessary correction.

Factor

Each l of 0.1N perchloric acid solution = 0.0195 g of chlorpheniramine maleate.

(ii) Alkalimetry

Weak acids can be determined by titration with metallic alkoxides using a protophilic solvent. End point can be detected by using indicator or by potentiometric method. For example, barbiturates are weak acid and cannot be estimated in the aqueous solution. They can be estimated by titration with standard sodium methoxide in dimethylformamide or in pyridine solution by using thymol blue as an indicator. The lithium methoxide solution is preferred over sodium or potassium methoxide which may form gelatinous precipitate.

Similarly, sulpha drugs can also be titrated in dimethylformamide or pyridine or ethylene-diamine by standard sodium methoxide.

Assay of Diphenylhydantoin (Phenytoin)

Phenytoin

Procedure

Dissolve diphenylhydantoin ($C_{15}H_{12}N_2O_2$) (0.5 g) in dimethylformamide, add 3 drops of saturated solution of azo-violet in benzene and titrate with 0.1N sodium methoxide solution to a blue end point. Perform a blank determination and make any necessary correction.

Factor

Each ml of 0.1N sodium methoxide solution = 0.02523 g of $C_{15}H_{12}N_2O_2$.

DIAZOTIZATION TITRATIONS

The substances containing primary aromatic amino group are converted into their respective diazonium salts by titration with sodium nitrite at low temperature in the presence of hydrochloric acid.

$$ArNH_2 + NaNO_2 \xrightarrow[\text{0–5°C}]{\text{HCl}} ArN \equiv N^+Cl^- + NaCl + 2H_2O$$

At the end point, a drop of nitrous acid (formed from $NaNO_2$ in acid medium) reacts with starch iodide paper and gives blue colour due to liberation of an iodine.

$$2I^- + 2HNO_2 + 2H^+ \longrightarrow I_2 + 2NO\uparrow + 2H_2O$$

$$I_2 \xrightarrow{\text{Starch mucilage}} \text{Blue colour}$$

Assay of Sulphanilamide

Procedure

Dissolve an accurately weighed sample of sulphanilamide (about 1.0 g), previously dried at 105°C for 2 hours in concentrated hydrochloric acid (40 ml) and water (100 ml). Cool the solution to about 5°C and titrate with 0.1M sodium nitrate dipping the tip of burette well in the solution. Add sodium nitrite slowly until an immediate blue colour is obtained on placing a drop of the solution to a starch iodide paper. The end point should be reproducible for a period of at least 1 minute.

Nitrous acid is formed from sodium nitrite in acidic medium which diazotizes sulphanilamide to form the diazonium salt.

$$NaNO_2 + HCl \longrightarrow HNO_2 + NaCl$$

$$\underset{\text{Sulphanilamide}}{H_2NSO_2-C_6H_4-NH_2} + HNO_2 + HCl \xrightarrow{0-5°C} \underset{\text{Diazotized sulphanilamide}}{H_2NSO_2-C_6H_4-N_2Cl} + 2H_2O$$

At the end point, a slight excess of nitrous acid reacts with starch iodide paper to give the blue colour.

Factor

Each ml of 0.1M $NaNO_2$ solution = 0.01722 g of sulphanilamide.

Assay of Dapsone

Dapsone (4,4′-diaminosulphone, DDS) is a used in the treatment of leprosy along with other drugs.

Dapsone contains not less than 98% and not more than 102.0% of $C_{12}H_{12}N_2O_2S$, calculated on the dried basis.

Principle

Dapsone is determined by diazotization method due to presence of primary aromatic amino group.

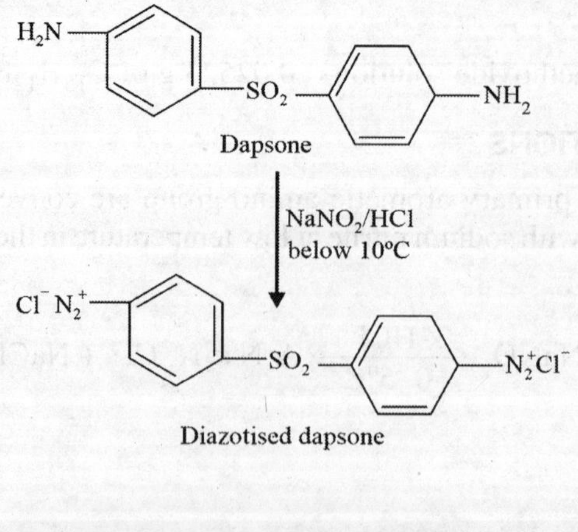

Dapsone

NaNO₂/HCl
below 10°C

Diazotised dapsone

On complete diazotization with nitrous acid (liberated from the reaction of $NaNO_2$ and HCl), a slight excess of nitrous acid react with starch iodide paper to give the blue colour (end point).

$$2KI + HNO_2 + 2HCl \rightarrow 2KCl + I_2 + 2NO + 2H_2O$$

$$I_2 + Starch \rightarrow Blue\ colour\ (end\ point)$$

Procedure

Dapsone powder: Weigh accurately about 0.3 g and dissolve in a mixture of 20 ml of water and 20 ml of hydrochloric acid. Cool the solution below 10°C temperature and carry out the titration with 0.1N $NaNO_2$ solution using starch iodide indicator paper. Perform a blank titration and make necessary correction.

Dapsone tablets: Weigh 20 tablets and reduce to fine powder. Carry out the assay described under dapsone powder, using an accurately weighed quantity of the powder equivalent to 0.25 g of dapsone.

Factor

Each ml of 0.1N $NaNO_2$ solution = 0.0124 g of dapsone.

Gravimetric Analysis

Gravimetric analysis is the measurement of weight of a substance in a simple analysis or calculation of weight of a substance from the weight of chemically equivalent amount of some other substance.

$$A + B \longrightarrow C + D$$

In the above general reaction, the weight of either reactant A or B can be calculated from the weight of either product C or D. For example, in the quantitative estimation of sodium chloride, the silver nitrate is added to precipitate the soluble chloride as insoluble silver chloride which is collected, washed and dried to a constant weight. From the weight of silver chloride, weight of sodium chloride is calculated.

$$NaCl + AgNO_3 \longrightarrow AgCl\downarrow + NaNO_3$$

In the simple gravimetric analysis, the organic compound is extracted by suitable a solvent from a mixture. The solvent is removed by evaporation/distillation and the residue so obtained is dried to a constant weight.

Gravimetric methods are not in use due to lack of accuracy. They are time consuming in comparison to volumetric methods. Some examples of gravimetrical assays, official in I.P. 1966 are illustrated here.

GENERAL OPERATION IN GRAVIMETRIC ANALYSIS

It involves the following operation:

(i) Solution
(ii) Precipitation
(iii) Filtration and washing of precipitate
(iv) Drying of precipitate
(v) Ignition of precipitate

(i) Solution

The substance to be estimated is first brought into solution in a vessel (usually a beaker). For this, weigh out exactly a suitable quantity (which will give about 0.2–0.3 g of ignited residue) of substance and dissolve in distilled water (about 50 ml) or dilute acid by gentle warming.

(ii) Precipitation

Precipitation is generally carried out in beakers. The precipitate obtained must either be of definite composition or must be capable of conversion into a substance of known composition on ignition. The precipitation must, of course, be as complete as possible. The precipitate should be granular and dense, as far as possible, so that it can be filtered in a reasonable time and also it may not pass through the filter paper. A dense and granular precipitate can be obtained by choosing suitable condition which are:

(a) Addition of the precipitant drop by drop so that the solution does not become supersaturated from the beginning.

(b) Constant stirring of the solution during the precipitation so that the initially formed crystals become bigger in size by deposition of more solid around them.

(c) Heating the solution and the precipitant before addition of the latter to the former so that solubility is increased at the time of precipitation.

(d) Allowing the precipitates to stand for some hours before filtering.

Impurities in precipitates

No discussion of gravimetric analysis would be complete without some discussion of the impurities which may be present in the precipitates.

Coprecipitation

This is anything unwanted which precipitates with the thing you do want. The soluble compounds from solution get removed during precipitation. Coprecipitation occurs to some degree in every gravimetric analysis (especially barium sulphate and those involving hydrous oxide). You cannot avoid it but you can minimize it by careful precipitation and proper washing.

Surface adsorption

Here, unwanted material is adsorbed into the surface of the precipitate. Digestion of a precipitate reduces the amount of surface area and hence the area available for surface adsorption.

Occlusion

This is a type of coprecipitation in which impurities are trapped within the growing crystal.

Postprecipitation

Sometimes, a precipitate standing in contact with the mother liquor becomes contaminated by the precipitation of an impurity on top of the desired precipitate. Examples include precipitation of copper sulphide in presence of zinc. Copper sulphide is formed first but if not directly filtered, zinc sulphide starts to precipitate on the top of it. The same is observed in the precipitation of calcium as the oxalate in presence of magnesium.

(iii) Filtration and washing of the precipitate

Gravimetrical filter papers (the weight of the ash of which is negligible and known) are used for filtration of the precipitate. The filter paper (or sintered glass crucible if used) must be of right porosity. Whatman No. 42 is suitable for fine precipitate while No. 40 should be used for gelatinous precipitate. It is most important that the folded filter paper should fit the funnel properly. This is done by properly adjusting the folds of filter paper so that the angle coincides with the angle of funnel. The folded filter paper is fitted into the funnel, moistened with distilled water and pressed against the sides of the funnel to which it should stick. This will prevent the entrance of air and thereby quicken filtration.

While filtering, the following points should be kept in mind:

(a) The liquid or precipitate must not more than about two-thirds fill of the filter to avoid creeping down of the precipitate from over the margin of the filter paper.

(b) To avoid loss by splashing, the system of the funnel must rest against the side of the receiving beaker.

Washing of precipitate

The precipitates is washed to remove soluble substances. Minimum amount of wash liquid should be used to avoid loss of traces of desirable precipitate by solution. The wash liquid chosen should have minimum solvent effect on the precipitate and should not peptise it even after all the electrolytes have been removed. Water is a suitable wash liquid for most of the precipitates but ammonium chloride or nitrate are sometimes added to it to avoid formation of a colloidal solution of the precipitates when all electrolytes have been removed.

To achieve best results, the precipitate must washed in a beaker itself by decantation using small quantities of wash liquid at a time. After shaking with about 20 ml of the wash liquid in the beaker, the precipitate is allowed to settle and the supernatant liquid is decanted off into the filter. After washing for or five times in this manner, the precipitate which is almost free from soluble electrolytes, transferred to the filter with the help of a glass rod. It is washed several times with the wash liquid till the filtrate gives no test for the particular impurity which is intended to be removed. Last traces of the precipitate sticking to the walls of the beaker should be removed by gentle rubbing with a policeman (a glass rod covered with about half an inch of the rubber tubing at the end) and washing with water. All the wash liquid must be transferred to the filter. While washing the precipitate on the filter paper, a jet of water should be directed at the top of the paper and not on the precipitate while rotating the funnel by hand.

(iv) Drying of the precipitate

The funnel containing the filter along with the precipitate is covered with a piece of paper having a few hole in it to enable water vapour to escape through them. The funnel is then kept in an air oven or a conc. containing precipitates is dried. In the case of the latter, the cone should be placed on a sand bath with a thin layer of sand on it or a wire gauze with asbestos for quick drying. If a wire gauze is used, a very small flame is put underneath not in the centre of the cone but at one side.

(v) Ignition and weighing of the precipitate

When the precipitate is dried, as much as possible, it is transferred to a clean and dry watch glass placed on a glazed paper. The watch glass is then covered with an inverted funnel. The particles of the precipitate which might fall on the glazed paper are transferred to the watch glass with the help of stout feather. Fold the filter paper several times into a narrow cone. Hold the upper edge with a pair of tongs and kindle the lower side over the crucible. The crucible should be placed on a watch glass which in turn is placed over a glazed paper. The ash is collected in the crucible and anything that may fall on the glazed paper or watch glass is transferred to the crucible with the help of feather. The crucible is now heated on a clay pipe triangle till the whole of the carbon is oxidized. It is then cooled and the precipitate is transferred into it. After this, the crucible is heated strongly on a Bunsen burner to a constant weight according to the direction given for the estimation concerned.

The crucible is then allowed to cool for a minute or two on the clay pipe triangle and then transferred to a desiccator. Knowing the weight of the crucible containing the precipitate and that of the empty crucible, the weight of the precipitates is detrmined by substraction. The weight of the precipitate is co-related with the weight of the substance to be analysed.

EXAMPLES OF GRAVIMETRIC ANALYSIS

Assay of Sodium Sulphate

Sodium sulphate IP contains not less than 99% and not more than the equivalent of 100.5% w/w of Na_2SO_4 calculated with reference to the substance dried to a constant weight at 105°C.

Weigh accurately sodium sulphate (about 0.5 g); dissolve in water (100 ml); add hydrochloric acid (1 ml); heat to boiling; add slowly a slight excess of hot solution of barium chloride and heat for half an hour on a water bath. Collect the precipitate, wash with water and ignite to a constant weight.

Sodium sulphate is precipitated by adding barium chloride solution as insoluble barium sulphate which is filtered and washed with water till filtrate is free from chloride. The precipitate is ignited to a constant weight.

$$Na_2SO_4 + BaCl_2 \longrightarrow BaSO_4 + 2NaCl$$
$$\quad\;\; 142\ g \qquad\qquad\qquad\qquad\quad 233.4\ g$$

Factor

Each g of the residue is equivalent to 0.6085 g of Na_2SO_4.

$$\% \text{ purity of the sodium sulphate} = \frac{0.6085 \times W}{a} \times 100$$

where W = weight of the precipitate
         a = weight of the sample of sodium sulphate

Note: The precipitate of barium sulphate is easily reduced to sulphide by the carbon of the filter paper above 600°C.

$$BaSO_4 + 4C \longrightarrow BaS + 4CO\uparrow$$

The reduction can be prevented by charring the filter paper slowly and then burning the carbon at a low temperature keeping the crucible open so as to allow free access of air. Treatment of the ash with few drops of sulphuric acid is sufficient to re-oxidize the reduced product. The excess of acid should then be removed by careful heating.

Assay of Zinc Sulphate

Zinc sulphate IP contains not less than 55.6% and not more than 61% w/w of $ZnSO_4$, corresponding to not less than 99.5% and not more than 104% w/w of the hydrated salt, $ZnSO_4.7H_2O$.

Weigh accurately zinc sulphate (about 1 g) and dissolve in water (100 ml). Heat the solution to about 90°C and then add solution of sodium carbonate to precipitate all the zinc as zinc carbonate, taking care to avoid a large excess of sodium carbonate. Boil for about five minutes and set aside to allow the precipitate to subside. Collect the precipitate in a tared Gooch crucible and wash with water until free from alkali. Dry the residue, ignite and weigh.

Zinc sulphate is precipitated as zinc carbonate by adding sodium carbonate solution. The precipitate of zinc carbonate is converted to zinc oxide on ignition. The constant weight of zinc oxide is correlated with the weight of zinc sulphate.

$$ZnSO_4 + Na_2CO_3 \longrightarrow ZnCO_3\downarrow + Na_2SO_4$$
$$ZnCO_3 \longrightarrow ZnO + CO_2\uparrow$$

Factor

Each gram of the residue is equivalent to 1.984 g of $ZnSO_4$.

Calculate the per cent purity as reported in sodium sulphate.

Note: Zinc oxide can be heated to bright redness without volatilisation, but in presence of carbonaceous matter such as filter paper, it is reduced to metal and it volatilises. In a accurate work, the precipitate is filtered in Gooch crucible which is then put in a nickel crucible and the heated until constant weight is attained.

Assay of Magnesium Sulphate

Magnesium sulphate IP contains not less than 99% and not more than 100.5% $MgSO_4$ calculated with reference to the substance dried to a constant weight at 300°C.

Weigh accurately magnesium sulphate (about 0.5 g), dissolve in water (50 ml), add hydrochloric acid (10 ml) and dilute with water to 150 ml. Cool to 0°C, add solution of ammonium phosphate (25 ml) and slowly with constant stirring dilute ammonia solution until the solution is just alkaline to phenol red. Add a further 10 ml of dilute ammonia solution. Stir well, allow to stand for 4 hours and filter. Wash the precipitate with a mixture of 1 volume of dilute ammonia solution and 19 volumes of water. Dissolve the precipitate in 1N hydrochloric acid (50 ml) and dilute to 150 ml with water. Add solution of ammonium phosphate (2 ml), add dilute ammonia solution until the solution is just alkaline to a solution of phenol red. Add a further dilute ammonia solution (10 ml), stir well and allow to stand for 4 hours and filter. Wash the precipitate with a mixture of 1 volume of dilute ammonia solution and 19 volumes of water until free from chloride dry and ignite to a constant weight at 1100°C.

Magnesium sulphate is precipitated as hydrated magnesium ammonium phosphate, $MgNH_4PO_46H_2O$ by addition of a solution of ammonium phosphate to an ice cooled acidified solution. The solution is then neutralized by addition of ammonia solution and made alkaline by adding an excess amount of the solution. The solution is allowed to stand for 4 hours, filtered and the precipitate washed with dilute ammonia solution.

The precipitate is redissolved in hydrochloric acid, reprecipitate as above, washed until free from chloride, dried and ignited. On ignition, magnesium ammonium phosphate is converted to magnesium pyrophosphate which is weighed.

$$2MgNH_4PO_4 \longrightarrow Mg_2P_2O_7 + 2NH_3 + H_2O$$

Magnesium   Magnesium
ammonium phosphate   pyrophosphate

Magnesium ammonium phosphate is very sparingly soluble in ammonical solution. Reprecipitation is recommended to avoid the coprecipitation.

Factor

Each g of the residue is equivalent to 1.082 g of $MgSO_4$.

Calculate the per cent purity as reported in the assay of sodium sulphate.

Assay of Alum, $KAl(SO_4)_2.12H_2O$

Weigh accurately alum (about 1.5 g) and dissolve in water. Add NH_4Cl (5 g) and do the precipitation with ammonia solution. Heat to boiling and filter the precipitate. Wash the precipitate with dilute ammonium nitrate solution till precipitates become free from chloride ion. Dry and ignite the precipitate at temperature of 1200°C to constant weight. Record the weight of the precipitate.

The alum is precipitated as aluminium hydroxide by means of ammonium hydroxide in the presence of ammonium chloride. The precipitate is then converted into the oxide by ignition and is weighed as Al_2O_3.

$$K \, Al(SO_4)_2.12H_2O \longrightarrow Al(OH)_3 \longrightarrow Al_2O_3$$

The estimation is subject to several errors. Aluminium hydroxide is amphoteric and dissolves slightly on addition of large excess of ammonia solution.

$$Al(OH)_3 + OH^- \longrightarrow AlO_2^- + 2H_2O$$

The concentration of OH⁻ ions should, therefore be carefully controlled. The addition of ammonium chloride reduces the concentration of OH ions and also help in coagulating the precipitate, which being gelatinous is difficult to filter.

Factor

Each g of Al_2O_3 is equivalent to 9.307 g of K $Al(SO_4)_2.12H_2O$.

Detection of Nitrogen, Sulphur and Halogen Elements in Organic Compounds

Organic compounds are non-ionic in nature. Therefore, they are fused with sodium metal for detection of these elements to convert them into water soluble inorganic compounds (ionized form). Based on this fact, Lassaigne's test was developed by French chemist, J.L. Lassaigne, in 1843.

LASSAIGNE'S TEST

Insert a small piece (in the size of pea) of freshly cut, clean and dry sodium metal into an ignition tube followed by addition of organic compound (50–60 mg). Heat the ignition tube in a bunsen flame till sodium melts and then strongly till it becomes red hot. Plung the red hot ignition tube immediately into a porcelain dish containing distilled water (50 ml). Add two or three ignition tubes into water in the same way. Crush the tube by gentle tapping, heat the solution to boiling for 10 minutes and then filter. This filtrate is known as sodium extract. The filtrate should be clear and alkaline. If it is dark in colour, it indicates incomplete fusion and so process should be repeated with fresh ignition tube. In this way, nitrogen is converted into water soluble inorganic cyanide while the halogens and sulphur formed water soluble halides and sulphide, respectively.

$$Na + C + N \longrightarrow NaCN$$

$$2Na + X_2 \longrightarrow 2NaX \ (X = Cl^-, Br^-, I^-)$$

$$2Na + S \longrightarrow Na_2S$$

The above sodium extract is alkaline in nature due to formation of sodium hydroxide.

$$Na + 2H_2O \longrightarrow 2NaOH + H_2 \uparrow$$

TEST FOR NITROGEN

Add about 0.2 g of ferrous sulphate crystals to the above sodium extract (2 or 3 ml) into a test tube to get dark greyish precipitate of $Fe(OH)_2$. If the solution remain clear, add few drops of NaOH solution. Boil the solution gently for few minutes to ensure the formation of ferrocyanide. Cool under tap, add one drop of $FeCl_3$ solution to form the ferric ferrocyanide and then acidify with dilute sulphuric acid. Formation of greenish blue colouration or somtimes prussian blue precipitate indicates the presence of nitrogen.

$$FeSO_4 + NaOH \longrightarrow Fe(OH)_2 \downarrow + Na_2SO_4$$
$$\text{Ferrous hydroxide}$$

$$Fe(OH)_2 + 6NaCN \longrightarrow Na_4[Fe(CN)_6] + 2NaOH$$
$$\text{Sodium ferrocyanide}$$

$$2Na_4[Fe(CN)_6] + 4FeCl_3 \longrightarrow Fe_4[Fe(CN)_6]_3 + 12NaCl$$
$$\text{Ferric-ferrocyanide}$$
$$\text{(Prussian blue)}$$

TEST FOR SULPHUR

(i) *Sodium Nitroprusside Test*: Add few drops of freshly prepared dilute solution of sodium nitroprusside, $(Na_2[Fe(CN)_5NO].2H_2O)$, to the sodium extract (2 ml). Formation of purple colour confirms the presence of sulphur.

$$Na_2S + Na_2[Fe(CN)_5NO] \longrightarrow Na_4[Fe(CN)_5NOS]$$

| Sodium extract | Sodium nitroprusside | Sodium thionitroprusside (purple colour) |

(ii) *Lead Acetate Test*: Acidify the sodium extract (2 ml) with acetic acid and then add lead acetate solution to it. Formation of black precipitate of lead sulphide confirms the presence of sulphur.

$$Na_2S + Pb(CH_3COO)_2 \longrightarrow PbS\downarrow + 2CH_3COONa$$

| | Lead acetate | Lead sulphide (black) |

TEST FOR NITROGEN AND SULPHUR

If the organic compound contains nitrogen and sulphur together, then sodium thiocyanate is formed during fusion with sodium. Sodium thiocyanate gives a blood red colour with ferric chloride solution.

$$Na + S + N + C \xrightarrow{\text{Fusion}} NaCNS$$
$$\text{Sodium thiocyanate}$$

$$3NaCNS + FeCl_3 \longrightarrow Fe(CNS)_3 + 3NaCl$$
$$\text{Ferric thiocyanate}$$
$$\text{(blood red colour)}$$

TEST FOR CHLORIDE, BROMIDE AND IODIDE

To the sodium extract (5 ml), add dilute HNO_3 solution and then boil the solution to expel H_2S or HCN, if present. Add few drops of silver nitrate solution.

(i) Formation of white precipitate, soluble in NH_4OH, indicates the presence of chloride in the organic compound.

(ii) Pale yellow precipitate, sparingly soluble but soluble in excess of NH_4OH, shows the presence of bromide.

(iii) Yellow precipitate, insoluble in NH_4OH, confirms the presence of iodide.

$$NaX + AgNO_3 \xrightarrow{\text{dil } HNO_3} AgX\downarrow + NaNO_3$$
$$\text{Silver nitrate} \quad \text{Silver halide}$$
$$(X = Cl^-, Br^-, I^-)$$

$$AgCl + 2NH_4OH \longrightarrow [Ag(NH_3)_2]^+Cl^- + 2H_2O$$

White   Ammonia   Silver aminochloride
precipitate   solution   (soluble)

$$AgBr + 2NH_4OH \longrightarrow [Ag(NH_3)_2]^+Br^- + 2H_2O$$

Pale yellow   Slightly soluble
precipitate

$$AgI + NH_4OH \longrightarrow No reaction$$

Yellow
precipitate

Determination of Melting and Boiling Points

Melting point of solid or boiling point of any liquid are determined in order:

(i) To check purity of the substances. Pure substances have sharp and definite melting /boiling point. The impure substance melts slowly. Similarly, boiling point of the impure liquid is high.

(ii) To identify the organic compounds. If the m.p. or b.p. of the given organic compound is determined with an accuracy of $\pm 2°C$, then possible compound can easily be guessed.

METHOD OF DETERMINATION OF MELTING POINT

A thin capillary tube of about 100 mm in length with uniform bore is sealed at one end by bringing it near to the flame. The pure, dry and fine powdered compound (nearly 2 mg) under identification is filled through open end of the capillary tube by gentle tapping the closed end.

Fix the assembly as shown in the Fig. 10.1 which consisted of a long necked flask (heating bath) containing concentrated sulphuric acid or glycerol or liquid paraffin (it is safer to use liquid paraffin). Moist the filled capillary with the liquid of flask and place it along side of thermometer with it sealed end near the bulb of thermometer. The capillary tube will cling to the thermometer by capillary attraction. Heat the flask gently by holding the burner in hand and rotating the flame round the bottom of flask so that the temperature of liquid rises uniformly. Observe the temperature and organic compound closely and record the temperature when substance begins to melt and become transparent. Repeat the experiment to determine the melting point as accurately as possible.

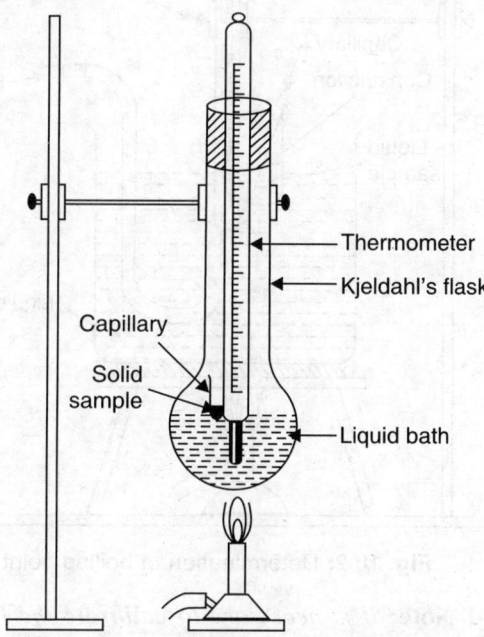

Fig. 10.1: Determination of melting point

(labels: Thermometer, Kjeldahl's flask, Capillary, Solid sample, Liquid bath)

METHOD OF DETERMINATION OF BOILING POINT

Take the liquid (0.5 ml) of which boiling point is to be determined in the ignition tube and tie with the thermometer with the help of rubber or thread. The thermometer along with ignition tube in the heating bath as shown in the Fig. 10.2. Put the sealed capillary tube, as in determination in melting point, into ignition tube containing liquid. Keep the fused end dipped in the liquid. Heat the bath gently and uniformly. The air bubbles from the end of the capillary tube start escaping at a slow rate but when the boiling point of the liquid is attained, a continuous escape of air bubbles will be observed. This temperature is recorded, and heating discontinued. The temperature is again recorded when the last air bubble appears. This temperature is the point at which the vapour pressure of the liquid is equal to atmospheric pressure. The mean of these two readings is the accurate boiling point of the liquid. This operation may be repeated for accuracy.

If the boiling point obtained is the same for second time also, the liquid is considered to be pure and easy to identify.

The melting point/boiling point can also be determined using Thiele tube as shown in Fig. 10.3. The Thiele tube is warmed using a microburner which heats elbow. This causes the oil to flow around the tube and past the sample and thermometer, thus warming the sample and thermometer.

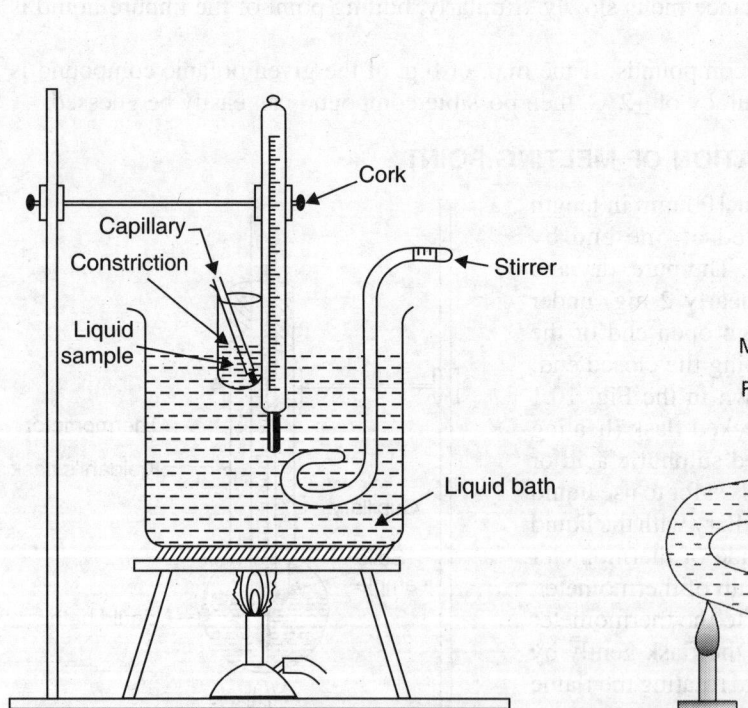

Fig. 10.2: Determination of boiling point

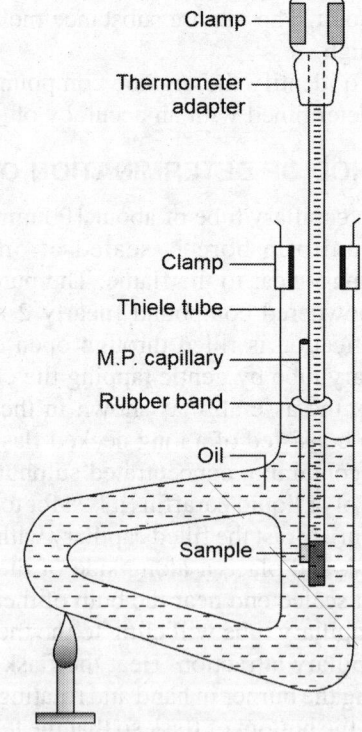

Fig. 10.3: Melting point using Thiele tube

Note: *It is necessary to calibrate the thermometer before making melting/boiling point determination. For calibration. test the 0°C point by dipping the thermometer into well-stirred mixture of crushed ice and water mixture. Put water (10 ml) in a 25 × 150 mm test tube, clamp the tube in a vertical position, add one unglazed porcelein piece to prevent bumping, boil gently, hold a thermometer and check the 100°C point.*

Qualitative Organic Analysis

Qualitative organic analysis includes the systematic identification of an organic compound. The identification of unknown organic compound includes the following steps:

1. Physical examination of the compound
2. Tests for unsaturation
3. Solubility tests
4. Detection of elements
5. Detection of functional groups
6. Determination of melting/boiling point of the compound.
7. Confirmatory tests of the inferred organic compound
8. Derivatization of unknown organic compound.

PHYSICAL EXAMINATION OF THE COMPOUND

The following physical characters are helpful in identifying the compounds:

(i) *Colour*: Organic compounds are coloured due to the presence of a chromophoric group. Sometimes compound can be guessed by observing the colour as shown below.
Pale yellow—nitro compounds, iodoform.
Orange—*o*-nitroaniline, alizarin, phenanthroquinone, azo compounds.
Red—1,2-napthaquinone.

(ii) *Odour*: The presence of characteristic odours is an indicative of a particular class of organic compounds.
Pleasant—esters, ether, lower aliphatic alcohols, chloroform.
Bitter almonds—nitrobenzene, benzaldehyde.
Phenolic—phenols, naphthols, some derivatives of salicylic acid.
Pungent—acetic acid, acetyl chloride, acetic anhydride, benzoyl chloride, benzyl chloride, formic acid and pyridine.
Moth balls—naphthalene.
Fishy—amines.
Rotten eggs—sulphur-containing compounds.

(iii) Ignition: Keep a small of compound on spatula and burn in a flame. Predict original compound on the basis of behaviour. Appearance of smoky flame indicates aromatic compounds while aliphatic compound burns with non-smoky flame. Polyhalogenated compound generally do not ignite. Compounds such as carbohydrates, tartaric acid and its salts are charred on ignition. Iodoform burns with violet vapours.

TESTS FOR UNSATURATION

To find out the unsaturation, perform the following tests:

(i) Bromine test: To a solution of compound, add the bromine solution dropwise with shaking. Disappearance of reddish brown colour of bromine solution indicates unsaturation.

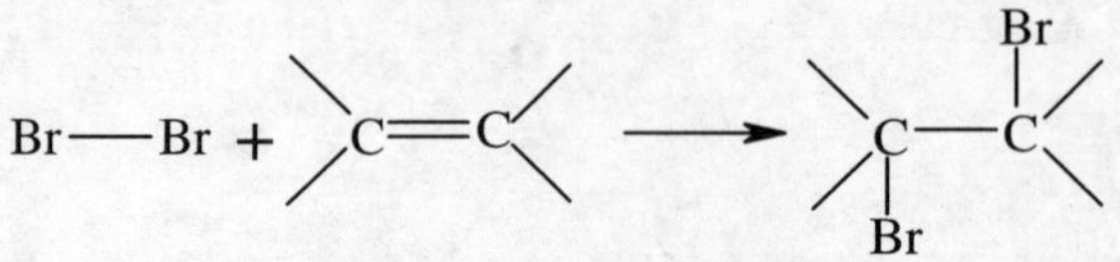

(ii) Baeyer test: To a solution of organic compound in water or ethanol, add Baeyer's reagent (1% w/v $KMnO_4$ solution) dropwise with continuous shaking. The disappearance of purple colour also indicates the presence of unsaturated compound.

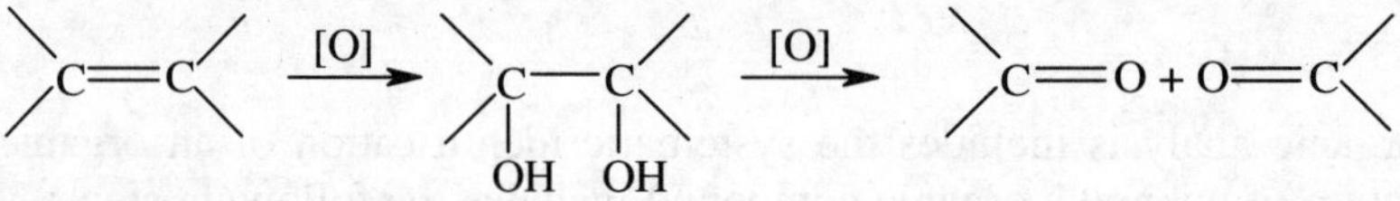

SOLUBILITY TESTS

Solubility behaviour of the organic compound can provide valuable information regarding the presence of certain classes of organic compounds. Therefore, it should be checked carefully.

Generally, the solubility test is performed in the following sequence:

(i) Dissolve the organic compound (0.10 g) in water (3–5 ml) with shaking. If the compound dissolves, then repeat the test with ether as solvent.

(ii) When the compound is insoluble in water, observe its solubility in 5% w/v NaOH solution. If it is soluble in sodium hydroxide, check its solubility in 5% w/v $NaHCO_3$ solution.

(iii) The compound insoluble in sodium hydroxide solution, is further checked for its solubility in 5% v/v HCl.

(iv) A organic compound, insoluble in water, NaOH and HCl solution, contains no nitrogen again is tested for its solubility in concentrated H_2SO_4 solution.

Flowchart 11.1 gives the solubility classes of various organic compound on which basis conclusion regarding the presence or absence of some classes can be drawn.

DETECTION OF ELEMENTS

Organic compounds are consisted of two or more elements. Generally, they contain carbon and hydrogen but the presence of nitrogen, sulphur and halogen is determined in certain compounds (see Chapter 9).

DETECTION OF FUNCTIONAL GROUPS

Functional group analysis is performed in the following order:

Compounds Containing C and H With or Without Oxygen

(a) Carboxylic Group, –COOH (e.g. formic, acetic, oxalic, succinic, lactic, tartaric, citric, benzoic, salicylic, phthalic and cinnamic acids)

General tests

These are mostly colourless crystalline solid except formic, acetic, lactic acid, etc. Formic and acetic acid have pungent odour while cinnamic acid has faint, pleasant and characteristic odour. Aliphatic acids are soluble in water. The aromatic acids are very sparingly soluble in cold water but readily soluble in boiling water.

Flowchart 11.1: Solubility

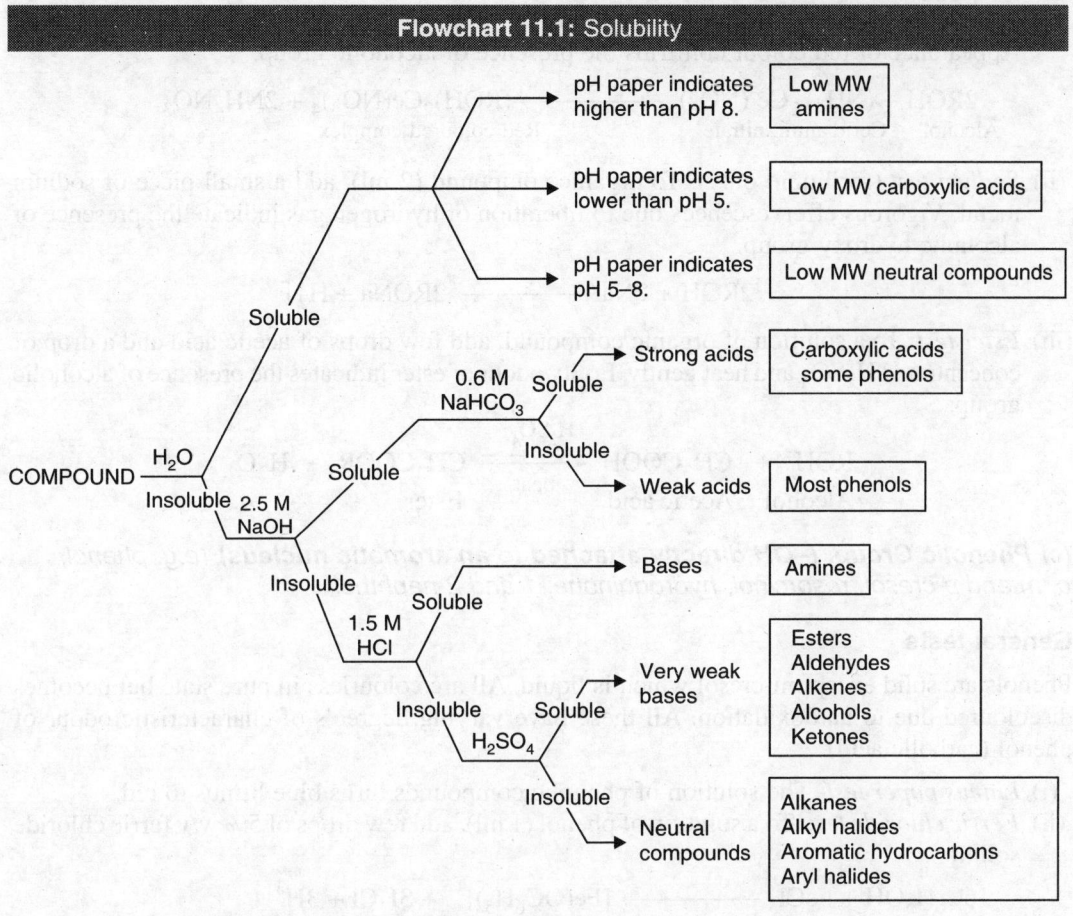

(i) *Litmus paper test*: Solution of organic compounds gives red colour with blue litmus paper.

(ii) *Sodium bicarbonate test*: To a saturated solution of sodium bicarbonate in a test tube, add a small quantity of the compound. Evolution of CO_2 with brisk effervescences indicates the presence of carboxylic group.

$$R–COOH + NaHCO_3 \longrightarrow R–COO^-Na^+ + H_2O + CO_2\uparrow$$
Carboxylic acid   Sodium salt

(iii) Ester formation: Heat gently ethanol (1 ml) with the compound (0.5 g or 1 ml) and a few drops of concentrated sulphuric acid for about one minute in a test tube. A fruity odour of ester indicates the presence of carboxylic group.

$$\underset{\text{Carboxylic acid}}{R – COOH} + \underset{\text{Ethanol}}{C_2H_5OH} \underset{\text{heat}}{\overset{\text{Conc. } H_2SO_4}{\rightleftharpoons}} \underset{\text{Ester}}{R – COOC_2H_5} + H_2O$$

(b) Alcoholic Group, –OH (e.g. methanol, ethanol, n-propanol, glycol, glycerol, benzyl alcohol, cyclohexanol)

General tests

Alcohols are colourless liquids, completely miscible with water except benzyl alcohol and cyclohexanol which are slightly soluble. Pure glycol and glycerol have high viscosity. Glycol and glycerol are odourless while other alcohols have faint odour.

(i) To a solution of organic compound, add few drops of ceric ammonium nitrate solution. Appearance of red colour confirms the presence of alcoholic group.

$$2ROH + (NH_4)_2Ce(NO_3)_6 \longrightarrow (ROH)_2Ce(NO_3)_4 + 2NH_4NO_3$$

Alcohol Ceric amm. nitrate   Red coloured complex

(ii) *Sodium test* (for liquid only): To organic compound (2 ml), add a small piece of sodium metal. Vigorous effervescences due to liberation of hydrogen gas indicate the presence of alcoholic hydroxy group.

$$2ROH + 2Na \longrightarrow 2RONa + H_2\uparrow$$

(iii) *Ester test*: To a solution of organic compound, add few drops of acetic acid and a drop of concentrated H_2SO_4 and heat gently. Fruity odour of ester indicates the presence of alcoholic group.

$$ROH + CH_3COOH \overset{H_2SO_4}{\underset{heat}{\rightleftharpoons}} CH_3COOR + H_2O$$

Alcohol Acetic acid   Ester

(c) Phenolic Group, (–OH directly attached to an aromatic nucleus) *(e.g. phenol, o, m and p-cresol, resorcinol, hydroquinone, 1 and 2-naphthol)*

General tests

Phenols are solid except m-cresol which is liquid. All are colourless in pure state but becomes discoloured due to autooxidation. All these have varying degree's of characteristic odour of phenol (carbolic acid).

(i) *Litmus paper test*: The solution of phenolic compounds turns blue litmus to red.

(ii) *Ferric chloride test*: To a solution of phenol (1 ml), add few drops of 5% w/v ferric chloride solution.

$$6C_6H_5OH + FeCl_3 \longrightarrow [Fe(OC_6H_5)]^{3-} + 3HCl + 3H^+$$

Complex ion (coloured)

(iii) *Liebermann's nitroso reaction:* Dissolve an organic compound (0.1 g) in concentrated sulphuric acid (1 ml) in a dry test tube and add few crystals of sodium nitrite. A blue-green

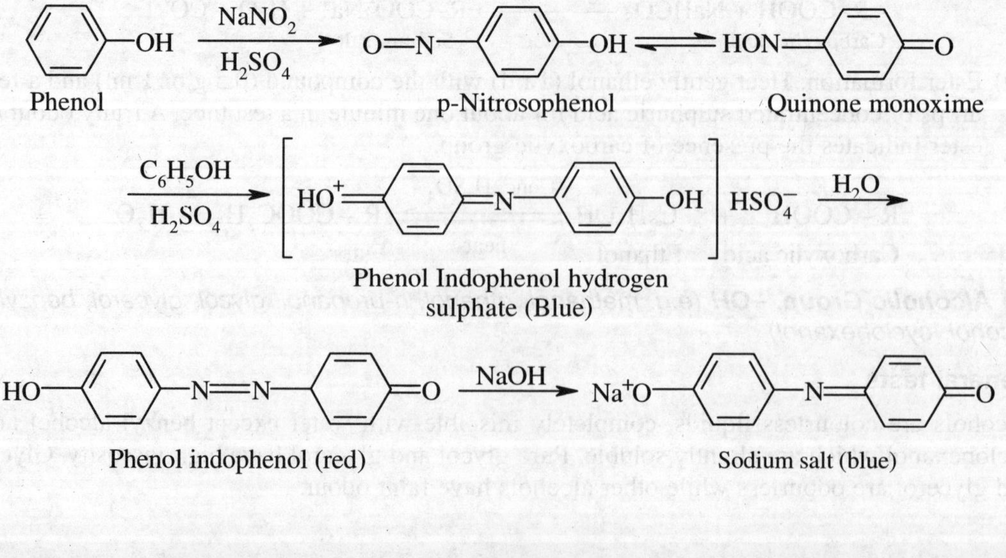

Phenol   p-Nitrosophenol   Quinone monoxime

Phenol Indophenol hydrogen sulphate (Blue)

Phenol indophenol (red)   Sodium salt (blue)

or blue-violet colour appears which changes to red on dilution with water. This colour changes to green, blue or violet on addition of sodium hydroxide solution. This reaction is termed Liebermann's nitroso reaction. *This test is only performed with the organic compound having free phenolic group at para position.*

(iv) *Phthalein test:* Heat the organic compound (0.2 g) and phthalic anhydride with concentrated sulphuric acid (2 drops) for one minute. Cool it and pour the contents into a beaker containing sodium hydroxide. The following characteristic colours are obtained: phenol—pink; *o*-cresol—pink or red-green; naphthols—light green; catechol, hydroquinone—blue. The colour disappears on adding excess of NaOH solution.

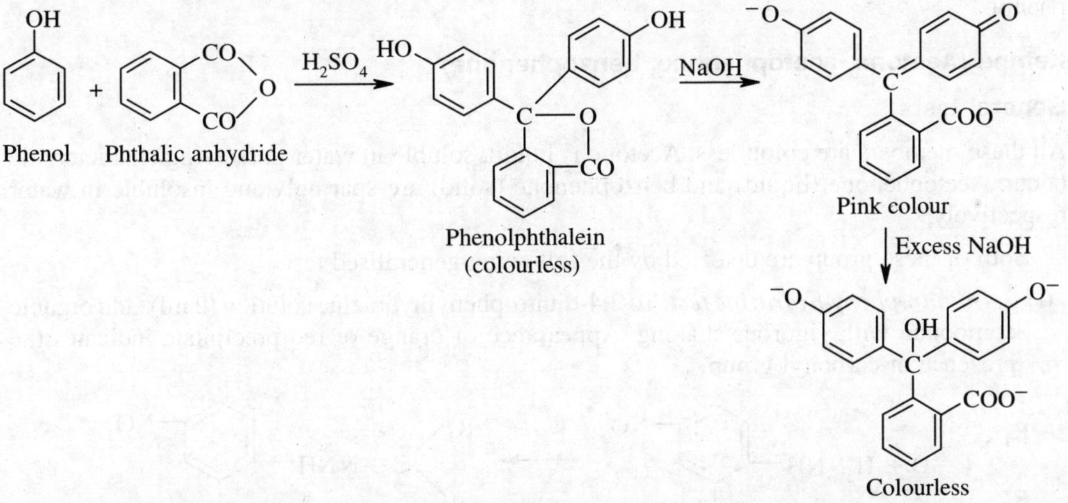

Phenol   Phthalic anhydride

Phenolphthalein
(colourless)

Pink colour

Excess NaOH

Colourless

(v) *Azo dye test:* Cool down a mixture of few drops of aniline, little sodium nitrite and dilute hydrochloric acid (1 ml) in freezing bath below 5°C. Add an alkaline solution of organic compound (phenol or β-naphthol) to it. Formation of yellow-orange and orange dye indicates the presence of phenol and β-naphthol, respectively.

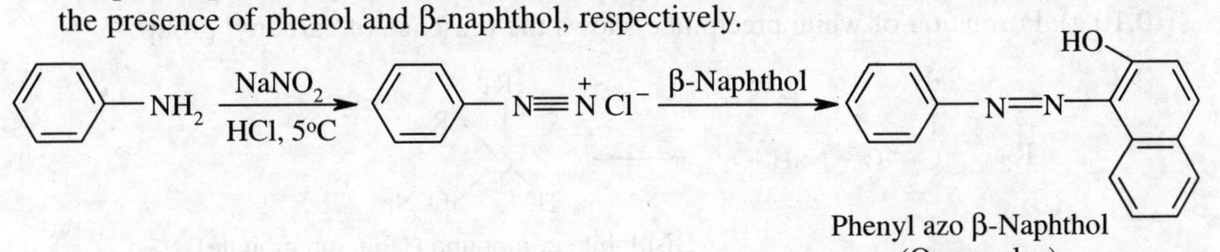

Phenyl azo β-Naphthol
(Orange dye)

(vi) *Bromine test:* To a concentrated aqueous solution of phenol, add bromine water gradually. Initially, bromine is decolourized and then on adding an excess, a white or yellow precipitate of polybromo derivative is produced with all (except catechol, hydroquinone, 1 and 2-naphthol).

(vii) Phenol (except those containing acidic group, e.g. nitrophenol) give no reaction with sodium carbonate solution.

(d) Carbonyl Group, C O

The carbonyl group is present in aldehyde, —C=O and ketone group, C=O.

Brady test: 2,4-dinitrophenylhydrazine can be used to qualitatively detect the carbonyl functionality of ketone or aldehyde functional group. A positive test is signalled by formation of a yellow, orange or red precipitate (known as a dinitrophenyl hydrazone).

Aldehyde

General tests

Most of the aldehydes are colourless. HCHO is a gas of which aqueous solution has pungent odour. Acetaldehyde is generally used in aqueous solution which has also a characteristic odour. Benzaldehyde and salicyldehyde are liquids insoluble in water. Benzaldehyde has a characteristic odour of bitter almond; salicyldehyde has a faint but also characteristic odour, resembling with phenol.

Ketone (Acetone, acetophenone, benzophenone)

General tests

All these members are colourless. Acetone is liquid, soluble in water possessing characteristic odour. Acetophenone (liquid) and benzophenone (solid) are sparingly and insoluble in water respectively.

Both of these group are detected by the following generalised test.

(i) *2,4-dinitrophenylhydrazine test*: To 2,4-dinitrophenylhydrazine solution (2 ml), add organic compound with vigorous shaking. Appearance of orange or red precipitate indicates the presence of carbonyl group.

2,4-Dinitrophenylhydrazine   2,4-Dinitrophenylhydrazone (orange coloured)

(ii) *Sodium bisulphite test*: To a sodium bisulphite solution (3 ml), add organic compound (0.10 g). Formation of white precipitate shows the presence of carbonyl group.

Bisulphite compound (white precipitate)

Differentiation Between Aldehyde and Ketone Groups

(i) *Schiff's reaction*: To Schiff's reagent (2 ml), add few drops of the organic compound. A deep violet-red or red colour indicates the presence of aldehyde group. The test is negative in ketones due to steric hinderance and some aromatic aldehydes (e.g. vanillin).

Schiff reagent (colourless)   Schiff adduct (violet red colour)

(ii) *Fehling's solution test*: Only aldehydes reduce Fehling's solution to red cuprous oxide. Mix Fehling's solutions A and B (1 ml each) in a test tube and add a small amount of organic compound to it. Boil the solution for 5 minutes on a water bath. Formation of reddish brown precipitate of cuprous oxide (Cu_2O) indicates the presence of aldehyde group.

$$R-\underset{\underset{\displaystyle H}{|}}{C} == O + 2CuO \longrightarrow ROOOH + Cu_2O$$
$$\text{Cuprous oxide}$$
$$\text{(red precipitate)}$$

Aldehydes that lack alpha (α) hydrogens, such as benzaldehyde, do not give positive Fehling's test.

(iii) *Tollen's test:* Add 10% w/v sodium hydroxide solution (1 ml) to a freshly prepared 10% w/v silver nitrate solution (1 ml) with shaking. To the mixture, add NH_4OH solution till the precipitated substance just dissolves. Add little organic compound along the sides of tube and then heat on a water bath for 5 minutes without disturbing the test tube. A silver mirror is deposited due to reduction of silver ion to metallic silver. The shining silver mirror indicates the presence of aldehyde group while ketones do not respond this test.

$$R-CHO + 2Ag(NH_3)_2OH \longrightarrow RCOONH_4 + 2Ag\downarrow + H_2O + NH_3$$

Only alpha hydroxy ketones that can tautomerize to aldehydes give a positive Tollen's test.

(iv) *Sodium nitroprusside test:* To an organic compound (0.10 g), add sodium nitroprusside solution (5 ml) followed by addition of excess of sodium hydroxide solution. Formation of red colour indicates the presence of ketonic group. This test is negative in case of aldehydes and aromatic ketones.

The nitroprusside ion acts as special carrier of nitrosonium ion and so forms coloured complex with methyl ketone, such as acetone is converted to $^-CH_2COCH_3$ ion which reacts with nitroprusside ion to give highly coloured ion.

$$CH_3COCH_3 \xrightarrow{OH^-} CH_2COCH_3 \xrightarrow{Na_2[Fe(CN)_5NO]} [Fe(CN)_5NO(CH_2COCH_3)]^{2-}$$
$$\text{Coloured ion}$$

(e) Ester Group (R $\overset{\overset{\displaystyle O}{||}}{C}$ OR^1)

(i) Fruity smell: All the esters have fruity smell.
(ii) *Phenolphthalein test*: To the organic compound (0.10 g), add dilute sodium hydroxide solution (3 ml) and phenolphthalein solution (1 ml). A pink colour is obtained due to the presence of sodium hydroxide which is discharged on heating the solution. *Ester is hydrolysed into an acid and alcohol. The acid neutralizes the sodium hydroxide and hence pink colour is discharged.*

$$R_1-COOR_2 + H_2O \xrightarrow{NaOH} R_1-COOH + R_2OH$$

(iii) *Hydroxyamic acid test*: Heat a small quantity (40 mg) of ester and hydroxylamine HCl solution (1 ml) in ethanol with 6M NaOH solution (0.2 ml). Acidify with HCl solution after cooling followed by addition of 1–2 drops of $FeCl_3$ solution. Appearance of red-violet colour indicates the presence of ester.

Esters react with hydroxylamine HCl to yield a compound which can make complex with ferric chloride to give coloured compound.

$$R-C\overset{O}{\underset{OR_1}{\big<}} + H_2NOH \longrightarrow R-C\overset{O}{\underset{NH-OH}{\big<}} + R_1-OH$$

Hydroxyamic acid

$$R-C\overset{O}{\underset{NH-OH}{\big<}} + FeCl_3 \longrightarrow \left[R-C\overset{O}{\underset{HN-O}{\big<}} \right]_3 Fe + 3HCl$$

Ferric Hydroxamate complex
Red-violet colour

Because other type of compounds may also give a positive tests, a preliminary test is used to help eliminate false positives.

(f) Carbohydrates

Carbohydrates are polyhydroxy aldehydes and ketones. They do not give all the tests of aldehydic or ketonic group as these groups are not present in free state in the carbohydrates. They are detected by following tests.

(i) *Molisch's test*: To a solution of organic compound in a test tube, add Molisch's reagent (10% alcoholic solution of α-naphthol) with shaking. Add concentrated sulphuric acid solution (2 ml) along the side of inclined tube carefully so that the acid forms a layer beneath the aqueous solution without mixing. Appearance of deep violet ring at the junction of two liquids indicates the presence of carbohydrate. This colour becomes violet-red on shaking the contents. It is a generalised test for carbohydrates.

   The acid dehydrates carbohydrates to give furfural or 5-hydroxy furfural which condense with α-naphthol to give violet colour.

(ii) *Fehling's solution test:* Heat the substance (0.5 g) with dilute hydrochloric acid. Neutralize reaction mixture by adding sodium hydroxide solution. Add equal quantities of Fehlings solutions A and B and then heat the mixture for 5 minutes. Red precipitate of cuprous oxide is produced on heating in case of reducing sugars (e.g. all monosaccharides and many cellobiose and gentiobiose).

   Non-reducing sugars include some disaccharides (sucrose and trihalose) which on boiling with acids are converted into reducing sugars and hence give this test. For example, sucrose (non-reducing sugar) on boiling with hydrochloric acid solution is hydrolyzed into fructose and glucose. Both are reducing sugars and give the red precipitates with Fehling solution in a usual way.

(iii) *Osazone formation:* A sugar on heating with phenylhydrazine hydrochloride, sodium acetate and acetic acid forms yellow crystals of osazone. Monosaccharides (reducing sugars only) form osazones.

   Take the compound (0.2 g), phenylhydrazine hydrochloride (0.5 g) and sodium acetate (0.5 g) in water (5 ml) in a test tube. Boil the reaction mixture on a water bath with shaking till precipitate appears (note the time of osazone formation). Cool, filter to collect the osazone and observe the shape of crystals under microscope. Also notice the time for osazone formation.

$$
\begin{array}{ccccc}
\underset{\text{Glucose}}{\begin{array}{c} \text{CHO} \\ | \\ \text{CHOH} \\ | \\ (\text{CHOH})_3 \\ | \\ \text{CH}_2\text{OH} \end{array}}
& \text{Or} &
\underset{\text{Fructose}}{\begin{array}{c} \text{CH}_2\text{OH} \\ | \\ \text{C}{=}\text{O} \\ | \\ (\text{CHOH})_3 \\ | \\ \text{CH}_2\text{OH} \end{array}}
& \xrightarrow[\substack{\text{Phenyl} \\ \text{hydrazine}}]{\text{C}_6\text{H}_5\text{NHNH}_2}
& \underset{\text{Osazone}}{\begin{array}{c} \text{C}{=}\text{N}{-}\text{NHC}_6\text{H}_5 \\ | \\ \text{C}{=}\text{N}{-}\text{NHC}_6\text{H}_5 \\ | \\ (\text{CHOH})_3 \\ | \\ \text{CH}_2\text{OH} \end{array}}
\end{array}
$$

(iv) *Resorcinol test for ketones (Selivanoff's test)*: Add some crystals of resorcinol to the solution of sugar and heat with an equal volume of concentrated hydrochloric acid. Appearance of pink colour indicates the presence of ketosis (e.g. fructose).

Differentiation Between Monosaccharides and Disaccharides

Heat the Barfoed's reagent with aqueous solution of organic compound (sugar) on a water bath. If red colour due to formation of cuprous oxide is developed readily, a monosaccharide (glucose, fructose) is present. Disaccharides, e.g. sucrose may develop the red colour on prolonged heating (about 10 minutes) due to partial hydrolysis into monosaccharides.

(g) Hydrocarbons

Hydrocarbons may be either saturated or unsaturated. Unsaturated hydrocarbon may be aliphatic or aromatic in nature. They are insoluble in water but soluble in many organic solvents. Due to lack of reactivity, their identification is based on result of preliminary tests (test of unsaturation, detection of elements), determination of melting point/boiling point, specific test for particular hydrocarbons and preparation of their derivatives.

(h) Ethers (Diethyl ether, anisole)

General tests

All these ethers are insoluble in water. The aliphatic ethers have characteristic odours, possess anaesthetic properties and are extremely inflammable. It the above tests are negative and the compound do not contain element, there may be possibility of ethers. These are tested as follows:

(i) *Feigl's test*: Heat the substance (2 ml) after covering the mouth of test tube with a filter paper moistened with a mixture of cupric acetate and benzidine hydrochloride; a deep blue colour appears on the filter paper:

$$
\underset{\text{Ether}}{\text{R}_1{-}\text{O}{-}\text{R}_2} + \tfrac{1}{2}\,\text{O}_2 \rightarrow \text{R}_1{-}\text{O}{-}\text{R}_2 \rightarrow \text{O}
$$

$$
\text{R}_1{-}\text{O}{-}\text{R}_2 \rightarrow \text{O} + \text{Cu}^{2+} \rightarrow \text{R}_1{-}\text{O}{-}\text{R}_2 + \underset{\substack{\text{Cupric} \\ \text{peroxide}}}{\text{CuO}_2}
$$

(Benzidine HCl) → (Benzidine blue)

(ii) Dissolve 2 or 3 drops of the substance in benzene (5 ml). Add very dilute solution of iodine in benzene (5 ml) and shake, a brown tint appears.

Compounds Containing C, H, N with or without Oxygen Atom

(a) Amino Group

It may be primary ($-NH_2$), secondary ($-NH$) and tertiary ($\diagdown N$) group.

(i) *Hinsberg test*: This test is performed to differentiate the primary, secondary and tertiary amines.

To any organic compound (0.1 g), add benzene sulphonyl chloride (0.2 g) and 10% w/v sodium hydroxide solution (5 ml) with vigorous shaking. Observe the formation of precipitate of benzene sulphonyl derivative. If no reaction occur, heat the contents on a water bath for 2–3 minutes and then cool in ice.

On cooling if no solid separates out, the organic compound may be tertiary amine. If a precipitate appears in alkaline medium, add water (5 ml) with shaking. If the precipitate does not dissolve, it indicates the presence of secondary amines.

In case of clear solution, acidify with dilute hydrochloric acid. Appearance of a precipitate indicates the presence of primary amine.

Primary amine:

$$C_6H_5SO_2Cl + H_2NR \xrightarrow{NaOH} C_6H_5SON(Na)R \xrightarrow{HCl} C_6H_5SO_2NHR$$

Benzene   Primary   Benzene sulphonyl   Benzene sulphonyl
sulphonyl chloride amine   derivative (water insoluble) derivative (water soluble)

Secondary amine:

$$C_6H_5SO_2Cl + HN\begin{matrix}R_1\\R_2\end{matrix} \xrightarrow{NaOH} C_6H_5SO_2N\begin{matrix}R_1\\R_2\end{matrix}$$

Secondary amine   Benzene sulphonyl derivative
                     (alkali insoluble)

Tertiary amine:

$$C_6H_5SO_2Cl + N\begin{matrix}R_1\\R_2\\R_3\end{matrix} \longrightarrow \text{No reaction}$$

Tertiary amine

This test can also be performed with *p*-toluene sulphonyl chloride.

(ii) *Carbylamine test:* Only primary aliphatic or aromatic amines respond this test.

Take a little organic compound in a test tube, add chloroform (1 ml) and alcoholic solution of potassium hydroxide (2 ml). Heat the contents. Evolution of an offensive smell of isocyanide (carbylamine) shows the presence of primary amine.

$$C_6H_5NH_2 + CHCl_3 + 3KOH \longrightarrow C_6H_5NC\uparrow + 3KCl + 3H_2O$$

Aniline   Phenyl isocyanide
                                 (carbylamine)

(iii) *Azo dye test*: If the carbylamine test is positive, then azo dye test is performed to determine whether the amine is primary aliphatic or aromatic one.

Dissolve organic compound (0.5 g) in dilute hydrochloric acid (5 ml). Cool down the solution in ice bath below 5°C. Add slowly sodium nitrite solution (5 ml) with shaking. Now add a few drops of an alkaline solution of β-naphthol. Formation of yellow, orange or red dye confirms the primary aromatic amine.

Aniline → (NaNO₂, HCl, 0-5°C) → Benzene diazonium chloride → (β-Naphthol) → Orange dye

(b) Amide Group *(e.g. formamide, acetamide, benzamide, salicylamide, urea)*

All are colourless solid except formamide which is a liquid. Formamide, acetamide and urea are readily soluble in water while benzamide and salicylamide are insoluble in water.

(i) Heat organic compound (0.2 g) with 10% w/v sodium hydroxide solution (2 ml) in a test tube. Evolution of ammonia indicates the presence of an amide group. Formation of ammonia is detected by dense white fumes with glass rod dipped in concentrated hydrochloric acid.

(c) Anilide Group (–NHCOR) *(e.g. acetanilide, benzanilide)*

General tests

All are colourless, odourless crystalline solids. Acetanilide and benzanilide are both sparingly soluble in cold water but acetanilide has the greater solibility in hot water.

(i) *Tafel's test:* Add concentrated sulphuric acid (3 ml) and potassium dichromate (0.3 g) to a little organic compound in a test tube. Red or violet colour changing to green shows the presence of anilide which do not contain substituent in the benzene nucleus.

(ii) *2,4-dinitrochlorobenzene test:* Organic compound having anilide group gives intense colour on a paper soaked with 2,4-dinitrochlorobenzene.

(iii) *Azo dye test:* It also undergoes diazotization and coupling in the same way as primary amines to form azo dye.

(iv) *Isocyanide test:* (If anilide is an acylated primary amine). Heat together gently the anilide (0.2 g), alc. NaOH solution (3 ml) and chloroform (1 ml). Hydrolysis of anilide occurs and the odour of the isocyanide can be detected after 2 minute's heating.

(d) Imides *(e.g. succinimides, phthalimides)*

Physical Properties

Both are colourless solid, succinimide is readily soluble and phthalimide sparingly soluble in cold water.

(i) Heats the organic compound (0.3 g) with 10% w/v sodium hydroxide solution (2 ml) in a test tube. Evolution of ammonia indicates the presence of an imide group.

$$R \begin{matrix} CO \\ \\ CO \end{matrix} NH + NaOH \longrightarrow R \begin{matrix} COONa \\ \\ COONa \end{matrix} + NH_3\uparrow$$

(e) Nitro Group (N) *(e.g. nitrobenzene, p-nitrotoluene, m-dinitrobenzene)*

(i) *Tollen's reagent test:* To the organic compound (0.5 g) in ethanol (10 ml) in a test tube, add ammonium chloride (0.5 g) and zinc dust (0.5 g) with shaking. Heat the contents on a water bath for 5 minutes. Cool the mixture, filter and add ammonical silver nitrate solution (Tollen's reagent) (1 ml). Formation of silver mirror indicates the presence of nitro group.

$$C_6H_5NO_2 \xrightarrow[\text{NH}_4\text{Cl}]{\text{Zinc}} C_6H_5NHOH + H_2O$$

Nitrobenzene   Phenyl hydroxylamine

$$C_6H_5NO_2 + 2[Ag(NH_3)_2]OH \longrightarrow C_6H_5NO + 2Ag^+ + 4NH_3 + 2H_2O$$

Silver
mirror

(ii) *Ferrous hydroxide test:* Add an organic compound (0.1 g) to a solution of 5% ferrous ammonium sulphate in a test tube. Then, add 2 drops of 6N sulphuric acid followed by 2N potassium hydroxide solution (2 ml) in methanol. Formation of red brown precipitate indicates the presence of nitro group. A negative test is indicated by green precipitate.

Ferrous ammonium sulphate $\rightarrow$ Fe(OH)$_2$

$$R - NO_2 + 6Fe(OH)_2 + 4H_2O \longrightarrow 6Fe(OH)_3 + R - NH_2$$

Blue green   Red brown precipitate

(iii) *Azo dye test:* To the organic compound (1 ml), add zinc dust and concentrated HCl and then boil the contents for 5 minutes in a boiling tube. Nitro group is converted into amino group and then perform the usual azo dye test as in the case of primary amino group.

$$C_6H_5NO_2 \xrightarrow[\text{HCl}]{\text{Zn}} C_6H_5NH_2$$

AMINO ACIDS

(a) Amino aliphatic carboxylic acid (e.g. glycine, tyrosine)

(i) Heat sodium carbonate solution with the compound, CO_2 is evolved slowly.
(ii) To a few ml of 20% w/v NaNO$_2$ solution, add a few drops of cold dilute acetic acid. Pour the mixture into a cold aqueous glycine solution, there is a brisk evolution of nitrogen.

$$NH_2.CH_2COOH + HNO_2 \longrightarrow HO.CH_2COOH + N_2\uparrow + H_2O$$

Glycine   Glycollic acid

(iii) *Sorensen's test*: Dissolve 0.2 g of glycine in few ml of water in test tube A, add 2 drops of phenolphthalein and then very dilute NaOH solution drop by drop until solution just turns pink. In a second test tube B, place 40% formalin solution (2 ml), add phenolphthalein (2 drops) and then dilute NaOH solution until the solution just turns pink. Pour the contents B into A and note the immediate decolourization of the phenolphthalein.

$$N^+H_3.CH_2COO^- + OH^- \rightleftharpoons NH_2CH_2COO^- + H_2O$$

$$CH_2O + H_2NCH_2COO^- \rightleftharpoons CH_2 = N-CH_2COO^- + H_2O$$

(b) Amino aromatic carboxylic acid (e.g. anthranilic acid)

(i) Add sodium carbonate solution, it dissolves with evolution of CO_2 gas.
(ii) Dissolve anthranilic acid (0.2 g) in dilute HCl solution (4 ml) and cool in ice water. To this, add slowly about cold 20% sodium nitrite solution (1 ml) and divide the cold diazonium solution into two parts—part A and B.
  (a) To part A, add cold alkaline solution of β-naphthol, brilliant red dye is formed.
  (b) Boil part B until evolution of nitrogen ceases, cool the solution and shake. Salicylic acid separates out.

$$NH_2C_6H_4COOH \xrightarrow[0-5^\circ C]{\text{NaNO}_2\text{-HCl}} ClN_2C_6H_4COOH \xrightarrow{\text{Boil}} HOC_6H_4COOH$$

Formation of salicylic acid can be identified by the formation of oil of winter green on heating with methyl alcohol.

(c) Amino aromatic sulphonic acid (e.g. sulphanilic acid)

(i) Dissolve in Na_2CO_3 solution with the evolution of CO_2.

(ii) Forms diazonium derivative which can be coupled with β-naphthol or with dimethylamine to form azo dyes.

Formation of methyl orange

Dissolve sulphanilic acid (0.3 g) in 10% aqueous sodium carbonate solution (2 ml). Cool in ice water, add 20% $NaNO_2$ solution (2–3 drops) and then add cold dilute HCl solution (1 ml) and shake. Meanwhile dissolve dimethyl aniline (1 drop) in dilute HCl (few drops), cool thoroughly in ice water and then add to cold diazo solution. Shake well and make alkaline with aqueous NaOH solution—note the formation of a deep orange yellow colouration or precipitate. On addition of HCl, a bright red colouration is produced.

Compounds Containing Halogen Atom (Halohydrocarbons)
(e.g. chloroform, iodoform, CCl_4, chlorobenzene, benzyl chloride)

These compounds are identified on the basis of:

(i) Presence of halogen (Cl^-, Br^-, or I^-).

(ii) Determination of boiling/melting point.

(iii) Preparation of suitable derivatives.

(iv) Determination of boiling/melting point of derivative.

The reactivity of halogen derivatives is tested by silver nitrate reagent. Heat the organic compound with an alcoholic solution of silver nitrate. If white or yellow precipitate is obtained, it indicates the presence of halogen in the side chain. A halogen atom directly attached to an aromatic nucleus like chlorobenzene does not react with silver nitrate solution.

$$\underset{\text{Benzyl chloride}}{C_6H_5CH_2Cl} + AgNO_3 \longrightarrow \underset{\text{White precipitate}}{AgCl\downarrow}$$

$$\underset{\text{Chlorobenzene}}{C_6H_5Cl} + AgNO_3 \longrightarrow \text{No precipitate}$$

Compounds Containing C, H and Sulphur with Oxygen or without Oxygen

(a) Sulphonic Acids (–SO_3H)

(i) Perform the test for this group if sulphur is present. The compound gives brisk effervescence with sodium bicarbonate solution.

$$\underset{}{C_6H_5SO_3H} + NaHCO_3 \longrightarrow C_6H_5SO_3Na + H_2O + CO_2\uparrow$$

(ii) *Potassium hydroxide fusion test*: Heat organic compound (0.5 g), solid potassium hydroxide (2 g) and 5 drops of water in a nickel crucible for about 10 minutes with occasional stirring. Acidify the solution with dilute sulphuric acid. Evolution of sulphur dioxide gas indicates the presence of sulphonic group. Sulphur dioxide may be detected by means of a filter paper moistened with acidified potassium dichromate solution which turns the paper green.

$$C_6H_5SO_3H + KOH \longrightarrow C_6H_5SO_3K + H_2O$$

$$C_6H_5SO_3H + KOH \longrightarrow C_6H_5OH + K_2SO_3$$

$$K_2SO_3 + H_2SO_4 \longrightarrow K_2SO_4 + H_2O + SO_2\uparrow$$

(b) Thiourea $\left(-NH-\overset{\displaystyle S}{\overset{\|}{C}}-NH-\right)$

(i) Heat an organic compound (0.10 g) with sodium hydroxide solution (2 ml) for about 1 minute. Cool down the solution and add 2 drops of aqueous lead acetate. Appearance of a dark brown or black colour indicates the presence of thiourea due to formation of lead sulphide.

$$R-NH-\overset{\displaystyle S}{\overset{\|}{C}}-NHR + 4NaOH \longrightarrow 2RNH_2 + Na_2CO_3 + Na_2S + H_2O$$

$$Na_2S + (CH_3COO)_2Pb \longrightarrow \underset{\text{Lead sulphide}}{PbS\downarrow} + 2CH_3COONa$$

(ii) Warm a small amount of organic compound with alcoholic solution of yellow mercuric oxide in a test tube. Appearance of black precipitate of mercuric sulphide indicates the presence of thiourea.

$$RNH-\overset{\displaystyle}{\underset{\displaystyle S}{\overset{\|}{C}}}-NHR + HgO \longrightarrow R-NH-\overset{\displaystyle S}{\overset{\|}{C}}-NHR + \underset{\text{Mercuric sulphide}}{HgS\downarrow}$$

(iii) Melt a small amount of organic compound in a test tube, cool and dissolve the products in water. Add aqueous ferric chloride solution. Appearance of red colour confirms the presence of thiourea.

$$S = C \overset{\Delta}{\longrightarrow} CNS^-$$

$$FeCl_3 + 3CNS^- \longrightarrow \underset{\substack{\text{Ferric thiocyanate} \\ \text{(blood red colour)}}}{Fe(CNS)_3} + 3Cl^-$$

(c) Mercaptans (Thiols)

Mercaptans, RSH (also thioether or sulphide $R_1–S–R_2$ and disulphides, $R_1–S–S–R_2$), are generally liquids and have an unpleasant odour.

Alkyl mercaptans are partially soluble in solution of caustic alkalies. Thiophenols are soluble in an alkali hydroxide solution.

Fusion with Caustic Alkali

Mix the organic compound (0.5 to 1 g) with potassium hydroxide (3 g) and 4–5 drops of water in nickel crucible. Heat the crucible gently with occasional stirring. Allow to cool and dissolve the solid mass in small amount of water by warming. Pour the solution in a test late and add cautiously 50% v/v sulphuric acid solution (2 ml); hydrogen sulphide is evolved (detected by lead acetate paper).

This test is given by all organic compounds of divalent sulphur (RSH, R_1–S–R and R_1–SS–R_2).

Compounds containing C and H only (e.g. Benzene, toluene, naphthalene, anthracene, phenanthrene, biphenyl)

These can be identified by determination of m.p./b.p., test for unsaturation, detection of elements. Identify these compounds on the basis of individual confirmatory test and formation of their derivatives.

All the above compounds can be nitrated, sulphonated and form picrates.

DETERMINATION OF MELTING POINT/BOILING POINT OF THE COMPOUND

See Chapter 10.

CONFIRMATORY TESTS OF THE INFERRED ORGANIC COMPOUND

After determining the functional groups and melting point/boiling point, one or two possible organic compounds are selected and specific confirmatory tests for these organic compounds are carried out.

Carboxylic Acids

1. Aliphatic carboxylic acid

(i) **Formic acid [HCOOH]** [b.p.100°C]:
  (a) Warm about 0.5 ml of formic acid with concentrated sulphuric acid (1 ml), carbon monoxide gas is evolved which burns with blue flame.
  (b) Add dilute solution of $KMnO_4$ drop by drop to the formic acid followed by addition of dilute sulphuric acid and observe the decolourization.
  (c) It gives red colour with ferric chloride solution.
  (d) Warm a neutral solution of a formate (dissolve free acid in dilute ammonia solution and remove the later by boiling) with ammonical silver nitrate solution. Silver separates out as a black precipitate or as a mirror from the dilute solution in a clean tube.
  (e) Add a small quantity of mercuric chloride solution to the formic acid, a white precipitate of mercurous chloride (insoluble in dilute HCl solution) is formed. The reduction may proceed further to produce grey coloured metallic mercury.

(ii) **Acetic acid [CH₃COOH]** [b.p.118°C]
  (a) Liquid smelling like vinegar.
  (b) To acetic acid (1 ml), add 10 drops of absolute ethanol and 10 drops of concentrated sulphuric acid. Heat gently for 5 minutes, cool and pour into water (5 ml) in a dish; a pleasant fruity smell of ethyl acetate is obtained.
  (c) It gives red colour with $FeCl_3$ solution.
  (d) It does not decolourizes potassium permanganate solution or mercuric chloride solution as formic acid.

(iii) **Oxalic acid [(COOH)$_2$]** [m.p.101°C]

(a) Take the aqueous solution of oxalic acid (2 ml) and neutralize it with dilute ammonium hydroxide solution.To this, add aqueous calcium chloride solution; white precipitate, insoluble in acetic acid but soluble in dilute hydrochloric acid is obtained. On adding calcium chloride solution, white precipitates of calcium oxalate are formed.

(b) Add 5 drops of concentrated sulphuric acid to a small amount of the compound in a dry test tube. Warm the contents gently by rotating the end of the tube over a small flame and turn the mouth of the tube periodically to the flame; characteristic blue flame of carbon monoxide appears.

(c) Heat the aqueous solution of the compound with acidic potassium permanganate solution; purple colour of the solution is discharged.

(iv) **Succinic acid [HOOC–CH$_2$–CH$_2$–COOH]** [m.p.185°C]

(a) To a small amount of the acid in a test tube, add a pinch of zinc dust and ammonium hydroxide. Heat the mixture and the place a matchstick soaked in concentrated hydrochloric acid in the vapours coming out of the tube which becomes red in colour.

(b) In a test tube, take the neutral solution of the acid (2 ml), add calcium chloride solution (2 ml), shake and boil for 2 minutes. On scratching the sides of test tube, a white precipitate of calcium succinate, soluble in acetic acid, is obtained.

(c) Add dilute hydrochloric acid to an aqueous solution of the acid. Now, add neutral aqueous ferric chloride solution, buff precipitate is obtained.

(d) In a test tube, take the acid (2 g) and twice its amount of resorcinol and add concentrated sulphuric acid (1 ml). Heat until the mixture becomes dark brown and then pour it in a beaker containing water. Make alkaline with sodium hydroxide solution, an orange green fluorescence is obtained.

Note: Phthalic acid also gives this test.

2. Aromatic Carboxylic Acids

(i) **Benzoic acid [C$_6$H$_5$COOH]** [m.p.121°C]

(a) To the acid (0.2 g) in a test tube, add the nitrating mixture (2 ml) (equal proportions of concentrated nitric and sulphuric acid). Heat carefully for 5–10 minutes, cool and pour in a beaker containing water, a pale yellow solid separates out.

(b) Heat the benzoic acid with sodalime, vapours of benzene are evolved.

(c) Gives buff precipitates with FeCl$_3$ solution in neutral solution.

(ii) **Phthalic acid** [ ][m.p.184°C]

(a) *Phthalein test:* Mix a rice grain of the substance with the double amount of phenol in a dry test tube. Add 2 drops of concentrated sulphuric acid and heat gently till the mixture attains red–brown colour. Cool, add few drops of water followed by gradual addition of aqueous sodium hydroxide solution with shaking till the solution becomes alkaline; reddish pink colour is produced due to formation of phenophthalein; the colour is discharged on adding an acid (see the general test for Phenol, page no. 148).

(b) *Fluorescein test:* Mix a rice grain of the substance with the double amount of resorcinol. Add 2 drops of concentrated sulphuric and heat gently till the mixture attains red brown colour. Cool, add few drops of water and then aqueous sodium hydroxide till the solution becomes alkaline. Take out this alkaline solution (1 ml) in another test tube and fill up the latter with water; yellow green fluorescence appears.

(iii) **Cinnamic Acid** [⟨benzene ring⟩—CH = CHCOOH] [m.p.133°C]

(a) Add a pinch of compound to a solution of potassium permanganate, the pink colour is discharged and a brown precipitate is produced accompanied by bitter almond smell of benzaldehyde.

(b) Add concentrated sulphuric acid to the compound, heat gently; a green colouration changing to brownish red is produced.

(c) To the neutral solution, add ferric chloride, a light yellow precipitate is produced.

(d) Dissolve cinnamic acid (0.2 g) in Na_2CO_3 solution (5 ml). Add bromine water drop by drop and note the separation of bromostyrene $C_6H_5CH=CHBr$ as colourless oil, having pleasant odour.

3. Hydroxy Carboxylic Acids

(i) **Lactic acid ($CH_3CHOHCOOH$)** [b.p.180°C]

(a) To a solution of lactic acid, add concentrated sulphuric acid and warm; brisk effervescence of carbon dioxide, sulphur dioxide and carbon monoxide appears.

(b) Warm 2–3 drops of the acid solution with concentrated sulphuric acid (2 ml) till the solution becomes pale yellow. Cool and add 2 drops of 5% guaicol solution in ethanol; intense red colour is developed.

(c) It decolourizes acidic potassium permanganate solution on warming.

(d) *Iodoform test:* To lactic acid (5 ml), add 10% NaOH solution, until alkaline to litmus, add 10% KI solution (5 ml) and sodium hypochlorite (10 ml) and mix well. A yellow precipitates of iodoform separates out.

(ii) **Citric acid** $\underset{\displaystyle CH_2COOH}{\overset{\displaystyle CH_2COOH}{C(OH)COOH.H_2O}}$ [m.p.100°C]

(a) To the neutral solution (2 ml) of the acid, add aqueous calcium chloride solution (2 ml). No precipitate is obtained in cold but on heating white shining crystals of calcium citrate separate out.

(b) To the aqueous solution (2 ml) of the acid, add Deniges reagent (1 ml) (mercuric oxide in sulphuric acid), boil and add potassium permanganate solution drop by drop. The purple colour disappears and a white precipitate is obtained.

(c) Take a mixture of small amount of acid and β-naphthol in a dry test tube and add concentrated sulphuric acid; a blue colour confirms the presence of citric acid.

(d) It does not reduce ammonical $AgNO_3$ solution and does not produce colouration with Fenton reagent (see tartaric acid).

(iii) **Tartaric acid** $\underset{\displaystyle CHOHCOOH}{CHOHCOOH}$ [m.p.169°C]

(a) It reduces ammonical silver nitrate solution.

Add dilute NaOH solution (1 drop) to $AgNO_3$ solution (5 ml) and add dilute NH_3 solution drop by drop until silver oxide is almost redissolved. Add $AgNO_3$ solution until faint but permanent precipitate is obtained. Then add neutral tartarate (0.5 ml) (make neutral with ammonium hydroxide solution) and place the tube in warm water; a silver mirror is formed in few minutes.

(b) Warm about 0.5 g of tartaric acid with concentrated sulphuric acid (1 ml), heavy charring takes place with the evolution of CO and SO_2 gas.

(c) To the acid solution, add cobalt nitrate solution followed by excess of sodium hydroxide solution. It shows no colour in cold, blue colour on warming, again colourless on cooling.

(d) It gives green colour with β–naphthol in concentrated sulphuric acid. The colour changes to orange on dilution.

(e) Take the neutral solution (3 ml) of the acid, add aqueous calcium chloride solution (1 ml) and shake vigorously. A heavy, white cystalline precipitate, soluble on boiling in glacial acetic acid (1 ml) appears.

(f) Heat the acid, (0.2 g), resorcinol (0.2 g) and concentrated sulphuric acid (2 ml) in a test tube. Violet colour appears.

(g) To the aqueous solution, add 5% solution of ammonium vanadate, acidify it with dilute acetic acid; orange colour appears.

(h) *Fenton's test*: To a solution of tartaric acid, add 1 drop of freshly prepared ferrous sulphate solution, 1 drop of hydrogen peroxide solution and the excess of NaOH solution, an intense violet colour is produced due to ferric salt of dihydroxy maleic acid HOOC.C (OH) = C (OH) COOH.

(iv) **Salicylic Acid [HOC$_6$H$_4$COOH] [m.p.158°C]**

(a) To 0.5 g of salicylic acid, add methanol (2 ml) and few drops of concentrated H_2SO_4 and warm carefully, a fragrant smell of methyl salicylate is given off.

(b) Acetylate by boiling salicylic acid (1 g) with acetic anhydride—acetic acid (4 ml) (equal volume) for 10 minutes. Pour into water. Filter off aspirin, m.p.136–137°C.

(c) Phthalein Formation: Heat together in a dry test tube a few crystals of salicylic acid with an equal quantity of phthalic anhydride moistened with drop of concentrated H_2SO_4. Cool, dissolve in water and add NaOH solution in excess, a red colouration is produced.

4. Amino Carboxylic Acid

(i) **Anthranilic acid** $\left[\begin{array}{c} \text{—NH}_2 \\ \text{COOH} \end{array} \right]$ (m.p. 146°C)

(a) Heat gently an equal small quantity of $CaCl_2$ and anthranilic acid. Dissolve the product in alcohol (2 ml)—red colouration with violet fluorescence is produced on keeping the tube.

(b) Fuse a small quantity of substance with $ZnCl_2$ by gentle heating. Dissolve the product in alcohol—yellow colour is produced.

(ii) ***p*-Aminobenzoic acid** [H$_2$N—〈 〉—COOH] (m.p. 188°C)

(a) Soluble in hot water.

(iii) **Glycine [H$_2$N–CH$_2$COOH] (m.p.232°C)**

(a) Soluble in water, insoluble in ethanol and ether.

(b) Add one or two drops of $FeCl_3$ to aqueous solution of the compound → red colour appears.

(c) Dissolve a small amount of the substance in water, add aqueous copper sulphate solution (2 ml)—blue colour (much deeper than the aqueous $CuSO_4$ solution) appears.

(d) Take aqueous solution (2 ml) of the compound in a test tube, add to it 2 drops of phenolphthalein solution, 2 drops of NaOH solution and neutralized ethanol (2 ml) → disappearance of red colour.

ALCOHOLS

1. Aliphatic Alcohols

(i) **Methyl alcohol [CH₃OH]** [b.p.65°C]

   (a) Heat a copper wire to redness and dip it in the methyl alcohol (2 ml) taken in a test tube. Pungent smell of formaldehyde is produced.

   (b) Methyl salicylate test. In a dry test tube, take the substance (1 ml), a pinch of salicylic acid and 2–3 drops of concentrated sulphuric acid. Heat the reaction mixture for 2 minutes, cool and pour in excess amount of water. A characteristic smell of oil of winter green (methyl salicylate) is produced.

   (c) On adding potassium dichromate and sulphuric acid to the substance in cold, formaldehyde is formed. The resultant solution, when warmed with a pinch of orcinol, gives a precipitate which is dissolved in sodium hydroxide with green fluorescence.

(ii) **Ethyl alcohol [C₂H₅OH]** [b.p.78°C]

   (a) *Ethyl acetate test*: To the substance (2 ml) in a test tube, add glacial acetic acid (2 ml) and concentrated sulphuric acid (1 ml). On heating a fruity smell of ethyl acetate is produced.

   (b) *Iodoform Test:* Add 3–4 drops of iodine solution and then sodium hydroxide solution drop by drop to the substance and then warm, the brown colour of iodine disappears and yellow precipitate of iodoform having characteristic smell is formed.

(iii) **Glycerol [CH₂OHCHOHCH₂OH]** [b.p.290°C]

   (a) To a small amount (0.5 g) of the compound, add finely powdered KHSO₄ (1 g). On strongly heating, an irritating pungent smell of acrolein (CH₂ = CH–CHO) is observed.

   (b) It reduces Tollen's reagent (ammonical silver nitrate solution).

   (c) *Phenol sulphuric test*: To equal amount of substance and phenol in a test tube, add few drops of concentrated sulphuric acid and gently warm. Cool and add excess of dilute ammonia solution (10 ml); a red colour is produced.

   (d) *Dunstan's test:* To borax solution (10%, 5 ml), add a drop of phenolphthalein solution when a pink colour is obtained. On addition of 2 or 3 drops of glycerol and shaking, the pink colour disappears. It reappears on warming and vanishes again on cooling.

(iv) **Glycol [HOCH₂–CH₂OH]** [b.p. 197°C]

   (a) *Oxalate test*: To a 0.5 ml of the compound in a test tube, add sodium carbonate solution (10% w/v) and pour this mixture into a boiling tube containing potassium permanganate (about 0.5 gm). Boil for 1–2 minutes and filter; if the colour of the filtrate is purple, decolourize with hydrogen peroxide. Acidify the filtrate (2 ml) with acetic acid, heat to boiling and add 2–3 drops of calcium chloride, a white precipitate of calcium oxalate confirms the presence of glycol.

2. Aromatic Alcohols

(i) **Benzyl alcohol [** ⬡ **—CH₂OH]** [b.p.205°C]

(a) To dilute nitric acid (2 ml) in a test tube, add 1–2 drops of substance and keep the tube in boiling water for 2 minutes. Pale yellow emulsion along with strong bitter almond smell is produced due to formation of benzaldehyde.

(b) On oxidation with potassium permanganate in aqueous solution, it yields benzoic acid, m.p.121°C.

(c) To the substance (1 ml) in a test tube, add concentrated hydrochloric acid (1 ml), shake and dip the tube in boiling water. The mixture becomes clear initially but within a minute white emulsion appears due to formation of benzyl chloride. On keeping the contents undisturbed, benzyl chloride forms, separated as colourless upper layer.

(d) Add concentrated H_2SO_4 (0.5 ml) to benzyl alcohol (0.5 ml) and shake. Heat is generated and gelatinous polymer gradually separates.

PHENOLS

(i) **Phenol [C_6H_5OH]** [m.p.42°C]

(a) Colour of phenol is slightly pink due to oxidation by atmospheric oxygen.

(b) It gives violet colour with ferric chloride.

(c) Heat a mixture of phenol and phthalic acid (2 : 1) after adding few drops of concentrated sulphuric acid. Pour few drops of the resultant product into a beaker containing dilute solution of sodium hydroxide. A pink red colour is obtained due to formation of phenolphthalein.

(d) To the small amount of phenol, add hot fuming nitric acid. Heat and then pour the contents in water; a pale yellow solid is obtained.

(e) *Liebermann's test*: To the compound (about 0.5 g) in a test tube, add few crystals of solid sodium nitrite and then few drops of concentrated sulphuric acid; a green or blue colour is obtained which changes to red on dilution and again turns blue green on making the solution alkaline with sodium hydroxide solution.

(f) Action of bromine water. To an aqueous solution of phenol, add bromine water gradually. First the colour of bromine is decolourized but on adding excess of bromine water, a white or yellowish white precipitates of tribromophenol is produced.

(ii) **Resorcinol** [ ] [m.p.110°C]

(a) It gives blue violet colour with neutral aqueous ferric chloride solution.

(b) *Phthalein test:* In a dry test tube, take the substance and phthalic acid in (2 : 1 ratio) and add concentrated sulphuric acid (2 ml). Heat the contents first gently and then strongly for 5 minutes. Then, pour the contents of the tube in a beaker containing dilute solution of sodium hydroxide; an intense yellow green fluorescence is produced due to formation of fluorescein.

(c) To small amount of the substance, add 2 drops of chloroform and sodium hydroxide solution (2 ml) and warm; red colour with green fluorescence is obtained.

(d) It does not reduces Fehling's solution or Tollen's reagent.

(iii) *o*-**Cresol** [ ] [b.p. 191°C]

(a) It responds to Liebermann reaction.

(b) It gives 'Phthalein test' described under phenol.

(c) It gives violet colour with aqueous ferric chloride.

(iv) *m*-Cresol [OH CH₃] [b.p. 203°C]

(a) Warm the mixture of original compound and phthalic anhydride and then add sodium hydroxide solution, a blue violet colour is formed.

(b) It gives blue violet colour with ferric chloride solution.

(c) It responds positively to Liebermann reaction.

(d) It gives 'Phthalein test' as described under phenol but instead of pink colour a blue-violet colour is obtained.

(v) *p*-Cresol [OH CH₃] [b.p. 202°C] [m.p. 35.5°C]

(a) Take a small amount of the substance in a dry test tube. Add to it few crystals of sodium nitrite and then few drops of concentrated sulphuric acid. Shake the test tube thoroughly; red colour appears.

(b) It gives blue colour with ferric chloride in water.

(c) It does not respond to Liebermann reaction.

(vi) *α*-Naphthol [OH] [m.p. 94°C]

(a) Insoluble in water.

(b) It does not give colour with neutral aqueous ferric chloride but gives white precipitate.

(c) Does not respond to bromine water and Liebermann's test.

(d) It gives green colour with titanic acid and concentrated sulphuric acid.

(e) Shake a small amount of the compound with a mixture having equal volume of iodine and potassium iodide and add excess of sodium hydroxide; violet colour appears which rapidly darken followed by a precipitate formation.

(f) Take a small amount of the compound in a test tube and add to it aqueous sodium hydroxide solution (2 ml) and one drop of chloroform; a blue colour appears on warming.

(g) To a small amount of compound in a test tube, add sodium hydroxide solution (2 ml), a drop of carbon tetrachloride and a pinch of copper powder and warm the contents. Blue colour is formed.

(vii) *β*-Naphthol [OH] [m.p.123°C]

(a) With alcoholic ferric chloride solution, a green colour is produced.

(b) With titanic acid in concentrated sulphuric acid, it gives red colour.

(c) Warm a mixture of the substance, sodium hydroxide and chloroform, blue colour appears.

(d) It gives yellow colour with sodium hypobromite solution (NaOBr).

(viii)   **Catechol** [ ] [m.p.105°C]

(a) Add aqueous ferric chloride solution, a green colour appears which changes into deep red colour on addition of ammonia.

(b) Solution of substance in sodium hydroxide turns brown on keeping in air.

(c) It reduces Fehling's solution and Tollen's reagent.

(d) To the aqueous solution (2 ml), add lead acetate solution (2 ml); a white precipitate is formed immediately.

(ix) **Quinol** [HO—〈 〉—OH] [m.p.170°C]

(a) It reduces ammonical silver nitrate solution in cold.

(b) Its aqueous solution gives brown colour on shaking with sodium hydroxide solution.

(c) Shake aqueous solution with ferric chloride solution. A blue colour appears which immediately changes to reddish brown.

(x) *m*-**Aminophenol** [ ][m.p.123°C]

(a) Slightly soluble in water and benzene.

(b) No colour with $FeCl_3$ solution in cold but on warming—darkening of solution occurs.

(xi) *o*-**Aminophenol** [ ][m.p.174°C]

(a) It gives dark brown precipitates with $FeCl_3$ solution.

(b) Yellow brown colour on warming with $AgNO_3$ solution.

(xii)*p*-**Aminophenol** [ ][m.p.186°C]

(a) It gives purple colour with $FeCl_3$ or $AgNO_3$ solution.

(b) Dissolve a small amount of the substance in dilute HCl (5 ml) on shaking or on warming. Cool it, add concentrated sodium hypochlorite solution ($NaOH + Cl_2$ water) and shake—yellow precipitate appears.

(c) Take a small amount of the substance in a test tube and add to it dichromate mixture (2 ml). Heat the contents to boiling—pungent odour of benzoquinone appears.

ALDEHYDES

1. Aliphatic Aldehydes

(i) **Formaldehyde [HCHO]** [b.p. 91–101°C], available as formalin (37% solution)

    (a) It is pungent in nature.

    (b) It gives reddish brown precipitate (charging to yellow green) with dilute solution of Nesseler's reagent.

    (c) On evaporation, a white residue of paraformaldehyde is obtained.

    (d) To aqueous solution of the substance (2 ml) in a test tube, add few crystals of resorcinol and then pour concentrated sulphuric acid (2 ml) carefully from side of the test tube. A red ring is formed at the junction of liquids and a white precipitate appears in the aqueous layer which turns violet red.

(ii) **Acetaldehyde [CH$_3$CHO]** [b.p. 21°C]

    (a) Nitroprusside reaction. To the aqueous solution of the substance (2 ml), add freshly prepared aqueous sodium nitroprusside solution (2 ml) and make alkaline with sodium hydroxide solution. A deep wine-red colour is produced.

    (b) On adding a few drop of aqueous solution of the substance to dilute solution of benzidine hydrochloride, a yellow colour is produced.

    (c) It reduces Tollen's reagent to yield a silver mirror and black precipitate.

    (d) It reduces Fehling's solution to yield a reddish brown precipitate of cuprous oxide.

    (e) A very dilute aqueous solution gives a light yellow precipitate with Nesseler's solution while concentrated solution gives a red precipitate turning grey.

    (f) To aqueous solution of the substance (2 ml), add 20% w/v potassium hydroxide solution (2 ml) and boil for 1 minute; the solution becomes yellow and finally a yellow precipitate changing to orange with a disagreable smell is obtained.

    (g) *Iodoform Test*: To aldehyde solution (1 ml), add 10% w/v KI solution (3 ml) and freshly prepared sodium hypochlorite solution, yellow crystals of iodoform soon separates out.

2. Aromatic aldehyde

(i) **Benzaldehyde [** ⬡—CHO **]** [b.p. 179°C]

    (a) It is insoluble in water.

    (b) It has odour of bitter almond.

    (c) Cannizzaro's reaction. To the compound (0.5 ml) in a test tube; add 30% solution of sodium hydroxide (2 ml) and heat the contents for 5 minutes. Dilute with water, filter and acidify the filtrate with dilute hydrochloric acid; a white precipitate of benzoic acid is obtained.

    (d) It does not reduce Fehling's solution.

    (e) Take the substance (1 ml), 5 drops of acetone, ethanol (5 ml) and dilute sodium hydroxide (2 ml) in a boiling tube and boil the contents for 2 minutes. Cool, shake vigorously and add water (20 ml). A yellow solid, dibenzyl acetone, separates out.

    (f) To the substance (1 ml), add dimethylaniline (1 ml) and small amount of fused zinc chloride. Heat the mixture; a dark green precipitate of benzaldimethylaniline is produced.

(ii) **Salicyldehyde [C$_6$H$_4$ (OH) CHO]** [b.p.196°C]

    (a) Add a few drops of FeCl$_3$ solution to a few drops of the aldehyde; an intense violet colouration is produced.

    (b) Add ammonia solution (1 ml) to aldehyde (1 ml), a precipitate of hydrosalicylamide (HOC$_6$H$_4$CH)$_3$N$_2$ is rapidly produced.

KETONES

1. Aliphatic Ketone

(i) **Acetone [CH$_3$COCH$_3$]** [b.p.56°C]

    (a) *Iodoform test*: Add 3–4 drops of iodine solution and then aqueous sodium hydroxide drop by drop to the compound and warm. The brown colour of iodine disappears and a pale yellow precipitate of iodoform having characteristic smell is formed.

    (b) Dissolve a small amount of *o*-nitrobenzaldehyde in original substance (2 ml) and pour in a beaker containing alkaline water. A blue colour due to formation of indigo is produced.

    (c) To saturated solution of sodium bisulphite (2 ml), add few drops of substance; white crystals of bisulphate adduct are formed with evolution of heat.

    (d) *m-Dinitrobenzene test*: Mix acetone (1 ml) with *m*-dinitrobenzene (0.1 gm). Add excess of sodium hydroxide solution and shake, a violet colouration is produced which fades slowly.

(ii) **Cyclohexanone** [⬡=O] [b.p.156°C]

    (a) Dissolve potassium dichromate (5 g) in dilute sulphuric acid (20 ml). Cool down and add cyclohexanone (1 ml) to it. Heat the mixture under reflux for 5 minutes, cool the flask, a white crystal of adipic acid separates out, m.p.153°C.

2. Aromatic Ketones

(i) **Acetophenone** [⬡—CO·CH$_3$] [b.p. 202°C]

    (a) It responds to iodoform test described under acetone.

    (b) Dissolve the substance in concentrated sulphuric acid, orange colour is produced.

    (c) To the substance (2 ml), add alkaline potassium permanganate solution (2 ml) and heat for 5 minutes. Cool, filter and acidify the filtrate with dilute hydrochloric acid; a white precipitate of benzoic acid is obtained.

    (d) Its aqueous solution gives wine red colour with alkaline sodium nitroprusside solution; on addition of acetic acid, the colour changes to blue.

    (e) It also responds to m-dinitrobenzene test as mentioned in acetone.

(ii) **Benzophenone [C$_6$H$_5$COC$_6$H$_5$]** [m.p. 48°C]

    (a) Dissolve the substances in concentrated sulphuric acid, a yellow solution is obtained.

    (b) Fusion of the substance with sodium produces deep blue colour.

    (c) To benzophenone (0.3 g), add naphthalene (1.0 g) and heat until completely molten. Add a small piece of sodium metal and heat again. The surface of the sodium metal becomes green.

    Note: It does not give the iodoform test.

ESTERS

1. Aliphatic ester

(i) **Ethyl Acetate [$CH_3COOC_2H_5$]** [b.p.77°C]

(a) It is sweet smelling colourless liquid with an apple like odour.

(b) It is slightly soluble in water.

2. Aromatic ester

(i) **Methyl Benzoate [$C_6H_5COOCH_3$]** [b.p.199°C]

(a) It is an aromatic, colourless liquid.

(b) Heat the compound with 10% aqueous sodium hydroxide solution, for 5 minutes. Cool the reaction mixture, filter the precipitate of benzoic acid, wash with cold water and dry it, m.p.122°C.

(ii) **Ethyl Benzoate [$C_6H_5COOC_2H_5$]** [b.p.213°C]

(a) Boil the ester with sodium hydroxide solution for few minutes. Cool and add ferric chloride solution; a buff coloured precipitate is formed.

CARBOHYDRATES

1. Monosaccharides

(i) **Glucose [$CH_2OH(CHOH)_4CHO$]** [m.p.90°C]

(a) It reduces Fehling's solution, Tollen's reagent and Barfoed's reagent.

(b) Add lead acetate (1 g) to aqueous solution (2 ml) of the substance, boil and add dilute ammonia solution (5 ml). Continue boiling for 5 minutes. A rose pink colour confirms the presence of glucose.

(c) *Rapid furfural test*: To the 1% solution of glucose (1 ml), add alcoholic solution of α-naphthol followed by addition of conc. HCl (6 ml). A violet colouration is produced after boiling for 1–2 minutes. (Fructose and sucrose give immediately on boiling.)

(d) It reduces Benedict's solution (solution of copper sulphate, sodium citrate and sodium carbonate) to yield yellow orange or orange red precipitate.

(ii) **Fructose [$CH_2OH.[CHOH]_3COCH_2OH$]** [m.p.95–105°C]

(a) It reduces Fehling's solution and Tollen's reagent.

(b) It gives blue colour on warming with ammonium molybdate solution.

(c) To a small amount of the compound, add equal amount of resorcinol and concentrated hydrochloric acid (1 ml). A red colour is obtained on warming the mixture.

(d) It reduces Barfoed's reagent (cupric acetate in acetic acid) on warming.

(e) It gives rapid furfural test as in glucose.

(f) Take a small amount of the compound in a test tube, add to it half the amount of sodium or selenium dioxide and dilute hydrochloric acid (2 ml). Heat the test tube in boiling water bath for 2 minutes. A red coloured precipitate of selenium is obtained.

2. Disaccharides

(i) **Sucrose [$C_{12}H_{22}O_{11}$]** [m.p.185°C]

(a) It does not react with Fehling's solution or with phenylhydrazine. However, after hydrolysis, by warming with dilute HCl, it reduces Fehling's solution and reacts with phenylhydrazine.

(b) On treatment with concentrated sulphuric acid, it is charred in cold.

(c) It gives red colour on boiling with saturated ammonical nickle sulphate solution followed by addition of dilute sulphuric acid.

(d) Warming the substance with cobalt nitrate and sodium hydroxide solution, a violet colour is produced.

(e) To aqueous solution of the substance (2 ml), add a pinch of resorcinol and concentrated hydrochloric acid (2 ml). Boil for 2 minutes. A deep wine red colour is produced.

(f) Add copper sulphate and sodium hydroxide solution, blue coloured solution is obtained.

(ii) **Lactose (milk Sugar) [$C_{12}H_{22}O_{11}$], m.p. 222°**

  (a) Reduces ammonical silver nitrate and Fehling's solution.

  (b) Forms yellow osazone, m.p. 208°C, soluble in hot water. If examined under microscope, characteristic clusters of hedge-hog crystal appears.

(iii) **Maltose (malt sugar) [$C_{12}H_{22}O_{11}$], m.p. 102–103° (monohydrate)**

  (a) Reduces the ammonical silver nitrate solution and Fehling's solution.

  (b) Form osazone, m.p. 206°C. If examined under microscope, sheaves of plates appears.

AMINES

1. Aliphatic amine

(i) **Ethylamine $C_2H_5NH_2$ [b.p.19°C]**

It gives white precipitate with Nessler's reagent.

2. Aromatic amines

(i) **Aniline [$C_6H_5NH_2$] [b.p.184°C]**

  (a) It is a colourless liquid when pure but turns brown when exposed to air.

  (b) On warming with alcoholic potassium hydroxide and chloroform, an unpleasant odour of phenylisocynate is produced.

  (c) Dissolve a drop of the compound in ether (2 ml) and add water (10 ml) to it. Add dilute solution (1 ml) of bleaching powder and shake. A purple colour is obtained.

  (d) Dissolve small amount of potassium dichromate in concentrated sulphuric acid and to this, add 1 drop of the substance. A blue or black colour is obtained.

  (e) Dissolve aniline (about 0.2 g) in concentrated HCl (2 ml) and then add a few drops of $FeCl_3$, a pale green colour develops.

(ii) **Benzylamine [$C_6H_5CH_2NH_2$] [b.p.185°C]**

  (a) On oxidation with alkaline potassium permanganate, it yields benzoic acid, m.p.121°C.

  (b) It is miscible with water.

(iii) **Diphenylamine [$(C_6H_5)_2NH$] [m.p.54°C] (also called Biphenyl)**

  (a) It is a colourless crystalline solid with pleasant odour.

  (b) To the solution of the compound in concentrated sulphuric acid, add one drop of aqueous sodium nitrite solution. A deep blue colour is produced.

(iv) **Dimethylaniline [$C_6H_5N(CH_3)_2$] [b.p.193°C]**

  (a) To the substance (1 ml), add oxalic acid (0.5 g) dissolved in ethanol (5 ml). A white precipitate of oxalate of dimethyl aniline is obtained.

(v) *o*-Toluidine [ ] [b.p. 199–200°C]

(a) Shake its ethereal solution with bleaching powder solution or sodium hypochlorite solution. The ethereal layer becomes brown.

(b) Add 2–3 drops of the compound to potassium dichromate solution. A blue colour is produced which changes to green on dilution.

(vi) **m-Toluidine [** (structure: benzene ring with NH_2 at top and CH_3 at meta position) **] [b.p. 203°C]**

(a) It is solution with HNO_3 gives red colour.

(b) Solution in 50% H_2SO_4 solution gives yellow brown colour with $K_2Cr_2O_7$.

(vii) **1-Naphthylamine[** (naphthalene structure with NH_2) **] [m.p. 50°C]**

(a) Solid, colourless when freshly crystallized but turns pink on exposure in air.

(b) Slightly soluble in hot water.

(c) Its hydrochloride solution gives blue precipitate with $FeCl_3$.

(viii) **2-Naphthylamine:** (naphthalene structure with NH_2) **[m.p. 113°C]**

(a) Pink coloured crystalline solid with characteristic odour.

(b) Sparingly soluble in hot water.

(c) Gives no colour with $FeCl_3$ solution (distinction from 1–naphthylamine).

(ix) **p-Toluidine[** (benzene ring with CH_3 at top and NH_2 at para position) **] [b.p. 200°, m.p. 43°C]**

(a) Dissolve the compound in 50% sulphuric acid solution and divide into two portion:

(i) To one portion add nitric acid. A blue colour is formed which changes gradually to violet red and then brown.

(ii) To another portion, add potassium dichromate solution—a yellow colour appears.

(b) Take a pinch of the compound in water (5 ml). Add 2–3 ml of concentrated hydrochloric acid and ferric chloride solution (1 ml) and heat the mixture. An orange reddish colour is produced.

NITRO COMPOUNDS

(i) **Nitrobenzene [$C_6H_5NO_2$] [b.p. 210°C]**

(a) Pale yellow liquid, immiscible with water and heavier than water.

(b) It possess characteristic smell of bitter almonds.

(c) To the compound (1 ml) in a boiling tube, add few pieces of tin (or a pinch of zinc dust or tin chloride) and concentrated hydrochloric acid (2 ml). Boil the mixture for 5 minutes; aniline is produced. Filter and divide the filtrate into two parts.

In the first part perform dye test; positive result is obtained.

In the second part perform carbylamine test; positive result is obtained.

(d) To a few drops of the compound, add a pinch of zinc dust, glacial acetic acid (2 ml) and boil. Add water (2 ml) and then a solution of sodium hydroxide drop by drop till the mixture is alkaline. Add 2 drops of this resultant solution to sodium hypochlorite solution (5 ml). Violet colour is produced.

(ii) **m–Dinitrobenzene** [ ] [m.p. 90°C]

  (a) It gives red–brown colour on boiling with sodium hydroxide solution.

  (b) Dissolve a pinch of the compound in acetone (2 ml) and add a drop of sodium hydroxide solution to it. A violet blue colour is produced which changes to violet red on adding acetic acid.

  (c) Dissolve a pinch of substance in dilute sodium hydroxide and boil. To this, add a very small amount of glucose (or tin chloride). Violet colour is produced.

AMIDES

1. Aliphatic Amides

(i) **Acetamide [CH_3CONH_2]** [m.p. 82°C]

  (a) Heat the compound with concentrated sulphuric acid, a strong smell of vinegar is produced due to formation of acetic acid.

  (b) Heat the compound with aniline, it yields acetanilide, m.p.114°C, with evolution of ammonia.

  (c) It does not evolve ammonia when heated alone (distinction from ammonia).

(ii) **Urea [H_2NCONH_2]** [m.p. 132°C]

  (a) *Biuret test*: Heat a small amount of the compound in a dry test tube. The solid melts and ammonia is evolved. Cool the tube when a white residue (biuret) is left in it. Dissolve it in water (2 ml), add a drop of copper sulphate solution and sodium hydroxide solution (2 ml) when violet colour is produced.

$$2NH_2CONH_2 \xrightarrow{\Delta} \underset{\text{Biuret}}{NH_2CONHCONH_2} + NH_3$$

  (b) Dissolve a small amount of the substance in dilute hydrochloric acid, cool and add a few drops of sodium nitrite solution to it. Nitrogen gas is evolved with effervescence.

  (c) Add 2 or 3 ml of concentrated nitric acid to the substance (0.5 g) and boil. On cooling white crystals of urea nitrate are obtained.

  (d) Mix concentrated solution of oxalic acid and urea, a white crystals of urea oxalate is formed.

2. Aromatic Amide

(i) **Benzamide [$C_6H_5CONH_2$]** [m.p. 129°C]

  (a) Sparingly soluble in water.

  (b) Heat a small amount of the compound with dilute sodium hydroxide for 5 minutes, cool and acidify with dilute hydrochloric acid; a white precipitate of benzoic acid, m.p. 121°C, is obtained.

(b) Mix a small amount of the compound with either sodalime or phosphorus pentachloride in a dry ignition tube and heat; smell of bitter almonds is produced due to formation of benzonitrile.

(ii) **Salicylamide [C_6H_5 (OH) $CONH_2$]** [m.p. 139°C]

(a) To a trace of the solid, add ferric chloride solution and shake; an intense violet coloration is produced.

IMIDES

(i) **Succinimide [$(CH_2CO)_2NH$]** [m.p. 125°C]

Fuse together in a dry test tube succinimide (0.1 g), resorcinol (0.1 g) and conc. H_2SO_4 (2 drops). Cool, add water and then NaOH solution in excess. A green fluorescent solution is produced.

(ii) **Phthalimide [** **NH]** [m.p. 233°C]

(a) *Phthalein test:* Heat gently in a dry test tube, phthalimide (0.1 g), phenol (0.1 g) and conc. H_2SO_4 (1 drop). Cool, add water and then NaOH solution in excess. An intense pink colouration is produced, decolorized by acids.

(b) *Fluorescein test:* Repeat the above test but the resorcinol instead of phenol and heat gently. A green solution is produced on addition of NaOH solution.

ANILIDE

1. Aliphatic Anilide

(i) **Acetanilide [$C_6H_5NHCOCH_3$]** [m.p. 114°C]

(a) Sparingly soluble in water.

(b) With concentrated nitric and sulphuric acids, it yields *p*-nitro derivative, m.p.216°C, on ignition.

(c) On bromination with bromine in acetic acid, it yields *p*-bromo derivative, m.p.168°C.

2. Aromatic Anilide

(i) **Benzanilide [$C_6H_5NHCOC_6H_5$]** [m.p. 162°C]

(a) With bromine in acetic acid, it yields *p*-bromo derivative m.p.204°C.

(b) On nitration in cold, it yield a mixture of *o*-nitro derivative, m.p.94°C, and *p*-nitro derivative, m.p. 199°C.

HALOGEN COMPOUND

(i) **Chloroform [$CHCl_3$]** [b.p. 61°C]

(a) It is a heavy liquid with sweet smelling odour.

(b) To a small amount of the substance, add few crystals of resorcinol and aqueous sodium hydroxide solution (2 ml) and boil; red colour is produced.

(c) *Carbylamine test*: To the substance (1 ml), add aniline (1 ml) and potassium hydroxide solution (4 ml). Boil for 2 minutes. Highly offensive odour of phenyl isocyanide is observed.

    (d) Boil a few drop of the substance with pyridine and sodium hydroxide solution and allow to stand, pyridine layer becomes red.

(ii) **Iodoform [CHI$_3$]** [m.p.119°C]

    (a) Heat the compound, violet vapours of iodine are produced.

    (b) To a small amount of compound, add resorcinol (1 gm) and alcoholic sodium hydroxide solution (2 ml) and warm. A red colour changing to violet is produced.

    (c) To the 20% sodium hydroxide solution (5 ml), add a pinch of compound and 4–5 drops of pyridine. Boil and allow to stand when pyridine layer becomes red in colour.

(iii) **Carbon Tetrachloride [CCl$_4$]** [b.p.78°C]

    (a) *Carbylamine test*: To 2–3 drops of the substance, add 2–3 drops of aniline and alcoholic potassium hydroxide solution (2 ml) and boil for 5 minutes. An obnoxious smell of phenyl isocyanide is produced but more slowly than chloroform.

    (b) Reduce the compound to chloroform by adding a pinch of zinc dust, dilute hydrochloric acid (1 ml) and boiling and then perform the carbylamine test as mentioned earlier.

(iv) **Chlorobenzene[** ⬡—Cl **]** [b.p.132°C]

    (a) It is an aromatic, colourless liquid with pleasant almond like odour, non-miscible with water.

    (b) It is inflammable.

(v) **Benzyl chloride[C$_6$H$_5$CH$_2$Cl]** [b.p.179°]

    (a) Boil benzyl chloride (1 ml), saturated aqueous KMnO$_4$ solution (50 ml) and anhydrous Na$_2$CO$_3$ (2 g) under reflux for 10 minutes. Acidify with concentrated HCl and then add 25% Na$_2$SO$_3$ solution until the brown precipitate of MnO$_2$ has dissolved. On cooling, benzoic acid crystallizes out.

    (b) It is inflammable.

SULPHONIC ACIDS

(i) **Benzene Sulphonic Acid [** ⬡SO$_3$H **]** [m.p.65°C]

It is freely soluble in water and ethanol; slightly soluble in benzene, insoluble in ether and carbon disulphide.

Derivatives:

    (a) Amide, m.p.153°C.

    (b) Anilide, m.p.110°C.

    (c) S–Benzyl iso-thiuronium salt, m.p.148°C.

(ii) *p*-**Toluene Sulphonic Acid [** CH$_3$—⬡—SO$_3$H **]** [m.p. 92°C]

It is soluble in dilute NaOH, ethanol and ether.

Derivatives:

    (a) Amide, m.p.137°.

    (b) Anilide, m.p. 103°C.

    (c) Chloride, m.p.69°C.

(iii) **Sulphanilic Acid (Amino Sulphonic Acid):** [NH$_2$—⟨benzene ring⟩—SO$_3$H] [m.p. 288°C]

  (a) It is a crystalline solid, soluble in water.

  (b) Heat with sodalime, it forms aniline, b.p. 183°C.

  (c) To a solution of NaHCO$_3$, add a pinch of substance. Carbon dioxide gas is evolved with effervescence.

  (d) On diazotization and then coupling with alkaline β-naphthol, an orange-red dye is produced.

  (e) Boil the compound (0.2 g) with potassium dichromate and concentrated sulphuric acid (1–2 ml), it forms p-benzoquinone having a characteristic pungent odour.

THIOUREAS

(i) **Thiourea [H$_2$NCSNH$_2$]** [m.p. 180°C]

  (a) It is a colourless crystalline solid, soluble in water.

  (b) Boil a small amount of the substance with sodium hydroxide. Ammonia gas is evolved.

  (c) Melt the compound (0.2 g) in a dry test tube, cool and add a few drops of ferric chloride. A blood red colour is produced due to formation of ferric thiocyanate.

  (d) Dissolve a small amount of the compound by heating in dilute acetic acid (2 ml). To the hot solution, add potassium ferrocyanide solution (2 ml). A green colour changing to blue appears.

  (e) Add lead acetate solution to the compound dissolved in sodium hydroxide solution, black precipitate appears.

(ii) **Phenyl thiourea [C$_6$H$_5$.NH.CS.NH$_2$]** [m.p. 154°C]

  (a) Boil with sodium hydroxide solution, ammonia gas evolves.

  (b) Boil with dilute hydrochloric acid, it produces pungent offensive odour of phenyl isocyanide.

  (c) Take a small amount of the compound in a dry test tube and add to it 5 drops of concentrated sulphuric acid. Heat for a moment, cool and carefully add water (5 ml). Again cool and then add aqueous sodium nitrite solution (5 ml). Add this solution (2 ml) to alkaline solution of β-naphthol (5 ml). A red-coloured solution is formed.

  (d) Repeat the above test up to the stage of dilution with water. Now make the solution alkaline by adding sodium hydroxide solution and then hold a strip of moistened red litmus paper near the mouth of the tube. The colour changes to blue.

HYDROCARBONS

(i) **Benzene [C$_6$H$_6$]** [b.p. 80°C]

  (a) Colourless liquid with characteristic aromatic odour, floats on water.

  (b) Take the substance (1 ml) in a boiling tube and to this, add concentrated nitric acid (2 ml) and then sulphuric acid (2 ml) drop by drop with shaking. Heat the contents for about 30 minutes, cool and pour the reaction mixture in ice-cold water. A yellow oily liquid is solidified on standing.

  (c) To the substance (2 ml), add ammonical solution of nickel cyanide (2 ml). A white coloured, violet tinted compound separates out.

(ii) **Toluene** [$\langle\!\!\!\bigcirc\!\!\!\rangle$—$CH_3$][b.p. 111°C]

   (a) To the substance (1 ml) in a boiling test tube, add nitration mixture (6 ml) (concentrated nitric acid and sulphuric acid, 3 ml each). Allow the reaction mixture to cool and pour in ice-cold water. A yellow solid of 2,4,6-trinitrotoluene separates out.
   (b) Heat the substance (1 ml) with a pinch of magnesium oxide and concentrated sulphuric acid (1 ml) in the presence of few crystals of copper sulphate. Benzaldehyde is formed which can be detected due to its bitter almond smell.

(iii) **Naphthalene:** [m.p. 80°C]

   (a) It is a colourless solid with characteristic odour, immiscible in water. Dissolve small amount of the substance in chloroform and add anhydrous aluminium chloride. A green colour develops.
   (b) Oxidation with concentrated sulphuric acid in the presence of mercuric sulphate yields phthalic acid, m.p. 195°C.

(iv) **Anthracene:** [m.p. 216°C]

   (a) Prepare a saturated solution of anthracene in xylene and keep it in sunlight for sometime when crystals of dianthracene appears.
   (b) Shake a small amount of the substance with saturated solution of picric acid (2 ml) in benzene. A deep red coloured solution is produced.
   (c) Heat chromium oxide (1 g) in water (1 ml) and glacial acetic acid (9 ml) in a 100 ml flask until all the chromium oxide has dissolved. Cool, add compound (0.5 g) and boil the contents under reflux gently for 10 minutes with occasional shaking. Cool the contents, add water (50 ml), shake and filter. Wash the anthraquinone with water until it is clear yellow in colour. Test the formation of anthraquinone as described below: Mix two rice grain of the compound with equal amount of zinc dust and add to it aqueous sodium hydroxide solution (5 ml). Boil the contents for about 30 seconds. A deep red colour is produced.

(v) **Phenanthrene:** [m.p. 100°C]

   (a) It dissolves in benzene with light blue fluorescence.

(vi) *o*-**Xylene:** [b.p. 144°C]

   (a) On oxidation alkaline with potassium permanganate solution, it produces phthalic acid, m.p.195°C.

(vii)*m*-**Xylene:** [m.p. 139°C]

(a) Warm it with the a mixture of concentrated nitric and sulphuric acids and then pour the reaction mixture in cold water, 2,4,6-trinitro derivative m.p. 182°C separates out.

(b) On oxidation with alkaline potassium permanganate, it yields isophthalic acid. m.p. 345–348°C.

(viii)   ***p*-Xylene:**   [b.p. 138°C]

(a) On oxidation with alkaline potassium permanganate, it yields terephthalic acid, $C_6H_4(COOH)_2$, m.p. 427°C.

(b) Heat it with a mixture of concentrated sulphuric and nitric acids and then pour the reaction mixture in cold water, 2,3,5-trinitroderivative, m.p. 139°C separates out.

(ix) **Diphenyl**   [m.p. 69°C]

(a) Pale yellow solid, insoluble in water.

(b) It gives positive nitration test.

DERIVATIZATION OF UNKNOWN ORGANIC COMPOUND

After concluding the organic compound, the appropriate derivative is prepared depending on the presence of the functional group (see Chapter 12). The determination of melting point of the derivative confirms the identity of the unknown organic compound.

Table 11.1: List of some important organic compounds with their common derivatives

Compound	State	m.p. or b.p., °C	Derivative, m.p., °C
A. Carboxylic acids			
1. Formic acid HCOOH	Liquid	b.p. 100	Amide, 195 Anilide, 47 Ammonium Salt, 114 Benzylthiouronium salt, 152
2. Acetic acid CH_3COOH	Liquid	b.p. 118	Amide, 82 Anilide, 113 Ammonium Salt, 66 Benzylthiouronium salt, 134
3. Propionic acid CH_3CH_2COOH	Liquid	b.p. 140	Amide, 79 Anilide, 105 Benzylthiouronium salt, 153
4. Oxalic acid HOOC–COOH	Solid	m.p. 101	Amide, 245 Toulidide, 267
5. Succinic acid $(CH_2COOH)_2$	Solid	m.p. 185	Amide, 242 Anilide, 226 Anhydride, 120 Benzylthiouronium salt, 154

(Contd.)

Compound	State	m.p. or b.p., °C	Derivative, m.p., °C
6. Tartaric acid $(CHOHCOOH)_2$	Solid	m.p. 169	Anilide, 126 Toluidide, 264
7. Acetylsalicylic acid 	Solid	m.p. 135	Amide,138 Anilide, 136
8. Citric acid (hydrated) CH_2COOH | $C(OH)COOH$ | CH_2COOH	Solid	m.p. 100	Anilide, 115 Amide, 210 Acetyl, 175
9. Benzoic acid C_6H_5COOH	Solid	m.p. 121	Amide, 129 Anilide, 162 m-Nitrobenzoic acid, 141 Acetylthiouronium salt, 167
10. Phthalic acid 	Solid	m.p. 184	Anhydride, 132 Amide, 220
11. Cinnamic acid 	Solid	m.p. 133	p-Nitro derivative 285 Anilide, 153° Amide, 147°
12. Salicylic acid 	Solid	m.p. 158	Aspirin, 135 Amide, 139
13. Gallic acid	Solid	m.p. 263	Anilide, 134
14. Phenyl acetic acid $C_6H_5CH_2COOH$	Solid	m.p. 76	Amide, 157 Anilide, 118
B. Amino carboxylic acid			
15. Glycine $NH_2CH_2–COOH$	Solid	m.p. 232	Acetyl, 206 Benzoyl, 187
16. Anthranilic acid 	Solid	m.p. 146°	Amide, 109 Anilide, 131 Benzoyl, 182
17. p-Aminobenzoic acid $p-NH_2C_6H_4–COOH$	Solid	m.p. 188	Acetyl, 252 Benzoyl, 278

(Contd.)

Compound	State	m.p. or b.p., °C	Derivative, m.p., °C
C. Alcohols			
18. Methyl alcohol CH_3OH	Liquid	b.p. 65	3,5-Dinitrobenzoate, 109 p-nitrobenzoate, 96
19. Ethyl alcohol C_2H_5OH	Liquid	b.p. 78	3,5-Dinitrobenzoate, 94 Iodoform, 120
20. *n*-Propyl alcohol $C_3H_5CH_2OH$	Liquid	b.p. 97	3,5-Dinitrobenzoate,75
21. *n*-Butyl alcohol $C_3H_7CH_2OH$	Liquid	b.p. 118	3,5-Dinitrobenzoate,64
22. Glycerol $HOCH_2–CHOH–CH_2OH$	Liquid	b.p. 290	Tribenzoate, 76 Trinitrobenzoate, 188
23. Glycol, $HOCH_2–CH_2OH$	Liquid	b.p. 197°	3,5-dinitrobenzoate, 169
D. Phenol			
24. Phenol C_6H_5OH	Solid	m.p. 42	Tribromophenol, 93 Toluene p-sulphonate,96 3,5-dinitrobenzoate, 146
25. *o*-Cresol	Liquid	b.p. 191	Bromoderivative, 56 Picrate, 88 p-nitrobenzoate, 94
26. *m*-Cresol	Liquid	b.p. 203 m.p. 12°	Bromo derivative, 84 Benzoyl derivative, 54 p-nitrobenzoate, 90
27. *p*-Cresol	Liquid	b.p. 202 m.p. 35.5	Benzoyl derivative, 71 p-Nitrobenzoate, 98
28. Catechol	Solid	m.p. 105	Diacetyl, 123 Dibenzoyl, 199
29. Resorcinol	Solid	m.p. 110	Benzoate, 117 *p*-Nitrobenzoate, 182

(Contd.)

Compound	State	m.p. or b.p., °C	Derivative, m.p., °C
30. Pyrogallol	Solid	m.p. 133	Triacetate, 161
31. Thymol	Solid	m.p. 51	p-Nitrobenzoate, 70
32. Hydroquinone	Solid	m.p. 172	Diacetyl, 123 Dibenzoyl, 199
33. o-Aminophenol	Solid	m.p. 174	Acetyl, 201 Dibenzoyl, 184
34. m-Aminophenol	Solid	m.p. 122	Acetyl, 148 Benzoyl, 174
35. p-Aminophenol	Solid	m.p. 184	Acteyl, 168 Benzoyl, 216
36. α-Naphthol	Solid	m.p. 96	Picrate, 189 Acetyl derivative, 46
37. β-Naphthol	Solid	m.p. 123	Picrate, 156 Acetyl derivative, 70
38. Picric acid	Solid	m.p. 122	Benzoate, 163

(Contd.)

Compound	State	m.p. or b.p., °C	Derivative, m.p., °C
39. *o*-Nitro phenol	Solid	m.p. 45	Benzoyl derivative, 142
			Picric acid, 122

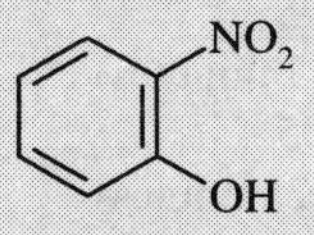

E. Aldehydes and Ketones

Compound	State	m.p. or b.p., °C	Derivative, m.p., °C
40. Formaline solution (40% aqueous solution of HCHO)	Liquid	b.p. 91–101	2,4-dinitrophenyl hydrazone, 166
41. Acetaldehyde CH_3CHO	Liquid	b.p. 21	2,4-dinitrophenyl hydrazone, 147
42. Crotonaldehyde	Liquid	b.p. 104	2, 4-dinitrophenyl hydrazone, 190
43. Benzaldehyde C_6H_5CHO	Liquid	b.p. 179	2,4-dinitrophenyl hydrazone, 237
44. Salicylaldehyde 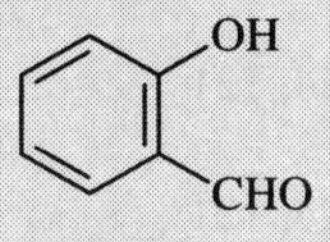	Liquid	b.p. 196°	Phenylhydrazone, 142
45. Vanillin 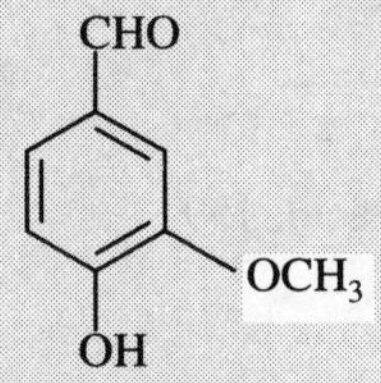	Soiid	m.p. 80	Phenylhydrazone, 105
46. Cinnamaldehyde $C_6H_5CH{=}CHCHO$	Liquid	b.p. 252	Phenylhydrazone, 168
47. Acetone CH_3COCH_3	Liquid	b.p. 56	2,4-dinitrophenyl hydrazone, 126
48. Acetophenone $C_6H_5COCH_3$	Liquid	b.p. 202	2,4-dinitrophenyl hydrazone, 250
49. Benzophenone $C_6H_5COC_6H_5$	Liquid	b.p. 49	2,4-dinitrophenyl hydrazone, 239
50. Ethylmethyl ketone $C_2H_5COCH_3$	Liquid	b.p. 80	2,4-dinitrophenyl hydrazone, 115
51. Cyclohexanone	Liquid	b.p. 156	hydrazone, 162
			Adipic acid, 152

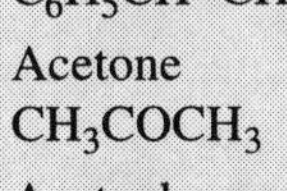

F. Ether

Compound	State	m.p. or b.p., °C	Derivative, m.p., °C
52. Ether $C_2H_5OC_2H_5$	Liquid	b.p. 35	—
53. Anisole $C_6H_5OCH_3$	Liquid	b.p. 154	—

(Contd.)

Compound	State	m.p. or b.p., °C	Derivative, m.p., °C
G. Carbohydrates			
54. D-Glucose	Solid	m.p. 90	Osazone, 205
($C_6H_{12}O_6.H_2O$)			(Formed in 5 minutes)
55. D-Fructose	Solid	m.p. 95–105	Osazone, 205
$C_6H_{12}O_6$			(Formed in 2 minutes)
56. Lactose (hydrates)	Solid	m.p. 203	Osazone, 208
$C_{12}H_{12}O_{11}.H_2O$			(Formed in 90 minutes)
57. Sucrose	Solid	m.p. 185	Octa-acetate, 67
$C_{12}H_{22}O_{11}$			
58. Starch	Solid	Decomp.	...
$(C_6H_{10}O_5)_n$		without melting	
59. Maltose	Solid	100 (decomp.)	Osazone, m.p. 206
$C_{12}H_{12}O_{11}$			
H. Esters			
60. Ethyl acetate	Liquid	b.p. 77	Anilide, 115
$CH_3COOC_2H_5$			
61. Methyl benzoate	Liquid	b.p. 199	Benzoic acid, 121
$C_6H_5COOCH_3$			
62. Ethyl benzoate	Liquid	b.p. 213	Benzoic acid, 121
$C_6H_5COOC_2H_5$			
63. Phenyl benzoate	Solid	b.p. 68	Benzoic acid, 121
64. Methyl salicylate	Liquid	b.p. 223	Salicylic acid, 159
65. Phenyl salicylate	Solid	m.p. 43	Benzoyl, 80
		b.p. 173	Salicylic acid, 159
I. Hydrocarbons			
66. Benzene	Liquid	b.p. 80	m-Dinitrotoluene, 90
			Picrate, 84
67. Toluene	Liquid	b.p. 111	2,4-Dinitrotoluene, 71
$C_6H_5CH_3$			
68. Diphenyl (Biphenyl)	Solid	m.p. 69	p,p-Dinitrodiphenyl, 237
C_6H_5–C_6H_5			

(Contd.)

Compound	State	m.p. or b.p., °C	Derivative, m.p., °C
69. Naphthalene 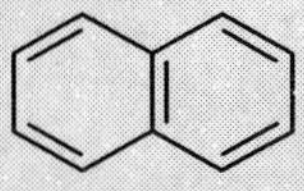	Solid	m.p. 80	Picrate, 152
70. Anthracene 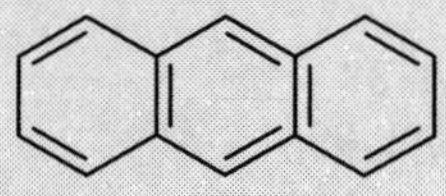	Solid	m.p. 216°	Picrate, 135°
71. Phenanthrene	Solid	m.p. 100	Picrate, 144
			9-Bromophenanthrene, 65

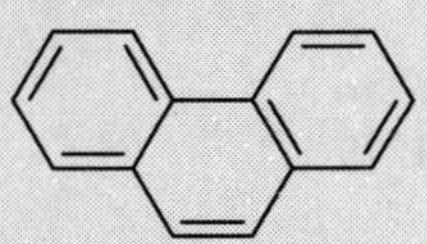

J. Amino compounds

Compound	State	m.p. or b.p., °C	Derivative, m.p., °C
72. Ethyl amine $C_2H_5NH_2$	Liquid	b.p. 19	Benzoyl, 71
			Picrate, 170
73. Benzyl amine $C_6H_5CH_2NH_2$	Liquid	b.p. 185	Acetyl, 60
			Benzoyl, 105
74. Ethyl aniline $C_6H_5NHC_2H_5$	Liquid	b.p. 205	Acetyl, 65
			Benzoyl, 60
75. Aniline $C_6H_5NH_2$	Liquid	b.p. 184	Acetyl, 114
			Benzoyl, 163
76. o-Toluidine	Liquid	b.p. 200	Acetyl, 112
			Benzoyl, 143
			Picrate, 214
77. m-Toluidine	Solid	b.p. 203	Acetyl, m.p. 66
			Benzoyl, m.p. 125
			Picrate, 195
78. p-Toluidine	Solid	m.p. 45	Acetyl, 148
		b.p. 200	Benzoyl, 158
79. o-Anisidine	Solid	m.p. 5	Acetyl, 88
			Benzoyl, 60
80. m-Anisidine	Liquid	b.p. 251	Acetyl, 81
			Picrate, 169
81. p-Anisidine	Solid	m.p. 57	Acetyl, 130
			Benzoyl, 153

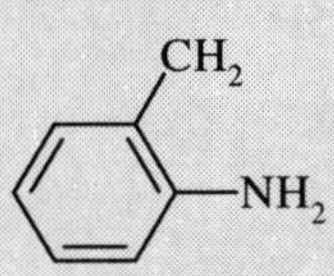

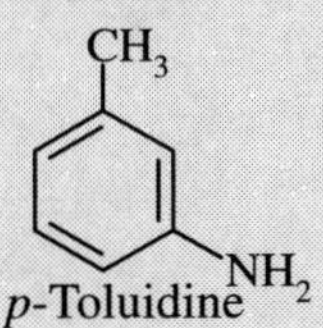

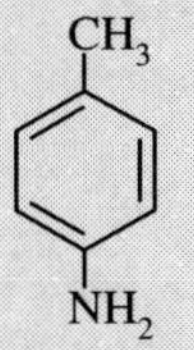

(Contd.)

Compound	State	m.p. or b.p., °C	Derivative, m.p., °C
82. α-Naphthylamine	Solid	m.p. 50	Acetyl, 160
			Benzoyl, 161
			Picrate, 163
83. o-Chloroaniline	liquid	b.p. 209	Acetyl, 88
			Benzoyl, 99
84. m-Chloroaniline 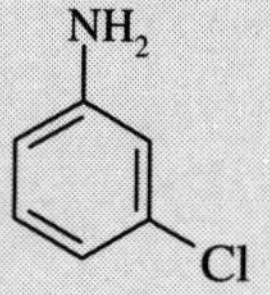	Liquid	b.p. 230	Acetyl, 79
85. β-Naphthylamine	Solid	m.p. 113	Acetyl, 134
			Benzoyl, 162
			Picrate, 195
86. Methyl aniline $C_6H_5NH-CH_3$	Liquid	b.p. 194	Acetyl, 103
			Benzoyl, 63
			Picrate, 145
87. Diethyl aniline $C_6H_5NH(C_2H_5)_2$	liquid	b.p. 216	Picrate, 142
88. Diphenylamine $C_6H_5-NH-C_6H_5$	Solid	m.p. 54	Acetyl, 103
			Benzoyl, 180
			Picrate, 182
89. Dimethylaniline $C_6H_5NH(CH_3)_2$	Liquid	b.p. 193	Picrate, 163
90. Pyridine C_5H_5N	Liquid	b.p. 115	Picrate, 167
91. Quinoline 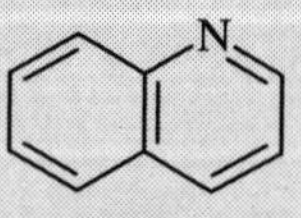	Liquid	b.p. 238	Picrate, 203

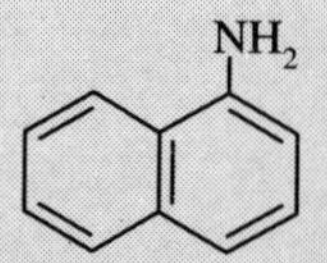

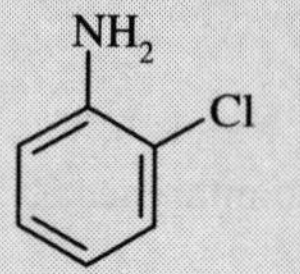

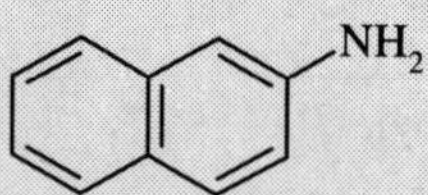

K. Nitro compounds

Compound	State	m.p. or b.p., °C	Derivative, m.p., °C
92. Nitrobenzene $C_6H_5NO_2$	Liquid	b.p. 210	*m*-Dinitrobenzene, 90
93. *m*-Dinitrobenzene 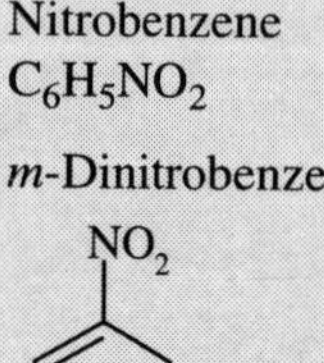	Solid	m.p. 90	*m*-Nitroaniline, 114

(*Contd.*)

Compound	State	m.p. or b.p., °C	Derivative, m.p., °C
94. *o*-Nitrotoluene	Liquid	b.p. 220	2,4-Dinitrotoluene, 70
			o-Nitrobenzoic acid,148

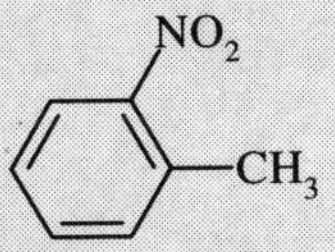

NO_2
CH_3

L. Amides

95. Acetamide CH_3CONH_2	Solid	m.p. 82	Anilide, 141
96. Benzamide $C_6H_5CONH_2$	Solid	m.p. 129	Anilide, 160
97. Urea $NH_2CO.NH_2$	Solid	m.p. 132	Urea nitrate, 163
			Anilide, 238
			Biuret, 192
			Oxalate,171
98. Salicylamide	Solid	m.p. 139	Acetyl, m.p.135
			Benzoyl, m.p.143

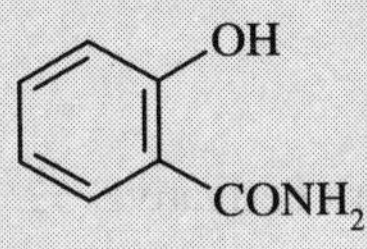

OH
CONH_2

M. Imide

99. Succinimide 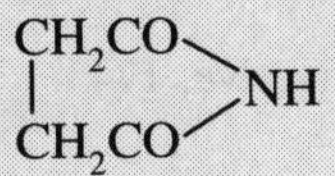	Solid	m.p. 125	Succinanil, m.p.156

CH_2CO
CH_2CO NH

100. Phthalimide 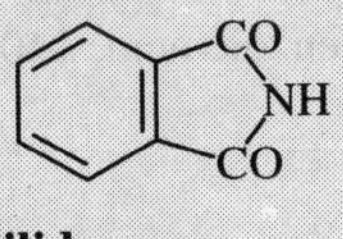	Solid	m.p. 233	Phthalic acid, m.p.196

CO
NH
CO

N. Anilides

101. Acetanilide C_6H_5-$NHCOCH_3$	Solid	m.p. 114	*p*-Bromoacetanilide, 168
102. Benzanilide C_6H_5-$NHCOC_6H_5$	Solid	m.p. 162	Benzoic acid, 121
			p-Bromoderivative, 204
103. *p*-Bromoacetanilide 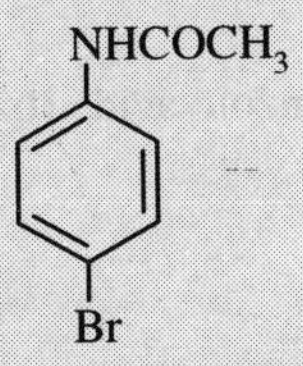	Solid	m.p. 168	*p*-Bromoaniline, 66

NHCOCH_3
Br

104. *p*-Nitroacetanilide 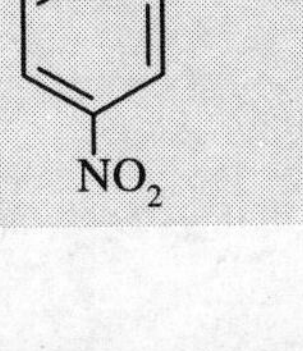	Solid	m.p. 216	*p*-aminoacetanilide, 163

NHCOCH_3
NO_2

(Contd.)

Compound	State	m.p. or b.p., °C	Derivative, m.p., °C
O. Quinones, anhydride			
105. Anthraquinone	Solid	m.p. 286	Monoximes, 224
106. Phthalic anhydride	Solid	m.p. 132	Phthalimide, 223
P. Compounds containing halogen atom (such compounds are immiscible with water)			
107. Chloroform $CHCl_3$	Liquid	b.p. 61	---
108. Iodoform CHI_3	Solid	m.p. 119	---
109. Carbon tetrachloride CCl_4	Liquid	b.p. 78	---
110. Chlorobenzene C_6H_5Cl	Liquid	b.p. 132	2,4-Dinitro derivative, 52
111. Bromobenzene C_6H_5Br	Liquid	b.p. 156	2,4-Dinitro derivative, 75
112. Iodobenzene C_6H_5I	Liquid	b.p. 188	*p*-Nitro derivative, 174
113. Benzyl chloride $C_6H_5CH_2Cl$	Liquid	b.p. 179	*p*-Nitro derivative, 71
114. *o*-Chlorotoluene	Liquid	b.p. 159	*o*-Chlorobenzoic acid, 140
115. *m*-Chlorotoluene	Liquid	b.p. 162	*m*-Chlorobenzoic acid, 153
116. *p*-Chlorotoluene	Liquid	b.p. 162	*m*-Chlorobenzoic acid, 162
Q. Sulphonic acids			
117. Benzene sulphonic acid $C_6H_5SO_3H$	Solid	m.p. 65	Amide, 153 Anilide, 110

(Contd.)

Compound	State	m.p. or b.p., °C	Derivative, m.p., °C
118. *p*-Toluene sulphonic acid CH₃—〈ring〉—SO₃H	Solid	m.p. 92	Amide, 137 Anilide, 103
119. Sulphanilic acid H₂N—〈ring〉—SO₃H	Solid	m.p. 288	2,4,6-Tribromo, 119 Sulphonamide, 164
R. Thioureas			
120. Thiourea H₂NCSNH₂	Solid	m.p. 180	Xanthyl, 136 Thiourea hydrochloride, 136
121. Phenylthiourea C₆H₅NH-CS-NH₂	Solid	m.p. 154	Thiocarbanilide, 153
S. Anhydrides			
122. Succinic anhydride (CH₂CO)₂O	Solid	m.p. 119	Anilide, 229
123. Maleic anhydride CH-CO ⟩O CH-CO	Solid	m.p. 130.5	Anilide, 187
T. Mercaptans			
124. Thiophenol C₆H₅SH	Liquid	b.p. 169	Benzoate, 149 2,4-Dinitrophenyl sulphone, 161
125. Benzyl mercaptan C₆H₅CH₂SH	Liquid	b.p. 194	Benzoyl, 30 2,4-Dinitrophenyl thioether, 130

Preparation of Derivatives

Derivatives are prepared on the basis of the functional group present in organic compounds. The derivatives are generally solid in nature and possess sharp melting point. It is the terminal step of qualitative analysis of organic compounds. The determination of melting point further confirms the presence of specific compound with particular functional group.

1. CARBOXYLIC ACIDS

(a) Amide

Shake the acid (0.5 g) with phosphorus pentachloride (1.5 ml) or thionyl chloride (1.5 ml) till the vigorous reaction ceases. Warm the solution gently for 30 minutes and then cool it. Now add cautiously concentrated ammonia solution (10.0 ml), stir, cool and filter the product (acid amide). Wash the acid amide with cold water, crystallize from water and dry it.

$$RCOOH + PCl_5 \longrightarrow RCOCl + POCl_3 + HCl$$
$$\text{Acid} \qquad\qquad\qquad \text{Acid chloride}$$

$$RCOCl + NH_4OH \longrightarrow RCONH_2 + HCl + H_2O$$
$$\text{Amide}$$

(b) p-Nitrobenzyl Ester

Dissolve a small amount of the compound in minimum amount of water or ethanol. Add a drop of phenolphthalein followed by addition of sufficient 20% aqueous potassium hydroxide solution till a permanent pink colour is obtained. Now add a little amount of the carboxylic acid till pink colour disappears and then evaporate the contents to dryness. Add p-nitrobenzyl chloride (0.5 g), water (2 ml) and ethanol (6 ml) to the solid mass. Reflux the contents for half an hour, cool and add water (5 ml). Filter the product, wash with cold water and crystallize from ethanol.

$$R\text{—}COOH + ClCH_2\text{—}\langle\text{—}\rangle\text{—}NO_2 \longrightarrow RCOOCH_2\text{—}\langle\text{—}\rangle\text{—}NO_2 + HCl$$

$$\text{p-Nitrobenzyl chloride} \qquad\qquad\qquad \text{p-Nitrobenzyl ester}$$

(c) Anilide or p-Toluidide

It is similar to amide derivative. If aniline or p-toluidine is added in place of ammonia solution, anilide or p-toluidide is obtained respectively. Shake the acid (0.5 g) with phosphorus pentachloride (0.5 ml) or thionyl chloride (1.5 ml) till the vigorous reaction ceases. Warm the solution gently and cool it. Add aniline or *p*-toluidine (1 ml) and shake the reaction mixture vigorously. If necessary, warm and then cool. Filter off the anilide or toluidide, wash it with cold water, crystallize from ethanol and dry it.

$$RCOOH + H_2NC_6H_5 \longrightarrow RCONHC_6H_5 + H_2O$$

Aniline — Anilide

$$RCOOH + H_2N\text{—}\bigcirc\text{—}CH_3 \longrightarrow RCONH\text{—}\bigcirc\text{—}CH_3 + H_2O$$

p-Toluidine — p-Toluidide

2. ALCOHOL

(a) Acetate

Take the alcohol (1 g), fused sodium acetate (0.5 g) and acetic anhydride (5 ml) in a conical flask. Shake and heat the mixture on a water bath for 30 minutes. Pour the hot solution into ice cold water (75 ml) with vigorous shaking. Keep the solution for sometime and filter the product. Wash with water and crystallize from ethanol.

$$ROH + (CH_3CO)_2O \xrightarrow{CH_3COONa} ROCOCH_3 + CH_3COOH$$

Alcohol   Acetic anhydride   Acetate

(b) Benzoate (Schotten-Baumann's method)

Take the alcohol (1 ml), acetone (10 ml), benzoyl chloride (5 ml) and aqueous sodium hydroxide solution (50 ml) in a small flask. Cool, cork and shake the flask vigorously till the odour of benzoyl chloride disappears. Filter off the solid compound, wash well with water and crystallize from ethanol.

$$ROH + ClCOC_6H_5 \longrightarrow ROCOC_6H_5 + HCl$$

Alcohol   Benzoyl
              chloride

(c) 3,5-Dinitrobenzoate

Dissolve the dry alcohol (0.5 g) in dry pyridine (5 ml). Add to this, solution of 3,5-dinitrobenzoyl chloride. Heat the mixture under refluxing condition for about 30 minutes, cool and pour into dilute hydrochloric acid (30 ml) when 3,5-dinitrobenzoate separates out. Wash the solid product with dilute sodium bicarbonate solution and then recrystallize from ethanol or aqueous ethanol or benzene.

$$ROH + \underset{\substack{O_2N \quad\quad NO_2 \\ \text{3,5-Dinitrobenzoyl Chloride}}}{\overset{COCl}{\bigcirc}} \longrightarrow \underset{\substack{O_2N \quad\quad NO_2 \\ \text{3,5-Dinitrobenzoate}}}{\overset{COOR}{\bigcirc}} + HCl$$

3. ESTERS

The most general derivatives of esters are their hydrolysed products, acids and alcohols or phenols.

A. *HYDROLYTIC PRODUCTS*

(i) Hydrolysis by Sodium Methoxide

Dissolve sodium metal (1 g) in pure methyl alcohol (10 ml) by warming in a dry flask fitted with a reflux condenser. Cool the solution and then treat it with the ester (1 g) and water (0.5 ml). A precipitate of carboxylic acid often separates out immediately; in case no precipitate is obtained, boil the reaction mixture for 30–60 minutes. Filter off the product, wash with little cold methyl alcohol and identify the acid as usual.

The alcoholic portion is isolated by careful distilling off the methanol from the filtrate. It is then characterized as usual.

(ii) Hydrolysis by Aqueous Alkali

Take the ester (5 g) in 30% potassium hydroxide solution (40 ml) in a conical flask. Boil the contents under reflux until hydrolysis is completed as indicated by a change in odour or appearance of mixture.

(a) Isolation of Alcohol

Distill off a test portion of the liquid, separate the distillate with potassium carbonate, in case a distinct layer of alcohol separates out on standing; remove this layer, dry it with anhydrous potassium carbonate and identify the alcohol.

(b) Isolation of Acid

Acidify the portion of the residue in the flask with dilute sulphuric acid, in case acid precipitates out, acidify whole of the residue. Filter off the acid, recrystallize and identify by melting point. In case no precipitate is obtained on acidification of reaction liquor, neutralize it to phenolphthalein and use the alkali salt of the acid for preparing a suitable derivative.

B. *HYDRAZIDE DERIVATIVE*

Heat the ester (0.5 g) with hydrazine hydrate (0.5 ml) on a water bath for 2–3 hours or until a test portion solidifies on cooling. Filter the solid and crystallize from water or ethanol.

$$R–COOR_1 + H_2N–NH_2 \longrightarrow RCONHNH_2 + R_1OH$$
$$\text{Hydrazide}$$

4. ALDEHYDES AND KETONES

A. *OXIME*

(i) For Aldehydes and Aliphatic Ketones

Dissolve $NH_2OH.HCl$ (0.5 g) and sodium acetate (0.5 g) in water (3 ml). Add to it carbonyl compound (0.5 g), heat the mixture on the water bath and add ethanol dropwise with shaking until a clear solution is obtained. Continue refluxing to complete the reaction. Cool down the contents to crystallize out the oxime derivative.

(ii) For Aromatic and Some Cyclic Ketones

Dissolve the ketone (1 g) and $NH_2OH.HCl$ (0.6 g) in a mixture of ethanol (3 ml) and water (1 ml). Add sodium hydroxide (1 g), shake the mixture, and reflux for 30 minutes. Cool down the reaction mixture, add water (20 ml) and shake. Filter the unchanged ketone, if any, and acidify the filtrate with dilute hydrochloric acid. Filter off the oxime.

B. *SEMICARBAZONE*

Dissolve semicarbazide hydrochloride (0.5 g) and sodium acetate (0.75 g) in water (5 ml). To the resulting solution, add the carbonyl compound (0.5 m) and shake well. In case a clear solution is not obtained, add methanol dropwise, with shaking. Shake the mixture and allow to stand when the precipitate of semicarbazone will be separated out, if not, heat the solution on water bath for 10 minutes and cool. Filter off the semicarbazone and recrystallize it from ethanol or glacial acetic acid or benzene.

$$\underset{\diagdown}{\overset{\diagup}{C}} = O + H_2NCONHNH_2 \longrightarrow \underset{\diagdown}{\overset{\diagup}{C}} = N - CONHNH_2$$

$$\text{Semicarbazide} \qquad\qquad\qquad \text{Semicarbazone}$$

5. CARBOHYDRATES

(a) Osazone

Take the powdered sugar (0.5 g) in a clean tube. In another test tube, dissolve phenylhydrazine hydrochloride (0.4 g) and crystalline sodium acetate (0.6 g) in cold water (4 ml) and add this solution to sugar. Loosely cork the test tube, immerse it in a boiling water bath with periodical shaking, and note the exact time required for the first appearance of a turbidity or precipitate of osazone. Cool the solution, filter the precipitate and recrystallize from ethanol.

(b) Acetate

Dissolve the carbohydrate (0.5 g), powdered anhydrous sodium acetate (0.5 g) and acetic anhydride (3 ml) in glacial acetic acid (5 ml) by refluxing on a water bath. Further heat the solution for 2 hours. Pour cautiously the hot reaction mixture in cold water (25 ml) and stir the solution vigorously to decompose the excess of acetic anhydride. Filter off the product, wash with cold water and recrystallize from ethanol.

(c) Oxime

See carbonyl aldehydes and ketones.

$$\underset{R}{\overset{CHO}{\underset{|}{\overset{|}{CHOH}}}} \quad \text{or} \quad \underset{R}{\overset{CH_2OH}{\underset{|}{\overset{|}{C=O}}}} \quad \xrightarrow{H_2NOH} \quad \underset{R}{\overset{CH=NOH}{\underset{|}{\overset{|}{CHOH}}}} \quad \text{or} \quad \underset{R}{\overset{CH_2OH}{\underset{|}{\overset{|}{C=NOH}}}}$$

6. PHENOLS

(a) Acetate

Since the acetate of monohydric phenols are usually liquids, acetates are prepared only in the case of polyhydric phenols and in naphthols.

Take the phenolic compound (1 g) in a clean dry test tube, add acetic anhydride (2.5 ml) and a drop of concentrated sulphuric acids. Cork the tube, shake it vigorously for 4–5 minutes and then transfer the reaction mixture to cold water (5 ml). Stir the contents with a glass rod till the oil solidifies. Filter, wash with water and recrystallize from hot water or dilute ethanol.

$$\underset{\text{Phenol}}{\langle\!\!\!\bigcirc\!\!\!\rangle\!-\!OH} + (CH_3CO)_2O \longrightarrow \underset{\text{Phenyl acetate}}{\langle\!\!\!\bigcirc\!\!\!\rangle\!-\!OCOCH_3} + CH_3COOH$$

(b) Benzoate

Dissolve the phenol (1.0 g) in acetone (5 ml) and add benzoyl chloride (2.5 ml) to it. Add aqueous sodium hydroxide (10 ml) gradually with cooling and shaking, then further add NaOH solution (40 ml). Stopper the tube or the flask and shake vigorously till the odour of benzoyl chloride has disappeared. The final solution should be alkaline to litmus. Filter the solid benzoyl derivative, wash first with dilute hydrochloric acid, then with cold water, and recrystallize from ethanol or acetone (in case of resorcinol and 2–naphthol) or benzene (in case of quinol and phloroglucinol).

$$\text{Phenol} \quad \text{Benzoyl chloride} \quad\quad\quad\quad \text{Phenyl benzoate}$$

Phenol—OH + C$_6$H$_5$COCl ⟶ Phenol—OCOC$_6$H$_5$ + HCl

(c) Bromo Derivative

Dissolve or suspend the phenol (2.0 g) in water (100 ml) and then add a solution of bromine (20 ml) in glacial acetic acid (10 ml) dropwise with vigorous shaking until faint yellow colour persists. Filter off the precipitated bromo derivative, wash thoroughly with water and recrystallize from ethanol.

$$\text{Phenol} + 3Br_2 \longrightarrow \text{Tribromophenol} + 3HBr$$

(d) Picrates

Dissolve the compound (0.1 g) in the minimum quantity of boiling ethanol and add this solution to a solution of picric acid (little more quantity). Shake, cool the reaction mixture and filter the solid which separates out. Crystallize with ethanol or benzene.

7. PRIMARY AND SECONDARY AMINES

A. ACETYL DERIVATIVE

(i) For Primary Amines

Heat the amine (0.5 g), glacial acetic acid (0.5 ml) and acetic anhydride (1.5 ml) with occasional shaking for 15 minutes. Cool the reaction mixture. If the oil does not solidify, stir with glass rod and cool in an ice bath. Filter the acetylated derivative and recrystallize from water or aqueous ethanol.

$$R{-}NH_2 \xrightarrow[CH_3COOH]{(CH_3CO)_2O} R{-}NHCOCH_3$$

(ii) For Secondary Amine

Warm a mixture of the amine (0.5 g) and acetic anhydride (0.5 g) on the water bath for 5–10 minutes. Cool, add water (3 ml) and stir the mixture until the derivative is solidified.

$$\begin{array}{c} R_1 \\ {>}NH \\ R_2 \end{array} + (CH_3CO)_2O \xrightarrow{Heat} \begin{array}{c} R_1 \\ {>}NCOCH_3 \\ R_2 \end{array} + CH_3COOH$$

(b) Benzoyl Derivative

Suspend the compound (0.5 g) in 5% sodium hydroxide solution (10 ml) in a small conical flask. Add dropwise benzoyl chloride (1 ml), stopper the flask and shake vigorously in cooling condition for 5–10 minutes. Filter the product, wash the derivative with water and recrystallize from ethanol.

$$R—NH_2 + C_6H_5COCl \longrightarrow R—NHCOC_6H_5 + HCl$$

$$\begin{array}{c} R_1 \\ \diagdown \\ \diagup \quad NH + C_6H_5COCl \longrightarrow \\ R_2 \end{array} \qquad \begin{array}{c} R_1 \\ \diagdown \\ \diagup \quad NCOC_6H_5 + HCl \\ R_2 \end{array}$$

(c) 2,4-Dinitro phenyl Derivative

Take the amine (1 g), 2,4-dinitro-chlorobenzene (1 g), ethanol (10 ml) and a slight excess of anhydrous potassium carbonate or sodium acetate in a conical flask. Reflux the contents after thorough mixing for 30 minutes. Pour the contents into cold water and filter off the product. Wash the derivative with water and recrystallize from ethanol.

Amine   2,4-Dinitro chlorobenzene   2,4-Dinitro phenyl derivative

(d) Bromo Derivative

A few aromatic amines give easily identifiable product on bromination (see phenols).

(e) Picrate

Make a concentrated solution of picric acid in acetone. To this solution (2 ml), add concentrated solution of amine in acetone (2 ml), shake and allow to stand, yellow precipitate of picrate is formed.

$$R–NH_2 + C_6H_2(NO_2)_3OH \longrightarrow R–NH_2C_6H_2(NO_2)_3.OH$$
$$\text{Picric acid}$$

8. TERTIARY AMINES

(a) Methiodide

Take the tertiary amine (0.5 g) in a test tube and treat it with methyl iodide (0.5 ml) at room temperature. Keep the reaction mixture undisturbed for 5 minutes, then heat under reflux on the water bath for 5 minutes and finally cool in ice cold water. The quarternary salt will be crystallized out and, if not, scratch the sides of the tube with a glass rod. Recrystallization may be done from absolute ethanol, acetone or glacial acetic acid.

$$\begin{array}{c} R_1 \\ \diagdown \\ R_2 \!-\! N + CH_3I \longrightarrow \\ \diagup \\ R_3 \end{array} \qquad \begin{array}{c} R_1 \\ \diagdown \\ R_2 \!-\! N^+\!\!-\!CH_3.I^- \\ \diagup \\ R_3 \end{array}$$

Tertiary Amine   Methiodide

(b) Picrate

See secondary amine, section 'e'.

$$R_2\!-\!\overset{R_1}{\underset{R_3}{N}} + C_6H_2(NO_2)_3OH \longrightarrow R_2\!-\!\overset{R_1}{\underset{R_3}{N}}\!\cdot\! C_6H_2(NO_2)_3\!\cdot\! OH$$

Picric acid   Picrate

(c) p-Nitroso Compound

Dissolve the amine (0.1 g) in an excess of 5N hydrochloric acid (3 ml) and cool to 0°C temperature in an ice bath. Add cold sodium nitrite solution dropwise until only a very slight excess of nitroso acid is present. Filter the crystalline product.

Dimethylaniline + HONO ⟶ p-Nitrosodimethylaniline

9. AMIDES, IMIDES AND ANILIDES

(a) Hydrolysis

Take the compound (0.5 g) and excess of 25% sodium hydroxide solution in a flask fitted with a reflux condenser. Reflux the contents until ammonia has been driven off completely and then cool. Add concentrated hydrochloric acid dropwise till the reaction mixture becomes strongly acidic. Filter the insoluble acid derivative and recrystallize from ethanol.

$$RONH_2 + H_2O \longrightarrow RCOOH + NH_3$$

$$RCONHR_2 + H_2O \longrightarrow RCOOH + R_2NH_2$$

(b) Xanthylamide

Add the substance (0.5 g) to 7% xanthydrol in glacial acetic acid (7 ml). Shake the contents well and then allow to stand for 10 minutes. If solid derivative is not obtained, heat the contents on a water bath for 30 minutes and then cool when solid xanthylamide is obtained. Filter it and recrystallize from acetic acid.

RCONH₂ + Xanthydrol ⟶ Xanthylamide + H₂O

(c) Miscellaneous

Derivative of urea: Make a concentrated solution of urea and oxalic acid in a separate test tube. Mix both the solution with shaking; a white precipitate of urea oxalate separate out, m.p. 171°C.

10. SULPHONIC ACIDS

(a) Sulphonamide

Mix dry sulphonic acid (1 g) and with phosphorus pentachloride (2 g). Heat the mixture on a oil bath at 150°C for about 30 minutes. When the reaction is completed, cool the contents and treat with cold water (15 ml). Stir and wash the sulphonyl chloride twice with cold water by decantation. Now add concentrated ammonia solution (5 ml) with stirring. Heat the reaction mixture on a water bath for 5–10 minutes and then cool. The amide will start crystallizing out. Recrystallize the derivative from water or aqueous ethanol.

$$SO_3H \quad + PCl_5 \longrightarrow SO_2Cl \quad + POCl_3 + HCl$$

Sulphonic acid   Sulphonyl chloride

$$SO_2Cl \quad + NH_3 \longrightarrow SO_2NH_2 \quad + HCl$$

Sulphonyl chloride   Benzenesulphonamide

(b) Sulphananilide

Prepare the sulphonyl chloride as above in method (a). Dissolve it in acetone and treat with pure aniline (0.5 ml) dissolved in acetone together with dilute sodium hydroxide solution (25 ml). Shake the mixture for 10 minutes and extract with ether to remove excess of aniline. Acidify the product, filter and recrystallize from ethanol.

$$SO_2Cl \quad \xrightarrow[\text{Aniline}]{H_2N-} \quad SO_2NH-$$

Benzene sulphonyl chloride   Sulphananilide

11. HYDROCARBONS

(a) Nitration of Halogen Hydrocarbons

Take the compound (1 g or 1 ml) in a dry test tube, add to it concentrated nitric acid (1.5 ml) and concentrated sulphuric acid (1.5 ml). Place the test tube in boiling water for 5 minutes with occasional shaking. Cool down, add water (1 ml) and shake. Filter off the product, wash with cold water and crystallize from ethanol.

(b) Picrate

Make a concentrated solution of picric acid in acetone. To this solution (2 ml), add concentrated solution of hydrocarbon (2 ml), e.g. naphthalene in acetone. Shake well, warm and allow to stand, a yellow precipitate of picrate is formed.

$$C_{10}H_8 + C_6H_2(NO_2)_3OH \longrightarrow C_{10}H_8C_6H_2(NO_2)_8OH$$

Naphthalene   Picric acid   Naphthalene picrate

(c) Oxidation products (by KMnO₄)

Add xylene (1.5 g) or ethyl benzene (1.5 g) or toluene (0.75 g) or a substituted toluene (0.75 g) of the compound to a solution of sodium carbonate (1 g) and potassium permanganate (3 g) in water (50 ml). Reflux the mixture until potassium permanganate colour disappears. Filter off precipitated manganese dioxide and acidify the filtrate with concentrated hydrochloric acid. Filter the precipitated acid and identify it.

Cl—C₆H₄—CH₃ $\xrightarrow{\text{KMnO}_4}$ Cl—C₆H₄—COOH

p-Chlorotoluene   p-Chlorobenzoic acid

12. NITRO COMPOUNDS

Aromatic hydrocarbons and most of their halogen and nitro derivatives can be nitrated with the help of suitable nitrating mixture. In fact, there is no general method for the preparation of nitro derivatives since the experimental conditions vary with the compound to be nitrated.

A. *NITRO DERIVATIVE*

(i) Nitration with Concentrated Nitric Acid

Add the compound (1 g) portion-wise with shaking to concentrated nitric acid (5 ml) at room temperature. Stir the mixture for 10 minutes and add some crushed ice when the product will be crystallized out either on standing or on scratching the sides of the test tube with a glass rod. Filter the product, wash with water and recrystallize.

[The above method is recommended for the mononitration of naphthalenes, alkyl-naphthalenes, halogen substituted naphthalenes and *p*-halogenophenols. For the mononitration of dihalogenobenzene and the dinitration of diphenyl, warm the mixture after adding the contents on a boiling water bath for 10 minutes, cool and then work as above.]

(ii) Nitration wtih Fuming Nitric Acid

Add the compound (1 g) portion-wise and with shaking to fuming nitric acid (5 ml) at 0°C. Stir the mixture at room temperature for 5–10 minutes, pour into ice and stir until the nitration product crystallizes out.

The method is recommended for the mononitration of dihalogenophenols, for the dinitration of mesitylene, dibenzyl and halogenophenols.

(iii) Nitration with a Mixture of Concentrated Nitric and Sulphuric Acids

Add the compound (1 g) dropwise with shaking to a mixture of concentrated sulphuric and nitric acids. Cool the solution either under tap or in ice cold water bath to 20–25°C. After standing for 10 minutes, pour the solution mixture onto ice and stir until the product solidifies.

The method is suitable for the dinitration of tetralin and anisole; for the mononitration of monohalogenobenzenes and for the dinitration of toluene, nitrophenols and *o*- and *p*-nitrotoluene and for the trinitration of dinitrophenols and *o*-nitroanisole.

(iv) Nitration with a Mixture of Fuming Nitric and Sulphuric Acids

Add the compound (1 g) dropwise to a mixture of fuming nitric acid (6 ml) and concentrated sulphuric acid (10 ml), with shaking. Heat the reaction mixture on a boiling water bath for 2–3 minutes, cool, pour into ice-water and stir until the product solidifies.

The method is suitable for the nitration for nitrobenzene, for the dinitration of benzene, mono- and di-halogenobenzenes and of o- and p-nitrotoluenes, for the trinitration of m-xylene and for tetranitration of diphenylmethane.

(B) *AMINO DERIVATIVE*

Nitro compounds can be easily reduced to the corresponding amino compounds in the presence of tin (or zinc) and hydrochloric acid, e.g. *p*-chloronitrobenzene.

Sn / HCl

p-Chloronitrobenzene   p-Chloroaniline

The corresponding amino derivative gives the derivatives of the amino group.

Place a small amount of the compound dissolved in ethanol in a conical flask. To this, add tin (Sn) pieces (2 g) and dilute hydrochloric acid (15–20 ml) in small portion with constant shaking after each addition. Reflux the mixture on a boiling water bath for 10–15 minutes. Decant off the hot solution, dissolve the tin hydroxide with the help of dilute (40%) sodium hydroxide solution and then extract the resulting solution several times with ether. Distill off the solvent ether and recrystallize the amino derivative with ethanol.

13. MISCELLANEOUS COMPOUNDS

DERIVATIVES OF THIOLS

Alkyl (or Aryl) 2,4-Dinitrophenyl Sulphides (or Thioethers)

Dissolve the mercaptan (0.5 g) in rectified spirit (10–15 ml) and add 10% sodium hydroxide solutions (2 ml). Mix the resulting sodium mercaptide solution with a solution of 2,4-dinitro-chlorobenzene (1 g) in rectified spirit (5 ml). Reaction may occur immediately with precipitation of the thioether. In any case, reflux the mixture for 10 minutes on a water bath in order to ensure the completeness of the reaction. Filter the hot solution rapidly; allow the solution to cool when the sulphide will crystallize out. Recrystallize from ethanol.

DERIVATIVES OF THIOUREA

S-Benzylisothiouronium Chloride

Place a mixture of benzyl chloride (2 g), thiourea (1 g) and rectified spirit (3 ml) in a 50 ml round bottomed flask fitted with a reflux condenser. Warm on a water bath. A sudden exothermic reaction occurs and all the thiourea passes into solution. Reflux the resulting yellow coloured solution for 30 minutes and then cool in ice. Filter the white crystals and dry in the air. Concentrate the filtrate to half of its original volume and thus obtain a further small crop of crystals. Recrystallize from 0.2N hydrochloric acid.

$$NH_2CSNH_2 + C_6H_5CH_2Cl \longrightarrow [C_6H_5CH_2\text{---}S\text{---}C\text{---}NH_2]^-\ Cl^-$$

Thiourea Benzyl chloride

$$^+NH_2$$

S-Benzyl isothiouronium chloride

Identification Test of Organic Drugs

The organic drugs are either obtained from natural sources or synthesized in laboratory. These drugs are identified on the bases of physical and chemical tests. Physical tests include determination of physical characters, e.g. shape, colour, solubility behaviour, specific rotation, refractive index and boiling or melting point. Chemical tests are carried out to perform some colour reactions which are based on functional groups present in the drug molecule.

In this chapter, identification tests are presented for some naturally occurring and synthetic organic drugs.

- Ascorbic acid
- Aspirin
- Analgin
- Acetazolamide

- Barbiturates
- Caffeine
- Chlorpromazine HCl
- Sulphacetamide

- Tannic acid
- Alkaloids
- Proteins
- Amino acid

- Chloramphenicol
- Chloroquine phosphate
- Procaine penicillin
- Paracetamol

ASCORBIC ACID OR VITAMIN C

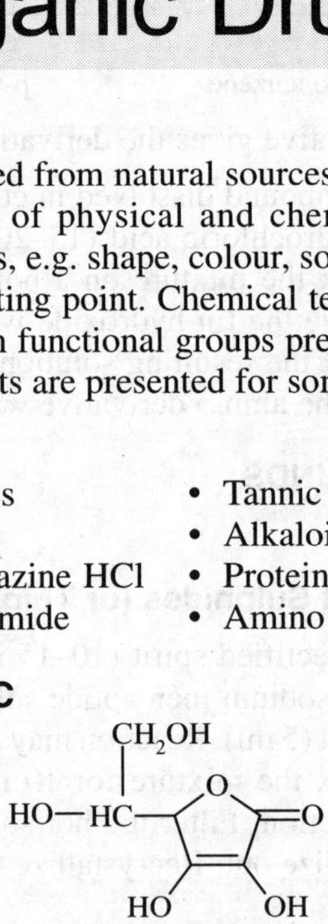

Ascorbic acid

Physical Properties

It is available as odourless, colourless crystals or white to pale yellow crystalline powder with acidic taste. It is freely soluble in water, slightly soluble in ethanol but insoluble in chloroform and ether.

Chemical Tests

(i) Add 2% w/v solution of ascorbic acid (2 ml) to a few ml of 2,6-dichlorophenol indophenol solution, the solution is decolourized.

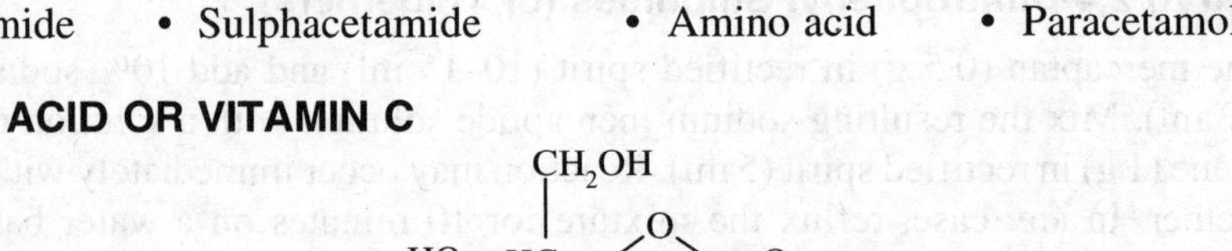

Dehydroascorbic acid

2,6-Dichlorophenol indophenol is blue-violet coloured dye and becomes colourless due to its reduction.

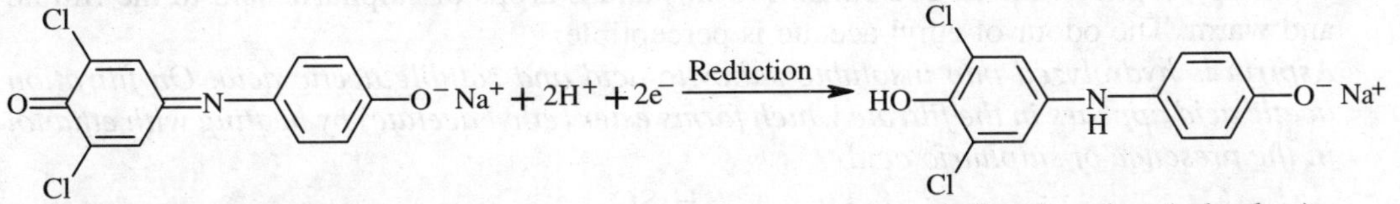

2,6-Dichlorophenol indophenol
(blue colour)

Reduced product (colourless)

(ii) Dilute 2% w/v solution of ascorbic acid (1 ml) with water (5 ml), add one drop of freshly prepared sodium nitroprusside and dilute sodium hydroxide solution (2 ml). Add hydrochloric acid (0.6 ml) dropwise with shaking. The yellow colour turns blue.

(iii) Dilute 2% w/v solution of ascorbic acid (2 ml) with water (2 ml), add sodium bicarbonate (100 mg) and ferrous sulphate (20 mg), shake well. A deep violet colour is produced which disappears on adding dilute sulphuric acid (5 ml).

(iv) Dissolve 0.10 g in 2.0 ml of water and add a few drops of nitric acid and a few drops of silver nitrate, a dark grey precipitate is produced.

Category

Antiscorbutic.

ASPIRIN
(Syn: Acetylsalicylic acid)

Chemical structure:

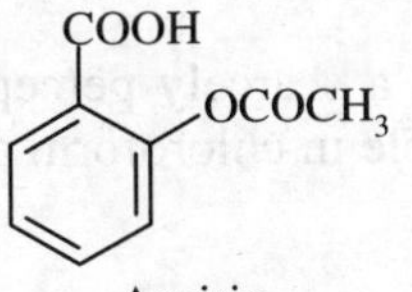

Aspirin
(2-Acetoxy benzoic acid)

Physical Properties

It is an odourless, colourless or white crystalline powder with slightly acidic taste. It is slightly soluble in water but soluble in ethanol, chloroform and ether.

Chemical Tests

(i) Boil aspirin (0.5 g) with sodium hydroxide solution (10 ml) for 5 minutes, cool and acidify with dilute sulphuric acid (10 ml). White precipitate is produced and the odour of acetic acid is perceptible. Filter the precipitate, dissolve in water and add ferric chloride solution; a deep violet colour is produced.

This test is based on the hydrolysis of aspirin into salicylic acid and acetic acid. Salicylic acid gives deep violet colour with ferric chloride solution due to the presence of phenolic group.

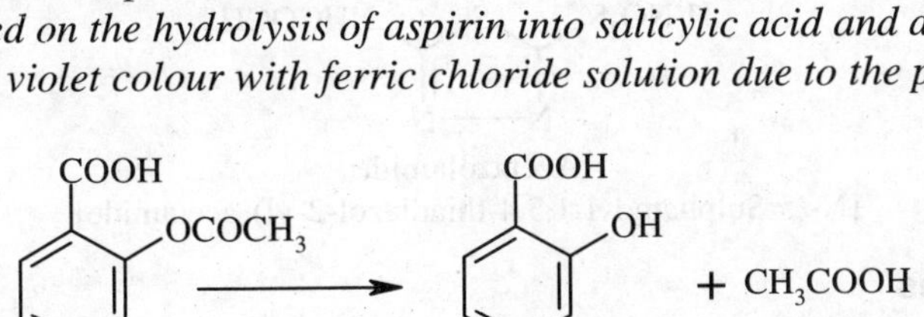

Aspirin

Salicylic acid

$+ CH_3COOH$

(ii) Boil aspirin (0.5 g) with sodium hydroxide solution (10 ml) for 3 minutes, cool and acidify with dilute sulphuric acid (10 ml). A white precipitate is produced and the odour of acetic acid is perceptible. Filter, add ethanol (3 ml) and 2 drops of sulphuric acid to the filtrate and warm. The odour of ethyl acetate is perceptible.

Aspirin is hydrolyzed into insoluble salicylic acid and soluble acetic acid. On filtration acetic acid appears in the filtrate which forms ester (ethyl acetate) by heating with ethanol in the presence of sulphuric acid.

$$CH_3COOH + C_2H_5OH \xrightarrow{\quad H_2SO_4 \quad} CH_3COOC_2H_5$$
$$\text{Ethyl acetate}$$

Category

Analgesic, antipyretic and anti-inflammatory and platelet aggregation inhibitor.

ANALGIN

Chemical structure:

Analgin
(1-Phenyl-2,3-dimethyl-5-pyrazolone-4-methyl aminomethyl sulphonate)

Physical Properties

It is a white crystalline powder with a scarcely perceptible yellowish tint, odourless, bitter taste. It is soluble in water but insoluble in chloroform and solvent ether.

Chemical Test

(i) Add a few drops of water to analgin powder (100 mg), then add ethanol (5 ml) and dilute hydrochloric acid (0.5 ml). To this solution, add potassium iodate solution (5 ml); crimson colour is produced which deepens on further addition of potassium iodate solution.

(ii) Boil analgin (200 mg) with dilute hydrochloric acid (2 ml), the characteristic odour of sulphur dioxide is produced followed by formaldehyde.

Category

Analgesic.

ACETAZOLAMIDE

Chemical structure:

Acetazolamide
[N-(5-Sulphamoyl-1,3,4-thiadiazol-2-yl) acetamide]

Physical Properties

It is white or yellowish white, odourless, tasteless crystalline powder. It is slightly soluble in water and ethanol but insoluble in chloroform and solvent ether.

Chemical Tests

(i) Triturate acetazolamide (0.5 g) with a mixture of water (5 ml), and 0.5 ml of sodium hydroxide solution (~ 80 g/litre). Add zinc powder (0.2 g), hydrochloric acid (0.5 ml) and mix well. Hydrogen sulphide gas is evolved which is recognized by its characteristic odour or by the use of lead nitrate paper which turns black on exposure.

(ii) To acetazolamide (25 mg), add water (5 ml), sodium hydroxide (4 ml) copper sulphate (2 ml). A bluish green colour or precipitate is produced.

Category

Diuretic, antiepileptic.

BARBITURATES

Barbiturates are cyclic ureides, used as hypnotic and sedative. They are found in two isomeric enolic and ketonic forms due to tautomerism.

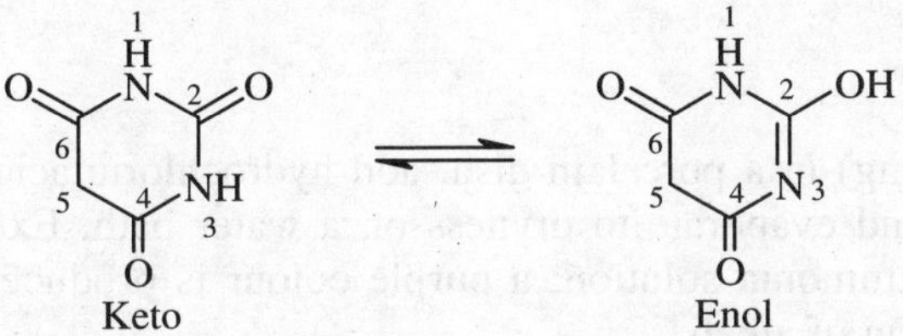

In alkaline solution, enolic form is favoured due to formation of salt. Substitution in barbituric acid at C-5 position by alkyl or aryl group gives the various types of barbiturates, differing in onset and duration of hypnotic action.

Physical Properties

Barbiturates are odourless, colourless or white crystalline powders with acidic character. They are slightly soluble in water but their corresponding sodium salt are soluble in water.

Chemical Test

(i) Boil a barbiturate (0.2 g) with sodium hydroxide solution (10 ml); ammonia is evolved.

(ii) Dissolve a barbiturate (0.18 g) in a mixture of sodium hydroxide (0.5 ml) and 10% w/v solution of pyridine (2 ml); add further pyridine solution (8 ml), copper sulphate solution (1 ml) with pyridine and set aside for 10 minutes, a specific colour is produced depending on barbiturate as shown above. For sodium salt, it is not necessary to add sodium hydroxide solution.

(iii) Barbiturates may be identified by preparation of their derivatives. For example, official identification test of amylobarbitone is based on preparation of its nitrobenzyl derivative by reaction with *p*-nitrobenzyl chloride.

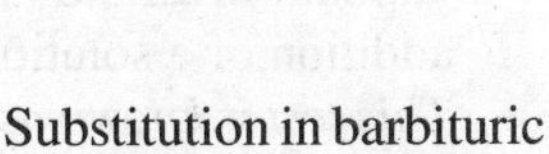

p-Nitrobenzyl chloride

Triturate amylobarbitone (0.6 g) with anhydrous sodium carbonate (0.15 g) and water (5 ml). Add a solution of *p*-nitrobenzyl chloride (0.45 g) in ethanol (10 ml) and warm on a water bath for 30 minutes. Cool, allow to stand for 1 hour, filter and wash the residue with sodium hydroxide (10 ml) and then with water. The residue after recrystallization melts at about 150°C or at about 168°C.

Category

Hypnotic and sedative.

CAFFEINE

Chemical structure:

Caffeine (1,3,7-Trimethylxanthine)

Physical Properties

It occurs as silky white crystals or white glistening needles or white crystalline powder, odourless with bitter taste. It is slightly soluble in water and ethanol but freely soluble in chloroform and boiling water.

Chemical Tests

 (i) Take caffeine (10 mg) in a porcelain dish, add hydrochloric acid (1 ml) and potassium chlorate (0.10 g) and evaporate to dryness on a water bath. Expose the residue to the vapours of dilute ammonia solution; a purple colour is produced which disappears on addition of a solution of alkali.

   This test is known as murexide test. A strong purple colour is produced due to formation of murexide (ammonium purpurate), a violet compound coloured.

 (ii) To a saturated solution of caffeine, add a few drops of tannic acid solution; a white precipitate is produced which is soluble in excess of the reagent.

Murexide

(iii) To a saturated solution of caffeine (5 ml), add 0.1N iodine solution (1.5 ml) until solution remains clear. Add a few drops of dilute hydrochloric acid; a brown precipitate is formed. Neutralize with sodium hydroxide solution, the precipitate is dissolved.

Category

CNS stimulant.

PHENOTHIAZINE

Phenothiazine is a tricyclic compound with two heteroatom, N and S present in central ring.

Phenothiazine is not sufficiently basic to form the stable salts with acid. Phenothiazine itself is used in veterinary practice as an anthelmintic and certain of its derivatives are of medicinal importance, e.g. chlorpromazine hydrochloride (antihistaminic drug).

Chlorpromazine Hydrochloride

Chemical structure:

Chlorpromazine hydrochloride

(3-(2′-Chlorophenothiazin-10yl) propyl-N,N-dimethyl ammonium chloride).

Physical Properties

It is a white or creamy white powder, odourless with very bitter taste.

Chemical Test

(i) Dissolve 10 mg in 5 ml of chloroform, add 1.0 ml of sodium metaperiodate (60 g/litre) and 2.0 ml of sulfuric acid. Shake vigorously and let the layers separate; a violet red colour that fades slowly on standing is produced in the aqueous layer, and the chloroform layer acquires a pink colour (distinction from promethazine).

(ii) Dissolve 10 mg in 5 ml of water, add 5 drops of ammonia solution, warm until oily drops separate and filter. To the filtrate add 1.0 ml of nitric acid and a few drops of silver nitrate solution—a white precipitate is produced. Separate the precipitate, wash it with water and add an excess of ammonia solution—the precipitate dissolves.

(iii) A solution (1 in 20) gives the reaction of chlorides as in ammonium chloride (Chapter 6).

Category

Central nervous system depressant, transquillizer and antiemetic.

SULPHONAMIDES

Sulphanilamide, *p*-aminobenzene sulphonamide, is the simplest sulphonamide.

The derivatives of sulphanilamide, used in medicine, may have variable substituents in place of hydrogen of sulphonamido group, e.g. sulphadiazine contains pyrimidine moiety.

Sulphadiazine

The *p*-amino group is essential for its activity and one of the hydrogen can be replaced only by such group which can provide again free amino group in the body. For example, phthalyl sulphathiazole and succinyl sulphathiazole.

Sulphonamides have the antibacterial activity.

Sulpha drugs containing free amino group can be identified by diazotization followed by coupling with alkaline β-naphthol solution to give dyes of orange-red colour.

Some sulphanilamides can be identified by the product of hydrolysis. For example, sulphacetamide on heating with 95% alc. solution in the presence of sulphuric acid gives the odour of ethyl acetate. Sulphaguanidine on alkaline hydrolysis forms ammonia.

Many sulphanilamide are characterized by the colours of copper complexes made by the action of copper sulphate in the alkaline solution.

SULPHACETAMIDE

Chemical structure:

$$CH_3CONHSO_2 \text{---} \bigcirc \text{---} NH_2$$

p-Acetylaminobenzene sulphonamide

Physical Properties

It is a white or yellowish white crystalline powder, odourless, with acidic and saline taste.

Chemical Test

(i) Dissolve sulphacetamide (50 mg) in warm dilute hydrochloric acid (2 ml) and pour the solution in β-naphthol (2 ml) containing sodium acetate (1 g). An orange precipitate is formed.

Sulphacetamide contains free aromatic amino group. Therefore, it is diazotized and coupled with β-naphthol to form an orange dye.

$$H_2N \text{---} \bigcirc \text{---} SO_2NHCOCH_3 \xrightarrow[0-10°C]{NaNO_2 \text{---} HCl} Cl^- N \equiv N^+ \text{---} \bigcirc \text{---} SO_2NHCOCH_3$$

Sulphacetamide   Diazotized sulphacetamide

(ii) Heat sulphacetamide with ethanol and sulphuric acid. Ethyl acetate, recognizable by its odour, is produced.

(iii) Place sulphacetamide (0.5 g) in a test tube, heat gently until it melts and then boil. An oily liquid, which has characteristic odour of acetamide, condenses on the wall of the test tube.

Category

Antibacterial.

TANNIC ACID

Tannic acid is obtained from the galls of various species of *Quercus* (Family: Fagaceae) or other vegetable sources.

Physical Properties

It is a yellowish white or light brownish powder with characteristic odour and astringent taste. It is soluble in water and ethanol but insoluble in glycerin.

Chemical Test

(i) A solution of tannic acid gives precipitates with a solution of gelatin, albumin and certain alkaloids.

(ii) A solution of tannic acid gives a bluish-black colour with solution of ferric chloride. On addition of dilute sulphuric acid, the colour disappears and a yellowish brown precipitate is formed.

Category

Astringent.

ALKALOIDS

Alkaloids are basic nitrogenous compounds with definite physiological and pharmacological activity. They contain at least one nitrogen in a ring except a few exceptions like ephedrine.

They differ considerably in chemical structure and behaviour. They are classified on the basis of basic skeleton present in the molecule. For example, quinine contains quinoline ring; atropine contains tropane ring. The alkaloids are colourless or white crystalline mass, insoluble in water but soluble in organic solvents. Alkaloidal salts are soluble in water and insoluble in organic solvent.

They are identified on the basis of their melting point and generalized chemical tests which are as follows:

 (i) Add a few drops of Dragendroff's reagent to a solution of alkaloid (2 ml) or its salt; orange-red precipitate is produced.
 (ii) Add a few drops of Mayer's reagent to a solution of alkaloid; a white-yellowish precipitate is produced.
(iii) Add a few drops of solution in potassium iodide to a solution of alkaloid, a brown precipitate is produced.
(iv) Add a few drops of saturated solution of picric acid to a solution of alkaloid, a pale yellow precipitate is produced.

PROTEINS

Proteins are complex molecules which contain carbon, hydrogen, nitrogen and sometime sulphur. They are made of basic units of amino acids which are linked together in chain or rings through peptide bonds. Carboxylic group of one amino acid is joined with amino group of another amino acid.

$$R_1-CH-COOH + NH_2-CH-R_2 \longrightarrow R_1-CH-CONH-CH-R_2$$

$$\underset{\text{Amino acid}}{\overset{|}{NH_2}} \quad \underset{\text{Amino acid}}{\overset{|}{COOH}} \quad \underset{\text{Peptide}}{\overset{|}{NH_2} \qquad \overset{|}{COOH}}$$

Proteins are amphoteric in nature. At some definite pH, characteristic of each protein, the positive and negative charges are exactly balanced and the molecules do not migrate in an electrical field. This condition is known as 'isoelectric point' and at this pH the protein has its least solubility.

Proteins are examined by the following colour reaction, e.g.

1. *Biuret reaction:* To alkaline solution of protein (2 ml), add dilute solution of copper sulphate. A red or violet colour is formed with peptides containing at least two peptide linkages. A dipeptide does not respond this test.
2. *Xanthroproteic reaction*: Proteins usually form a yellow colour on warming with concentrated nitric acid. This colour becomes orange when the solution is made alkaline. The colour is due to nitration of aromatic ring containing amino acids like phenylalanine and tyrosine.
3. *Ninhydrin test:* To an aqueous solution of a protein, add alcoholic solution of ninhydrin and then heat. Red to violet colour is formed.

Ninhydrin   Amino acid   Coloured compound

4. *Nitroprusside test*: Proteins containing sulphur atom form red colour with nitroprusside solution.
5. *Lead sulphide test:* Alkaline solution of sulphur containing protein, on addition of lead acetate, produces a black precipitate.

AMINO ACIDS

An amino acid is the hydrolytic product of protein. They are characterized by the presence of amino and carboxylic groups together. They are either aliphatic or aromatic in nature. They are detected by following chemical test.

1. Amino acids give red to violet colour with ninhydrin.
2. Phenolic amino acids give red colour on addition of ferric chloride solution.
3. Aromatic amino acids undergo diazotization with nitrous acid which couple with alkaline β-naphthol solution to give red coloured aze dye.
4. *Sorensen test* (only for aliphatic amino acid): Dissolve the compound (0.5 g) in water or ethanol. Add two drops of phenolphthalein and then dilute sodium hydroxide solution till pink colour is obtained. In the other test tube, take the similar things in a similar order only with the difference that the amino acid is replaced by 40% formalin solution. Add the solution from the second test tube to the first; the disappearance of the pink colour is the indication of amino acid.

GLYCINE H_2N—CH_2—$COOH$

Physical Properties

Glycine is the simplest amino acid. It is a colourless solid. It is readily soluble in water.

Chemical Test

1. Glycine contain the basic group, –NH_2 as well as the acidic group –$COOH$, hence it forms salt with both alkalies and acids.
2. Its aqueous solution gives red colour on addition of 2 or 3 drops of ninhydrin solution.
3. To the compound (2 ml), add 2 drops of phenolphthalein solution, 2 drops of dilute aqueous sodium hydroxide solution and 2–3 ml of neutralized ethanol (3 ml). The pink colour disappears.
4. Glycine reacts with nitrous acid like primary amines, the NH_2 group is displaced by hydroxyl group and glycolic acid is formed.

$$NH_2CH_2COOH + HNO_2 \longrightarrow HOCH_2COOH + N_2 + H_2O$$
$$\text{Glycolic acid}$$

CHLORAMPHENICOL

$$O_2N-\langle\bigcirc\rangle-\overset{1}{C}H-\overset{2}{C}H-\overset{3}{C}H_2OH$$
$$| \qquad |$$
$$OH \quad NHCOCHCl_2$$

Chloramphenicol
(D-Threo-N-dichloroacetyl-1-*p*-nitrophenyl-2-amino-1,3-propanediol)

Physical Properties

It occurs as a fine, white to greyish white or yellowish white, crystalline powder. It is odourless with bitter taste.

Chloramphenicol is slightly soluble in water; freely soluble in ethanol and in acetone; slightly soluble in solvent ether.

Chemical Test

1. Dissolve 10 mg in 5 ml of water, add 0.10 g of zinc powder, heat the mixture for 10 minutes in a water-bath and filter. To the filtrate add a few drops of nitric acid and a few drops of silver nitrate solution—a white, curdy precipitate is produced. Separate the precipitate, wash it with water and add an excess of ammonia solution—the precipitate dissolves.
2. Dissolve 10 mg in 5 ml of water and add 1.0 ml of sulphuric acid and 0.05 g of zinc powder. Heat the mixture for a few minutes in a water-bath and filter. To the cooled filtrate add 2 or 3 drops of sodium nitrite solution—and, after a few minutes, add 1.0 g of urea and a solution of 10 mg of 2-naphthol in 2.0 ml of sodium hydroxide solution—a red colour is produced.
3. Add 10 mg to a mixture of 5 drops of liquefied phenol and 0.20 g of potassium hydroxide. Heat to boiling over a small flame and shake; a brown-red colour is produced. Add 2.0 ml of water; the colour turns dark green.
4. To the substance (20 mg), add sodium hydroxide solution (5 ml) and pyridine (2 ml). Shake well and heat on a water bath. A brownish red colour is developed in the pyridine.

Category

Antibacterial

CHLOROQUINE PHOSPHATE

Chloroquine phosphate
[7-Chloro-4-(5-diethylamino-2-pentylamino)quinoline]

Physical Properties

It is available as a white, or almost white, crystalline powder; odourless or almost odourless. Melting point: About 87–89.5°C.

Chemical Test

1. To 10 mg of sample, add 2 ml of sulphuric acid; no colour is produced. Add 1 drop of potassium dichromate solution—a brownish-red colour is produced.
2. Dissolve 20 mg in 2.0 ml of water and add 5 drops of potassio-mercuric iodide; a white, curdy precipitate is produced.
3. Dissolve 10 mg in 2.0 ml of water, add 2 drops of ammonia solution and 2.0 ml of silver nitrate (40 g/litre) and heat; a yellow precipitate is produced. To a portion of the precipitate add a few drops of nitric acid, a clear solution is produced. To another portion of the precipitate add a few drops of ammonia solution and shake well; a clear solution is produced.

Category

Antibacterial.

PROCAINE PENICILLIN

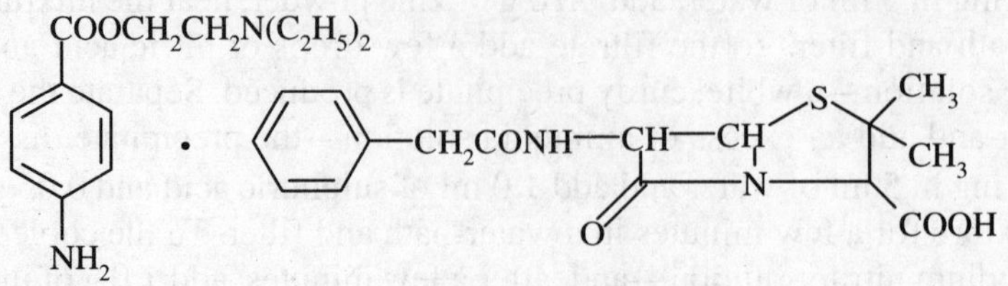

$$COOCH_2CH_2N(C_2H_5)_2$$

—CH$_2$CONH—CH—CH

S

CH$_3$

CH$_3$

N

O

COOH

NH$_2$

Physical Properties

It is a white crystalline powder; slightly soluble in water.

Chemical Test

Diazotization test: This test depends upon the presence of the aromatic primary amino group which is a part of the procaine molecule.

Dissolve the substance (0.1 g) in dilute hydrochloric acid with gentle warming, if necessary, cool in an ice and add 1% w/v sodium nitrite solution (4 ml). Pour the solution into a mixture of β-naphthol solution (2 ml) containing sodium acetate (1 g). A bright orange red precipitate is produced (dye formation).

Category

Antibacterial.

PARACETAMOL

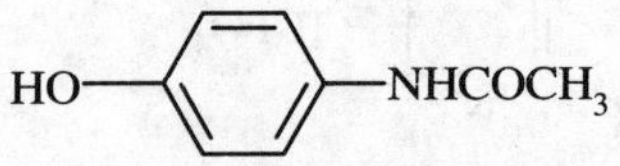

HO—⟨ ⟩—NHCOCH$_3$

Paracetamol
(*p*-Acetyl aminophenol)

Physical Properties

It is white crystalline, odourless powder.

Melting point: About 170°C.

Eutectic temperature: With benzanilide, about 137°C; with phenacetin, about 114°C.

Chemical Test

1. Dissolve 0.10 g in 10 ml of water and add 1 drop of ferric chloride solution—a violet-blue colour is produced.
2. Boil 0.10 g in 1.0 ml of hydrochloric acid for 3 minutes, add 10 ml of water and cool; no precipitate is formed. Add 1 drop of potassium dichromate solution—a violet colour is slowly produced which does not turn red (distinction from phenacetin).

Category

Analgesic and antipyretic.

Basic Laboratory Techniques

CRYSTALLIZATION TECHNIQUE

The most common method of purifying solid organic compounds is recrystallization method. In this technique, an impure solid compound is dissolved in a solvent under hot condition and then allowed to slowly crystallize out as the solution cools. As the compound crystallizes from the solution, the molecules of the other compounds dissolved in solution are excluded from the growing crystal lattice, giving a pure solid.

Crystallization of a solid is not the same as precipitation of a solid. In crystallization, there is a slow, selective formation of the crystal framework resulting in a pure compound. In precipitation, there is a rapid formation of a solid from a solution that usually produces an amorphous solid containing many trapped impurities within the solid's crystal framework. For this reason, experimental procedures that produce a solid product by precipitation always include a final recrystallization step to give the pure compound.

The process of recrystallization relies on the property that for most compounds, as the temperature of a solvent increases, the solubility of the compound in that solvent also increases. For example, much more table sugar can be dissolved in very hot water (just below the boiling point) than in water at room temperature. What will happen if a concentrated solution of hot water and sugar is allowed to cool to room temperature? As the temperature of the solution decreases, the solubility of the sugar in the water also decreases and the sugar molecules will begin to crystallize out of the solution. (This is how rock candy is made.) This is the basic process that goes on in the recrystallization of a solid.

The steps in the recrystallization of a compound are:

1. Selection of a suitable solvent for the recrystallization.
2. Dissolving the impure solid in a minimum volume of hot solvent.
3. Removal of any insoluble impurities by filtration.
4. Crystallization of the desired compound from the solution.
5. Isolation of the purified solid compound.

1. Selection of a suitable solvent for the recrystallization

The first consideration in purifying a solid by recrystallization is to find a suitable solvent. There are four important properties that you should look for in a good solvent for recrystallization.

(a) The compound should be very soluble at the boiling point of the solvent and only sparingly soluble in the solvent at room temperature. This difference in solubility at hot versus cold temperatures is essential for the recrystallization process. If the compound is insoluble in the chosen solvent at high temperatures, then it will not dissolve. If the compound is very soluble in the solvent at room temperature, then getting the compound to crystallize in pure form from solution is difficult. For example, water is an excellent solvent for the recrystallization of benzoic acid. At 10°C only 2.1 g of benzoic acid dissolves in 1 liter of water, while at 95°C the solubility is 68 g/L.

(b) The unwanted impurities should be either very soluble in the solvent at room temperature or insoluble in the hot solvent. This way, after the impure solid is dissolved in the hot solvent, any undissolved impurities can be removed by filtration. After the solution cools and the desired compound crystallizes out, any remaining soluble impurities will remain dissolved in the solvent.

(c) The solvent should not react with the compound being purified. The desired compound may be lost during recrystallization if the solvent reacts with the compound.

(d) The solvent should be volatile enough to be easily removed from the solvent after the compound has crystallized. This allows for easy and rapid drying of the solid compound after it has been isolated from the solution.

Finding a solvent with the desired properties is a search done by trial and error. First, test the solubility of tiny samples of the compound in test tubes with a variety of different solvents (water, ethanol, methanol, ethyl acetate, diethyl ether, hexane, toluene, etc.) at room temperature. If the compound dissolves in the solvent at room temperature, then that solvent is unsuitable for recrystallization. If the compound is insoluble in the solvent at room temperature, then the mixture is heated to the solvent's boiling point to determine if the solid will dissolve at high temperature, and then cooled to see whether it crystallizes from the solution at room temperature.

2. Dissolving the impure solid in a minimum volume of hot solvent

Once a suitable solvent is selected, place the impure solid in an Erlenmeyer flask and add a small volume of hot solvent to the flask. Erlenmeyer flasks are preferred over beakers for recrystallization because the conical shape of an Erlenmeyer flask decreases the amount of solvent lost to evaporation during heating, prevents the formation of a crust around the sides of the glass, and makes it easier to swirl the hot solution while dissolving the solid without splashing it out of the flask.

Keep the solution in the Erlenmeyer flask warm on a hot plate or in a water bath, and add small volumes of hot solvent to the flask until all of the solid just dissolves. Swirl the solution between additions of solvent and break up any lumps with a stirring rod or spatula. Occasionally there will be impurities present in the solid that are insoluble in the chosen solvent even at high temperature. If subsequent additions of solvent to the solution do not seem to dissolve any of the remaining solid, stop adding solvent to the solution (as this will decrease the percent recovery of the desired compound) and filter or decant the hot solution to remove the insoluble impurities.

3. Removal of any insoluble impurities by filtration

Insoluble impurities are simply removed by filtration. The soluble coloured impurities can be removed by using decolourizing carbon. Coloured impurities are sometimes difficult to remove from solid mixtures. These coloured impurities, often due to the presence of polar or polymeric compounds, can cause a colourless organic solid to have a tint of colour even after recrystallization. Decolourizing or activated carbon is used to remove the coloured impurities from the sample. Decolourizing carbon is very finely divided carbon that provides high surface area to adsorb the coloured impurities.

Very little decolourizing carbon is needed to remove the coloured impurities from a solution. You must be judicious in your use of decolourizing carbon: if too much is used, it can adsorb the desired compound from the solution as well as the coloured impurities. After the impure solid sample is dissolved in hot solvent, a small amount of decolourizing carbon, about the size of a pea, is added to the hot solution. This must be done carefully to avoid a surge of boiling from the hot solution. The solution is stirred and heated for a few minutes and then filtered hot to remove the decolourizing carbon. The resulting filtrate should be colourless and the recrystallization process continues as before.

4. Crystallization of the desired compound from the solution

After the insoluble impurities have been removed, cover the flask containing the hot filtrate with a watch glass and set it aside undisturbed to cool slowly to room temperature. As the solution cools, the solubility of the dissolved compound will decrease and the solid will begin to crystallize from the solution. After the flask has cooled to room temperature, it may be placed in an ice bath to increase the yield of solid. Do not rapidly cool the hot solution by placing the flask in an ice bath before it has cooled to room temperature—this will result in a rapid precipitation of the solid in an impure form because of trapped impurities.

Sometimes the dissolved compound fails to crystallize from the solution on cooling. If this happens, crystallization can be induced by various methods. One way to induce crystallization is by scratching the inner wall of the Erlenmeyer flask with a glass stirring rod. This is believed to release very small particles of glass which act as nuclei for crystal growth. Another method of inducing crystallization is to add a small crystal of the desired compound, called a seed crystal, to the solution. Again, this seed crystal acts as a template on which the dissolved solid will begin crystallizing. If neither of these two techniques results in crystallization, the compound was probably dissolved in too much hot solvent. If you believe that you may have too much solvent for the amount of dissolved compound, reheat the solution to boiling, boil off or distill some of the solvent, and then allow the solution to cool to room temperature again to effect crystallization.

5. Isolation of the purified solid compound

Once the compound has completely precipitated from the solution, it is separated from the remaining solution (also called the mother liquor) by filtration. Typically, this is done by vacuum or suction filtration using a Buchner funnel. Line the bottom of the Buchner or Hirsch funnel with a piece of filter paper that is large enough to cover the holes in the bottom plate of the funnel without curling up on the sides of the funnel. Place a neoprene adapter on the stem of the funnel and insert it in the top of a filter flask (a thick-walled Erlenmeyer flask with a side-arm) that has been securely clamped to a ring stand.

Using a piece of thick-walled vacuum tubing, connect the side-arm of the filter flask to a water aspirator. Turn the water to the aspirator on full force to create a vacuum through the system. If necessary, carefully adjust the piece of filter paper so that it covers all of the holes in the funnel, and then dampen it with a small volume of cold solvent; this will create a better seal between the filter paper and the plate in the funnel, preventing any solid from getting under the filter paper and passing through the funnel. Slowly pour the recrystallization solution into the funnel and allow the suction to pull the mother liquor through. Rinse the Erlenmeyer flask with a small volume of cold recrystallization solvent to remove any remaining solid. Add this solvent to the funnel and then wash the solid in the funnel, called the filter cake or residue, with a few milliliters of fresh, cold recrystallization solvent to remove any remaining mother liquor and dissolved impurities.

Leave the aspirator on for a few minutes and allow air to pass through the crystals to dry them. After pulling air through the crystals for a brief time, remove the vacuum from the system by disconnecting the vacuum tubing from the aspirator before turning the water off. If you turn the aspirator water off first, water can be sucked into the filter flask and may contaminate the product. The filter cake is removed from the funnel by carefully prying it from the filter using a spatula. The cake of crystals will still be slightly wet with solvent and should be allowed to dry thoroughly before measuring the weight or melting point of the solid material.

Experiment 14.1: To prepare crystals of pure benzoic acid from an impure sample by crystallization

Theory

Benzoic acid is a crystalline solid has high solubility in hot water. An impure sample of benzoic acid is dissolved in hot water and then filtered to remove insoluble impurities.

Requirements

Crude sample of benzoic acid, 250 ml measuring flask, funnel, a glass rod, and a beaker.

Procedure

It involves the following steps:

1. Take about 2–3 g of the crude sample of benzoic acid in a 250 ml beaker, in another take about 150 ml of water and keep it for boiling.
2. Add slowly with stirring least amount of boiling water to the beaker containing crude sample of benzoic acid to dissolve it.
3. Add 0.5 g of animal charcoal to the solution and boil for a minute.
4. Filter the solution while hot using filter paper placed in a funnel.
5. Collect the clear filtrate in a beaker.
6. Allow the filtered solution to cool at room temperature. Now cool it by placing it in a beaker/container filled with cold water.
7. Separate the crystals by suction using Buchner funnel.
8. Wash the crystals with water, dry the crystals.
9. Record the weight of the crystals.

Result

Yield = ... %.

Physical appearance

Shining white crystals of benzoic acid.

Experiment 14.2: To prepare crystals of pure copper sulphate from an impure sample by crystallization

Theory

Copper sulphate, blue stone, blue vitriol are all common names for pentahydrated cupric sulphate, $CuSO_4.5H_2O$, which is the best known and the most widely used copper salt. This form is characterized by its bright blue colour. However, its anhydrous form is white in colour.

Requirements

Crude sample of copper sulphate, funnel, a glass rod, and a beaker.

Procedure

It involves the following steps:

1. Take about 10 g of the crude sample of copper sulphate in a 100 ml beaker.
2. In another take about 150 ml of water and keep it for boiling.
3. Add slowly with stirring least amount of boiling water to the beaker containing crude sample of copper sulphate to dissolve it.

    Note: The solubility of copper (II) sulphate pentahydrate in water is around 35 g/100 g of water. When heated to 90°C, solubility increases to 100 g/100 g of water.
4. Filter the solution while hot using filter paper placed in a funnel.
5. Concentrate the solution, cover the solution with foil and leave in a dark place for 24 hours.
6. Filter or decant the solution into another beaker and take out the crystals that have formed. It is important to choose a crystal with the right form, without cracks and other defects.
7. Dry the crystals.
8. Record the weight of the crystals.

Result

Yield = ... %.

Physical appearance

Triclinic blue coloured crystals of copper sulphate.

HEATING UNDER REFLUXING CONDITION

The rate of organic reactions is generally temperature dependent—run faster at higher temperatures and slower at lower temperatures. Many reactions commonly run in an organic Chemistry lab. need to be heated in order to proceed at a satisfactory rate. The most convenient way to heat a reaction is by boiling it in a solvent in a conical vial or round bottom flask. It is easy to observe whether or not a liquid is boiling, and because of the laws of thermodynamics, once boiling begins the temperature cannot rise any higher. To control the temperature of the reaction, simply choose a solvent with a boiling point at this temperature. To prevent the solvent from boiling away, a reflux condenser is used. This is a glass column with a second column surrounding it through which cool water flows. If there is a high boiling solvent, then there is no need of water flow. As vapor from the boiling solvent rises into inside column of the reflux condenser, it is cooled by the jacket of water on the outside and condenses. It then falls back into the solution. In this way, you can maintain a reaction at the boiling point of the solvent indefinitely, as long as the water in the reflux condenser is cool enough to condense all of the vapor. Any time you heat a liquid, you should always stir it to avoid bumping. Bumping occurs when only the liquid at the very bottom is hot enough to boil, and it builds up pressure and bursts suddenly, sometimes spattering out of the container. Also, you should never heat a closed system—pressure can build up and burst the glassware. The reflux condenser is open at the top to prevent pressure build-up. If you need to protect a reaction from moisture, a drying tube filled with calcium carbonate is used so that water cannot get in but air can get in and out to prevent pressure build-up.

Procedure

1. To reflux a reaction, add all of the reagents including solvent to a round bottom flask as directed.
2. Fix a reflux condenser, securing it with a clamp (attach the clamp to the condenser).

3. Attach tubing to the condenser so that water flows from the tap into the bottom of the condenser, and out of the top and into the drain. (If you attach the tubing backwards, the water will just run down part of the inside of the condenser instead of filling it up, and will not do a good job of cooling.)

4. Turn on the stirrer and the water (not too fast—all you need is for the water to be moving through the condenser fast enough to cool the vapor—no need to waste it), and then gradually heat the reaction until you can see the solvent refluxing. You should observe liquid forming in the condenser and flowing back into the reaction. It may appear as droplets or as a continuous stream.

5. When you finish refluxing, allow the reaction to cool, turn off the water, and proceed as per instruction.

DISTILLATION

Distillation is one of the most useful methods for the separation and purification of liquids. It is perhaps the oldest separation technique known. It is most commonly used to purify a liquid from either liquid or solid contaminants by exploiting differences in their boiling points.

Types of Distillation

- **Simple distillation** can separate compounds cleanly if the difference in boiling points between the compounds is greater than 70°C. The process is useful to further purify relatively pure liquids, to get rid of volatile organic solvents, or to separate the liquid from polymerization products and mineral impurities.

- **Fractional distillation** is a separation technique that is used when the boiling point differences of the compounds in a mixture to be separated are not large enough to employ the simple distillation technique. The components to be separated are collected in different fractions, whose identity are usually then confirmed via spectroscopy or TLC (thin layer chromatography). The first fraction (or the first mixture between fractions), usually just a few drops, is called the forerun. It contains any highly volatile substances that were present in the sample, and is a kind of first rinse of the distillation glassware. It may be combined with the next fraction if analysis warrants.

- **Vacuum distillation** is used to purify compounds that can decompose before reaching their boiling point at atmospheric pressure. By lowering the gas pressure above a liquid, that liquid can be encouraged to boil at a lower temperature. This is important if it would breakdown at a higher one.

- **Steam distillation** is also used for high boiling point substances that decompose before the boiling point is reached. In this case, instead of using a vacuum, the liquid in question is mixed with another, immiscible liquid. The presence of the second liquid causes both to boil at a temperature lower than the regular boiling points of either liquid. For example, naphthalene, a solid at room temperature that boils at 218°C, can be melted and mixed with water. Because the two are immiscible, they will steam distill at a temperature around 90°C, less than 100°C (the boiling point of water) and well below 218°C. In all steam distillations, the distillate collected will be a mixture of both liquids, but since they are immiscible, they can generally be separated easily via extraction.

Similarly, attempting to distill these essential oils directly from the plant material is generally not feasible. In general, most of the oils' constituents are high boiling and will decompose under the high heat needed to bring them to a boil. Steam distillation is a much gentler method of separating the oil at lower temperature than the normal boiling point of either component of the mixture. It means, mixture will boil at a temperature slightly less than the normal boiling point of water.

In steam distillation, the distilling pot is infused with steam (indirect method), which carries the oil's vapor into the distilling head and then into the condenser, where the oil and water co-condense. As an alternative, steam is generated *in situ* in the distilling pot itself (direct method) (Fig. 14.1).

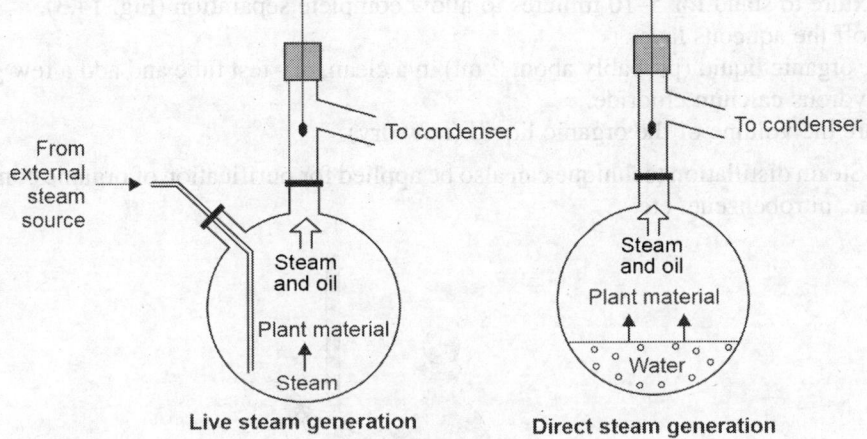

Fig. 14.1

Experiment 14.3: Isolation of orange oil by steam distillation

The purpose of this experiment is to demonstrate the ability to distill an organic liquid at a temperature considerably below that of the boiling point of the pure liquid.

Procedure

1. Transfer small pieces of orange peel of 2–3 medium size oranges in a 500 ml round bottom flask.
2. Add a few boiling chips to the flask.
3. Set up a steam distillation apparatus as shown in Fig. 14.2.
4. Add 250 ml of distilled water to the flask. Heat the flask at a steady rate, approximately 1 drop per second of distillate.

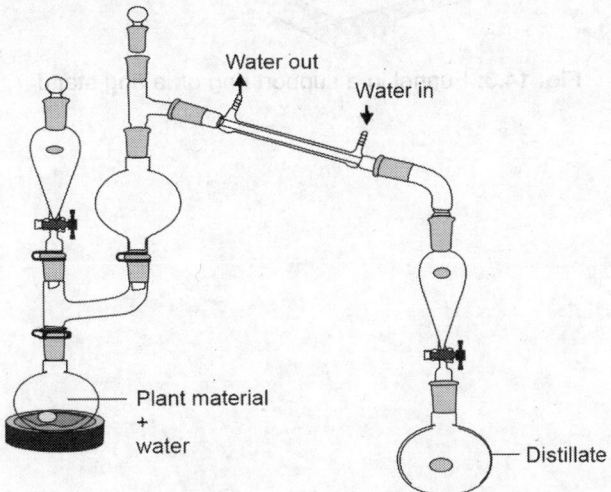

Fig. 14.2: Steam distillation setup

5. At the first drop of distillate, record temperature and volume of distillate collected. Repeat this every 4 ml, until 50 ml of distillate has been collected.
6. Stop the distillation. The distillate should have two layers. The top layer should be oil and the bottom one should be aqueous. Transfer the distillate to a separatory funnel and allow the mixture to stand for 5–10 minutes to allow complete separation (Fig. 14.3).
7. Drain off the aqueous layer.
8. Put the organic liquid (probably about 2 ml) in a clean, dry test tube and add a few granules of anhydrous calcium chloride.
9. Measure the volume of the organic liquid (now dry).

Note: Steam distillation technique can also be applied for purification of organic compounds like aniline, nitrobenzene, etc.

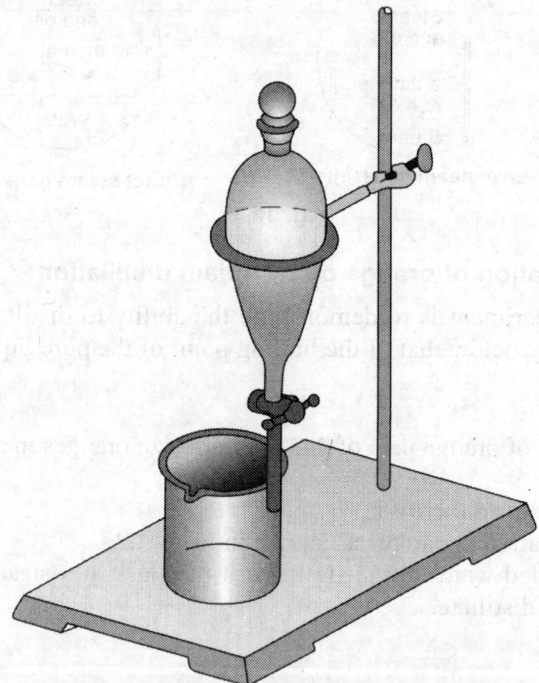

Fig. 14.3: Funnel in a support ring on a ring stand

List of Organic Preparations

Single Step Preparations

1. Preparation of aspirin from salicylic acid
2. Preparation of *m*-dintrobenzene from nitrobenzene
3. Preparation of aspirin from salicylic acid
4. Preparation of benzoic acid from alkyl benzoate (ethyl benzoate)
5. Preparation of benzoic acid from benzoyl chloride
6. Preparation of salicylic acid from alkyl salicylate (methyl salicylate)
7. Preparation of 2,4,6-tribromoaniline from aniline
8. Preparation of picric acid (2,4,6-trinitrophenol) from phenol
9. Preparation of 2,4,6-tribromophenol) from phenol
10. Preparation of iodoform from ethanol or acetone
    Method I (from ethanol)
    Method II (from acetone)
11. Preparation of benzoic acid from benzamide
12. Preparation of Schiff's base from benzaldehyde and aniline
13. Preparation of benzimidazole from *o*-phenylendiamine
14. Preparation of *para*-iodobenzoic acid from para amino benzoic acid
15. Preparation of 1,3,4-tetrahydrocarbazole
16. Preparation of benzalacetophenone from acetophenone
17. Preparation of 3-methyl-1-phenyl pyrazol-5-one
18. Preparation of *p*-acetylaminophenol (paracetamol)
19. Preparation of phenacetin from acetaminophen
20. Preparation of α-phenylthiourea
21. Preparation of glucosazone from glucose
22. Preparation of phenolphthalein from phenol
23. Preparation of urotropine (hexamethylenetetramine) from formaldehyde
24. Preparation of barbituric acid from urea
25. Preparation of phenyl azo-β-naphthol (an azo dye)
26. Preparation of dibenzalacetone (dinbenzylidene acetone)
27. Preparation of cinnamic acid from benzaldehyde
28. Preparation of *m*-nitrobenzoic acid from benzoic acid
29. Preparation of 5-nitrosalicylic acid from salicylic acid
30. Preparation of methyl salicylate (oil of wintergreen)

31. Preparation of benzocaine
32. Preparation of 3,5-dimethylpyrazole from acetylacetone
33. Preparation of phenothiazine from diphenylamine
34. Preparation of 2,5-diphenyl oxazole
35. Preparation of chlorobutanol from acetone and chloroform
36. Preparation of benztriazole from o-phenylenediamine
37. Preparation of 2,4,5-triphenyl-1H-imidazole from benzyl

Two steps preparations

38. Preparation of p-nitroacetanilide from aniline
39. Preparation of p-bromoacetanilide from aniline
40. Preparation of p-bromobenzanilide from aniline
41. Preparation of methylorange from aniline
42. Preparation of tetrabromofluorescein (eosin) from resorcinol
43. Preparation of benzilic acid from benzoin
44. Preparation of 2,3-diphenyl quinoxaline from benzoin
45. Preparation of 5,5-diphenylhydantoin from benzoin
46. Preparation of 4-benzylidene-2-phenyl oxazole-5-one from glycine
47. Preparation of 7-acetoxy-4-methyl coumarin from resorcinol
48. Preparation of isatin from chloral hydrate
49. Preparation of p-bromoaniline from acetanilide
50. Preparation of 2-phenyl indole from acetophenone
51. Preparation of antipyrine

Three steps preparations

52. Preparation of acridone from anthranilic acid
53. Preparation of succinanil from succinic anhydride
54. Preparation of anthrone from o-benzoyl benzoic acid
55. Preparation of acetanilide from benzene
56. Preparation of diphenic acid from phthalic anhydride
57. Preparation of sulphanilamide from acetanilide
58. Preparation of tolbutamide from toluene
59. Preparation of 3-hydroxycoumarin from benzoyl glycine

█ SINGLE STEP PREPARATIONS

1. Preparation of aspirin from salicylic acid

Method I

Requirements

Salicylic acid	10 g
Acetic anhydride	14 ml
Conc. H_2SO_4	2 ml

Chemical Reaction

Salicylic acid   + $(CH_3CO)_2O$ $\xrightarrow[\Delta]{H_2SO_4}$ Aspirin   + CH_3COOH

Reaction Mechanism

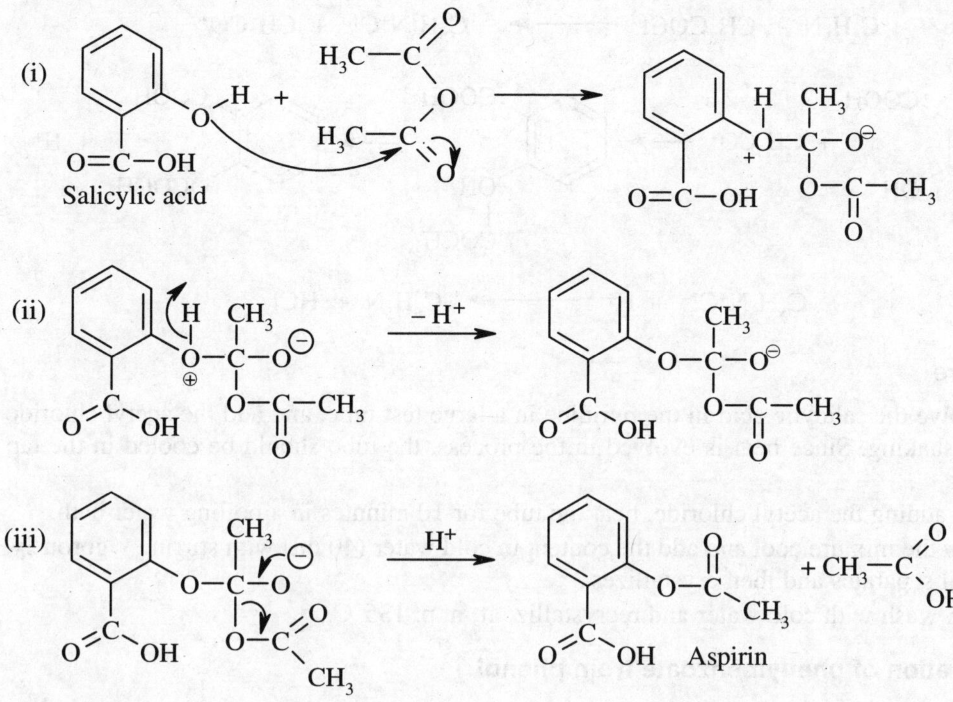

(i)

(ii)

(iii)

Procedure

(i) Heat gently the mixture of salicylic acid (10 g), acetic anhydride (20 ml) and concentrated sulphuric acid (4–5 drops) for half an hour on a water bath with frequent stirring.

(ii) Pour down the contents into cold water (150 ml) with continuous stirring and filter the crude aspirin.

(iii) For recrystallization, dissolve the product in ethanol (30 ml) and pour the solution into warm water (75 ml). If a solid separates, warm the mixture to dissolve the solid.

(iv) Allow the clear solution to cool slowly to get needle shaped crystals of aspirin, m.p. 136–137°C.

Method II

Requirements

Salicylic acid	2 g
Acetyl chloride	1.5 ml
Pyridine	1.0 ml

Chemical Reaction

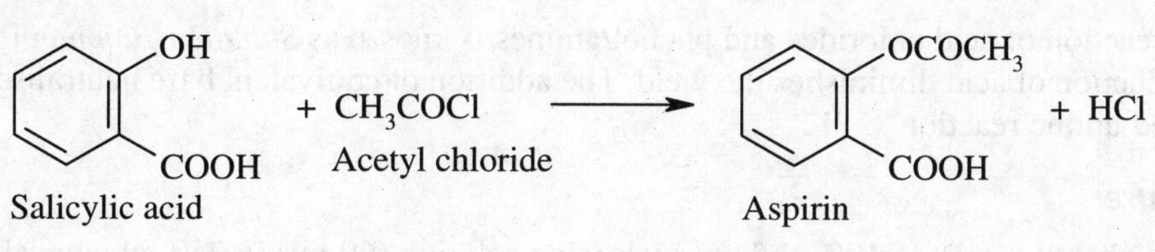

Salicylic acid   + CH$_3$COCl   →   Aspirin   + HCl
                  Acetyl chloride

Reaction Mechanism

$$C_5H_5N + CH_3COCl \longrightarrow C_5H_5N^+Cl^- + CH_3CO^+$$

$$C_5H_5N^+Cl^- + H^+ \longrightarrow C_5H_5N + HCl$$

Procedure

(i) Dissolve the salicylic acid in the pyridine in a large test tube, and add the acetyl chloride with shaking. Since heat is evolved in the process, the tube should be cooled in the tap water.

(ii) After adding the acetyl chloride, heat the tube for 10 minutes in a boiling water bath.

(iii) Allow the mixture cool and add the content in cold water (40 ml) with stirring vigorously. An oil separates and then crystallizes.

(iv) Filter, wash with cold water and recrystallize it, m.p. 135°C.

2. Preparation of phenylbenzoate from phenol

Requirements

Phenol	4 g
Benzoyl chloride	8 ml
10% Sodium hydroxide solution	60 ml

Chemical Reaction

Reaction Mechanism

The reaction of acid chlorides and phenol/amines is known as *Shoutten-Baumann reaction*. The production of acid diminishes the yield. The addition of equivalent base neutralise the acid and speed up the reaction.

Procedure

(i) Add phenol (4 ml) to 10% sodium hydroxide solution (60 ml) in 250 ml conical flask.

(ii) Add redistilled benzoyl chloride (8 ml) slowly with continuous shaking.

(iii) Cork the flask and shake it vigorously till the odour of benzoyl chloride can no longer be detected.

(iv) Filter the crude product, wash with cold water and recrystallize from hot ethanol, m.p. 69°C.

3. Preparation of *m*-dinitrobenzene from nitrobenzene

Requirements

Nitrobenzene	12.5 ml
Conc. sulphuric acid	21 ml
Conc. nitric acid	15 ml

Chemical Reaction

Nitrobenzene   Conc. HNO₃ / Conc. H₂SO₄ / Δ 2 hr.   *m*-Dinitrobenzene

Reaction Mechanism

$$HNO_3 + 2H_2SO_4 \rightleftharpoons NO_2^+ + H_3O^+ + 2HSO_4^-$$

Nitronium
electrophile

Procedure

(i) Place concentrated sulphuric acid (21 ml) and concentrated nitric acid (15 ml) in 250 ml round bottomed flask containing few small pieces of unglazed porcelain to prevent bumping.

(ii) Attach reflux condenser, add slowly nitrobenzene in a portion of 2–3 ml with shaking and heat it with frequent shaking for 2 hours.

(iii) Cool the mixture and then pour it into ice cold water with stirring.

(iv) Filter the crude *m*-dinitrobenzene with suction, wash with cold water and recrystallize from hot methylated (or rectified) spirit to obtain yellow crystalline substance, m.p. 90°C.

4. Preparation of benzoic acid from alkyl benzoate (ethyl benzoate)

Requirements

Ethyl benzoate	2 ml
10% w/v sodium hydroxide solution	15 ml
Hydrochloric acid	q.s.

Reaction

Ethyl benzoate   Sodium benzoate   Benzoic acid

When ethyl benzoate is shaken with water two liquid layers form. The upper layer is ethyl benzoate (less dense) and the lower layer is water. There is no clear indication of any reaction taking place. In this condition, ethyl benzoate reacts very slowly with water and is hydrolyzed to give benzoic acid and ethanol but the reaction does not go to completion. However, ethyl benzoate is found to react much faster with aqueous sodium hydroxide, the reaction going to completion, to give sodium benzoate (water soluble) and ethanol (miscible with water).

This process is called base hydrolysis (or saponification) of an ester and is used in this experiment to first obtain sodium benzoate solution, and then benzoic acid from sodium benzoate. The ethanol may be recovered by simple downward distillation from the reaction mixture and collected as a solution in water. But this step is omitted in this experiment to allow it to be completed in the available time. The sodium benzoate is non-volatile and remains in solution. Treatment of this solution with hydrochloric acid (step 2) releases the free benzoic acid as a white crystalline solid that is washed with ice cold water and then recrystallized from hot water.

Reaction mechanism

Procedure

1. To the round bottom flask, add about 5 g of ethyl benzoate.
2. To the ethyl benzoate (2 ml), add 10% sodium hydroxide solution (15 ml) and a few anti-bumping granules.
3. Set up the apparatus for heating under reflux. Using a heating mantle, reflux the reaction mixture until all the oily drops of the ester have disappeared. This may take 45–60 minutes.
4. Allow the apparatus to cool and then transfer the reaction mixture to a 100 ml glass beaker.
5. Slowly and with stirring add hydrochloric acid to the reaction mixture to precipitate out the benzoic acid. Continue adding the acid until no more precipitation takes place and the mixture turns acidic (test with blue litmus paper or pH paper).
6. Allow the mixture to cool to room temperature and filter off the precipitate at the water pump. Wash the crude benzoic acid with a small volume of water.

7. Transfer the crude benzoic acid to a 100 ml beaker and recrystallize it from hot water.
8. Filter off the crystals of benzoic acid at the water pump and wash them with a small volume of water. Allow air to be drawn through the crystals for a few minutes in order to partially dry them.
9. Dry the crystals in an oven at about 70°C and weigh it.
10. Calculate the percentage yield of benzoic acid.
11. Determine the melting point of the benzoic acid product, m.p. 122°C.

5. Preparation of benzoic acid from benzyl chloride

In this reaction a side chain oxidation is performed. In order to achieve this, benzyl chloride is mixed with sodium carbonate solution and is oxidized with potassium permanganate solution. The sodium salt of benzoic acid is formed, this is acidified with concentrated hydrochloric acid to crystallize out benzoic acid.

Reaction

Benzyl chloride   Benzoic acid

Reaction mechanism

Benzyl cation formed due to heterolytic bond fission of C–Cl bond in benzyl chloride, is resonance stabilized. Hence benzyl chloride may follow S_N^1 mechanism. It is two stepped, first step involves formation of benzyl cation. Second step involves attack of nucleophile on cation from either side.

Benzyl chloride   Benzyl alcohol

Benzoic acid

Requirements

Benzyl chloride	2 ml
Anhydrous sodium carbonate	2 g in 20 ml of water
Potassium permanganate	8 g in 80 ml water
Sodium sulphite	4 g
HCl solution	q.s.

Procedure

1. Add about 2 ml of benzyl chloride to a solution of anhydrous sodium carbonate (2 g dissolved in 20 ml of distilled water) in round bottom flask, fitted with a water reflux condenser.
2. Heat the solution and potassium permanganate solution (4 g dissolved in 80 ml of water), added in small quantities through the water condenser until a permanent pink colour persists even after continuous boiling.
3. Boil the content for about an hour.
4. Transfer the mixture to a beaker. Add about 4 g of sodium sulphite to this mixture.
5. Now add concentrated hydrochloric acid to this solution until the solution is acidic.
6. Cool down the solution, filter the precipitated benzoic acid and wash the precipitate.
7. Recrystallize from boiling water.
8. Determine its melting point, 121°C.

6. Preparation of salicylic acid from alkyl salicylate (methyl salicylate)

Requirements

Methyl salicylate	3 ml
6M NaOH solution	50 ml
Hydrochloric acid solution	q.s.

The alkaline hydrolysis of esters is referred as saponification. In this reaction, one mole of methyl salicylate reacts with 2 moles of sodium hydroxide solution to form sodium salicylate with methanol and water. The resulting sodium salicylate is acidified to get the salicylic acid.

Reaction

Methyl salicylate   Salicyclic acid

$+ CH_3OH + Na_2SO_4$

Reaction mechanism

Procedure

1. Take methyl salicylate (oil of winter green) (3 ml) and 50 ml of 6M NaOH solution in round bottom flask with couple of boiling chip.
2. Heat the content under refluxing condition for 30–45 minutes or till clear solution is obtained (there is no smell of oil of winter green).
3. Remove the boiling chip and transfer the content in 250 ml beaker and cool down.
4. Acidify the content with stirring with hydrochloric acid solution (check with litmus paper).
5. Cool down the solution in a ice bath for 15 minutes.
6. Filter the product and wash with ice cold water.
7. Recrystallize the product from hot water and dry it.
8. Determine the melting point of resulting product, m.p.158–159°C.

7. Preparation of 2,4,6-tribromoaniline from aniline

Requirements

Aniline	20 ml
Glacial acetic acid	20 ml
Acetous bromine solution	8.4 ml dissolved in 20 ml of glacial acetic acid

Chemical Reaction

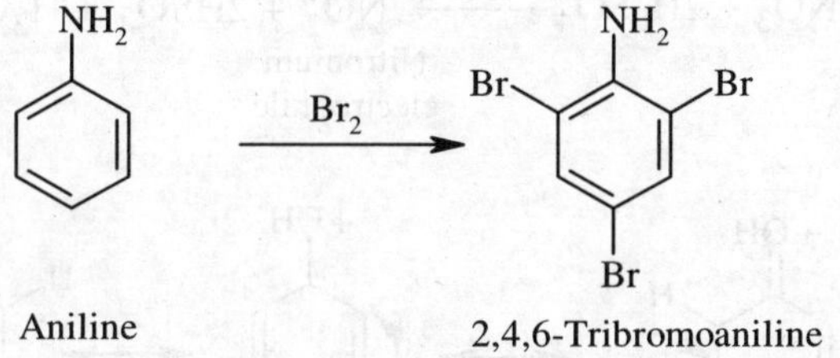

Aniline   2,4,6-Tribromoaniline

Reaction Mechanism

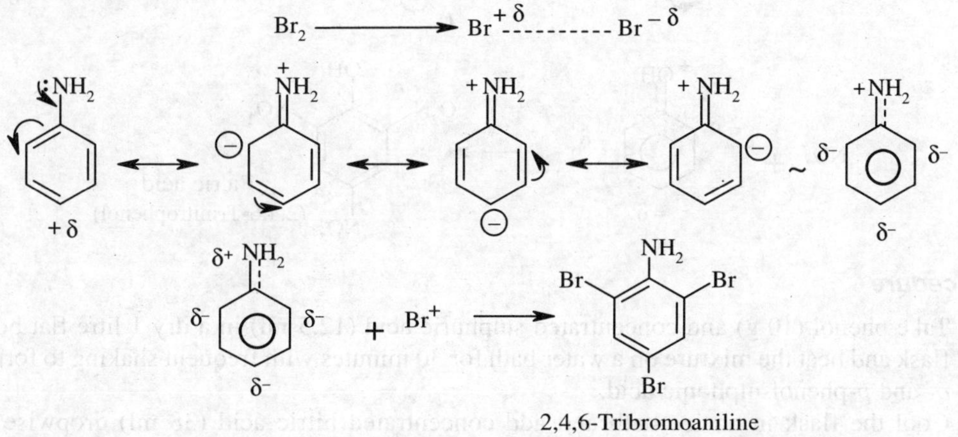

2,4,6-Tribromoaniline

Procedure

(i) Take aniline (5 ml) and glacial acetic acid (20 ml) in a 250 ml conical flask.
(ii) Add to it dropwise bromine solution (8.4 ml) dissolved in 20 ml of glacial acetic acid with constant stirring while keeping the flask in an ice bath.
(iii) Filter the solid mass so obtained, wash with cold water and recrystallize from dilute ethanol to obtain colourless crystals, m.p. 120°C.

Caution: Bromine must be handled with great care and in the fuming chamber.

8. Preparation of picric acid (2,4,6-trinitrophenol) from phenol

Requirements

Phenol	10 g
Conc. HNO_3	38 ml
Conc. H_2SO_4	12.5 ml

Chemical Reaction

Reaction Mechanism

$$HNO_3 + 2H_2SO_4 \longrightarrow NO_2^+ + 2HSO_4^- + H_3O^+$$

Nitronium
electrophile

Picric acid
(2,4,6-Trinitrophenol)

Procedure

(i) Take phenol (10 g) and concentrated sulphuric acid (12.5 ml) in a dry 1 litre flat bottom flask and heat the mixture on a water bath for 30 minutes with frequent shaking to form the *o-* and *p-*phenolsulphonic acid.

(ii) Cool the flask in an ice bath and add concentrated nitric acid (38 ml) dropwise with continuous shaking (this step should be carried in funning cupboard).

(iii) Allow the reaction mixture to stand for sometime and when evolution of red fumes are stopped, heat the flask on a water bath for 2 hours with occasional shaking.

(iv) Add cold water (100 ml), chill thoroughly in ice water, filter the yellow coloured crude product on suction, wash with water till free from acid and recrystallize from dilute ethanol (ethanol : H_2O, 1 : 2), m.p. 122°C.

9. Preparation of 2,4,6-tribromophenol from phenol

Requirements

Phenol   5 g
Bromine solution   8 ml

Chemical Reaction

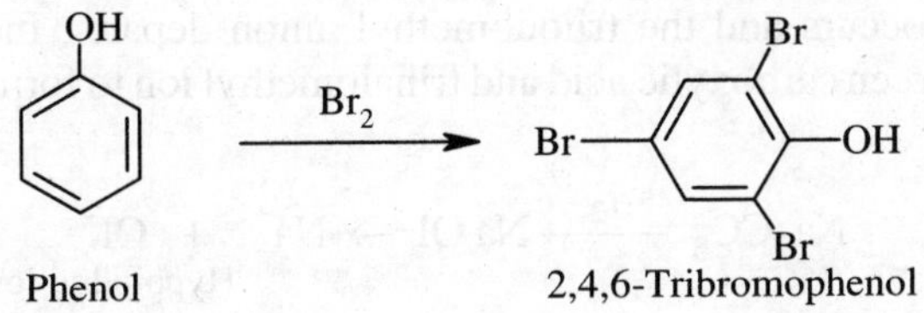

Phenol   2,4,6-Tribromophenol

Reaction Mechanism

$$Br_2 \longrightarrow Br^{\delta+} + Br^{\delta-}$$

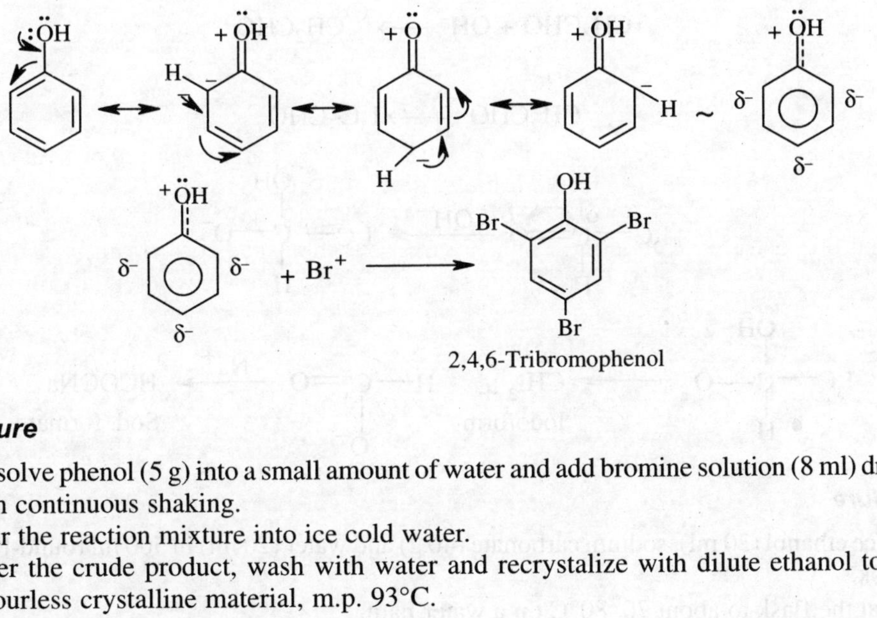

2,4,6-Tribromophenol

Procedure

(i) Dissolve phenol (5 g) into a small amount of water and add bromine solution (8 ml) dropwise with continuous shaking.

(ii) Pour the reaction mixture into ice cold water.

(iii) Filter the crude product, wash with water and recrystalize with dilute ethanol to obtain colourless crystalline material, m.p. 93°C.

10. Preparation of iodoform from ethanol

Requirements

Ethanol   20 ml
Iodine   3 g
Sodium carbonate   40 g

Chemical Reaction

$$C_2H_5OH + 4I_2 + 3Na_2CO_3 \longrightarrow CHI_3 + 5NaI + HCOONa + CO_2 + 2H_2O$$
Ethanol   Iodoform

Reaction Mechanism

The ethanol is oxidized by iodine to give ethanol. The hydrogen atom on the methyl group is slightly acidic and can be removed with hydroxide. The carbanion formed then react with iodine molecules to give an organic iodo compound. Introduction of the first atom (owing to its electronegativity) makes the remaining hydrogens of methyl group more acidic. Hence, a base-catalyzed iodination of monohalogenated compound occurs at the carbon that is already substituted. The next step is a nucleophilic attack by hydroxide on the carbonyl carbon atom. A carbon bond cleavage occurs and the triiodomethyl anion departs. In the last step, a proton transfer takes place between carboxylic acid and trihalomethyl ion to form ultimately carboxylate ion and iodoform.

$$Na_2CO_3 \xrightarrow{I_2} Na\,OI \rightarrow Na^+ + OI^-$$
$$\text{Hypoiodite ion}$$

$$OI^- + I + H_2O \rightleftharpoons I_2 + 2OH^-$$

$$C_2H_5OH + I_2 \longrightarrow CH_3CHO$$

$$CH_3CHO + OH^- \longrightarrow {}^{\ominus}CH_2CHO$$

$$^{\ominus}CH_2CHO \xrightarrow{I^-} I_3C\text{--}CHO$$

Procedure

(i) Place ethanol (20 ml), sodium carbonate (40 g) and water (20 ml) in 500 ml round-bottomed flask.

(ii) Heat the flask to about 70–80°C on a water bath.

(iii) To the warm solution, add small amount of iodine at a time with constant shaking. Add more iodine so that the reaction product should have a pale yellow colour.

(iv) Allow to stand for 5 minutes. Add dropwise a dilute solution of sodium hydroxide if any brown colour of iodine persists.

(v) Filter the crude iodoform, wash with cold water and recrystallize from hot ethanol to obtain the yellow crystals, m.p. 119°C.

Method I (from acetone)

Reaction

$$CH_3COCH_3 + 4I_2 + 4NaOH \rightarrow CHI_3 + 3NaI + CH_3COONa + 2H_2O$$

Reaction mechanism

Requirements

Acetone	15 ml
Iodine	5 g
5% NaOH solution	q.s.
Methylated spirit	q.s.

Procedure

1. Dissolve 5 g of iodine in 5 ml acetone in a conical flask.
2. Add sufficient 5% sodium hydroxide solution slowly with shaking until the colour of iodine is discharged.
3. Allow contents of flask to stand for 10–15 minutes.
4. Filter the yellow precipitate of iodoform through Buchner funnel. Wash the precipitate with cold water.
5. Dry precipitate between filter paper and weigh it.
6. Determine its melting point, 121°C.

11. Preparation of benzoic acid from benzamide

Requirements

Benzamide	1 g
Sodium hydroxide (10%) solution	15 ml

Chemical Reaction

Reaction Mechanism

Benzamide   Benzoate

Procedure

(i) Place benzamide (1 g) and 10% aqueous sodium hydroxide solution (15 ml) in 100 ml conical flask and boil the mixture for 30 minutes under refluxing condition to evolve out the ammonia gas.

(ii) Now, cool the solution in a ice water. Then, add concentrated hydrochloric acid to make acidic.

(iii) Filter the separated solid of benzoic acid and recrystallize from hot water, m.p. 120–121°C.

12. Preparation of Schiff's base from benzaldehyde and aniline

Requirements

Aniline	10 ml
Benzaldehyde	10 ml

Chemical Reaction

Benzaldehyde   Aniline   Schiff base

Schiff's bases are condensation products of aldehydes and primary aromatic amines.

Reaction Mechanism

Benzaldehyde   Schiff's base

Procedure

(i) Place purified benzaldehyde (10 ml) and redistilled aniline (10 ml) in a flask and heat on boiling water bath for 15 minutes with stirring.

(ii) Cool the contents, stirr well, filter the Schiff's base and crystallize it from ethanol, m.p. 55°C.

13. Preparation of benzimidazole from o-phenylenediamine

Requirements

o-phenylenediamine	1 g
Formic acid	2.0 ml

Chemical Reaction

o-Phenylenediamine   HCOOH   Benzimidazole

Reaction Mechanism

$$- 2H_2O$$

Procedure

(i) Place o-phenylenediamine (1 g) and formic acid (2 ml) in a dry test tube.

(ii) Plug the mouth of test tube and heat it on a boiling water bath for 1.5 hours.

(iii) Cool down the test tube under tap water.

(iv) Basify it, with 10% sodium hydroxide solution with constant stirring, filter the product, wash with cold water and crystallize with hot water, m.p. 175°C.

14. Preparation of *para*-iodobenzoic acid from *para*-aminobenzoic acid

para-iodobenzoic acid is used as anti-infective, contraceptive agent and X-ray contrast medium for diagnostic radiology.

Requirements

para-aminobenzoic acid	1.374 g
3M HCl solution	10 ml
NaNO$_2$	0.70 g
Potassium iodide	1.66 g
Urea	Minimum
Ethanol (95%)	Enough for recrystallization

para-iodobenzoic acid is prepared via Sandmeyer reaction from diazotized *para*-amino-benzoic acid.

Reaction

para-Amino benzoic acid   *para*-Iodo-benzoic acid

Reaction mechanism

(i) Formation of the nitrosonium ion

(ii) Formation of the benzenediazonium ion

(iii) Formation of para-iodobenzoic acid

para-Iodobenzoic acid

Procedure

1. Place *para*-aminobenzoic acid (PABA) (1.374 g) into a 100 ml Erlenmeyer flask.
2. Add 10 ml 3M HCl solution.
3. Warm gently while stirring until PABA dissolves.
4. Dissolve NaNO$_2$ (1.66 g) in 10 ml water.
5. Cool both solutions in ice baths until both are below 5°C temperature
6. Add sodium nitrite solution to Erlenmeyer flask, keep below 10°C.
7. Test with starch-iodide paper, add minute amounts of urea to give a negative test.
8. Dissolve KI (1.66 g) in 100 ml of water.
9. Pour diazonium salt solution into 600 ml beaker with the KI solution, and stir.
10. Heat gently, pop foam with glass rod.

11. Collect product with vacuum filtration, cold water wash.
12. Recrystallize with 80% ethanol/20% water.
13. Dry the product and determine its melting point, 270–273°C.

15. Preparation of 1,2,3,4-tetrahydrocarbazole

Requirements

Cyclohexanone	9 ml
Phenylhydrazine	8 ml
Glacial acetic acid	25 ml

Chemical Reaction

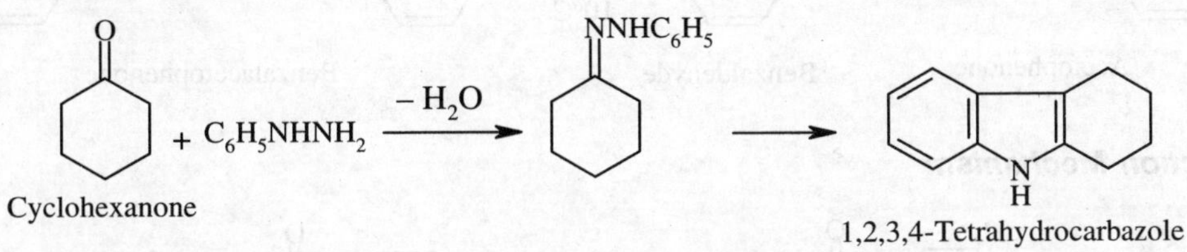

Cyclohexanone

1,2,3,4-Tetrahydrocarbazole

Reaction Mechanism

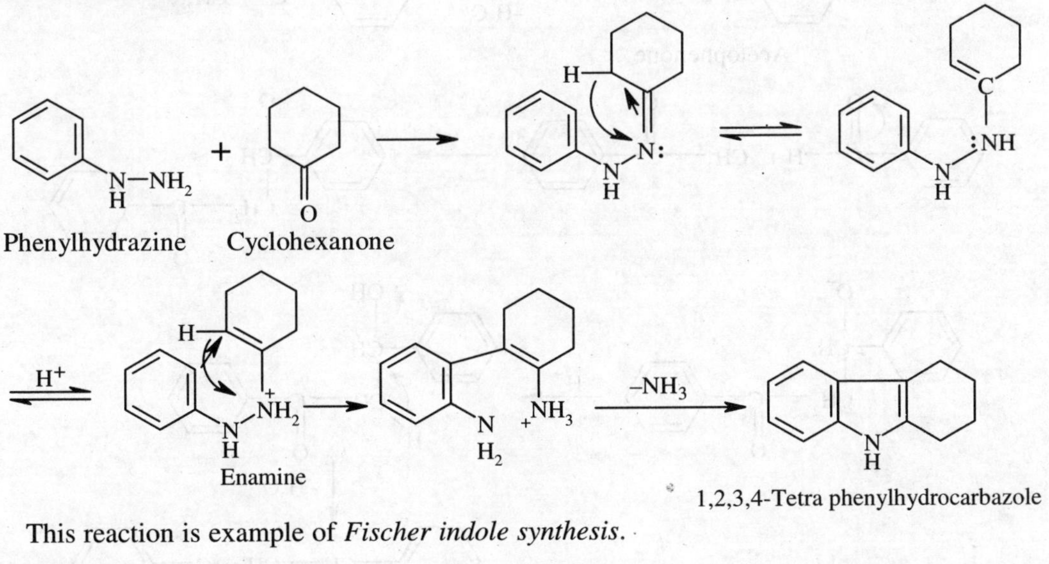

Phenylhydrazine   Cyclohexanone

Enamine

1,2,3,4-Tetra phenylhydrocarbazole

This reaction is example of *Fischer indole synthesis*.

Procedure

(i) Dissolve cyclohexanone (9 ml) in glacial acetic acid (25 ml) in a two-necked flask attached with refluxing condenser and separatory funnel.
(ii) Place redistilled phenylhydrazine (8.0 ml) in a separatory funnel.
(iii) Heat the contents of flask to gentle reflux and add the phenyl hydrazine slowly for 30 minutes.
(iv) Heat the contents for further 30 minutes.
(v) Cool down the solution in a ice bath to get crystals of tetrahydracarbazole.
(vi) Filter the solid, drain well and recrystallize with aqueous ethanol, m.p. 120°C (its picrate, m.p. 148°C).

Note: Picrate derivative is prepared by mixing cold saturated solution of tetrahydrocarbazole and picric acid.

16. Preparation of benzalacetophenone from acetophenone

Requirements

Acetophenone	12 ml
Benzaldehyde	10 ml
Ethanol	30 ml
Sodium hydroxide	0.5 g

Chemical Reaction

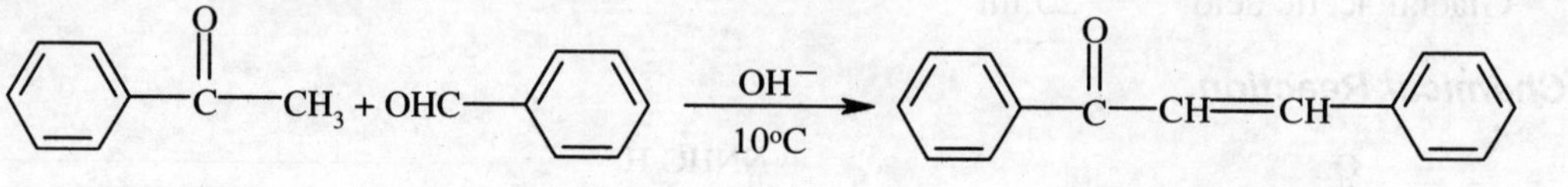

Acetophenone   Benzaldehyde   Benzalacetophenone

Reaction Mechanism

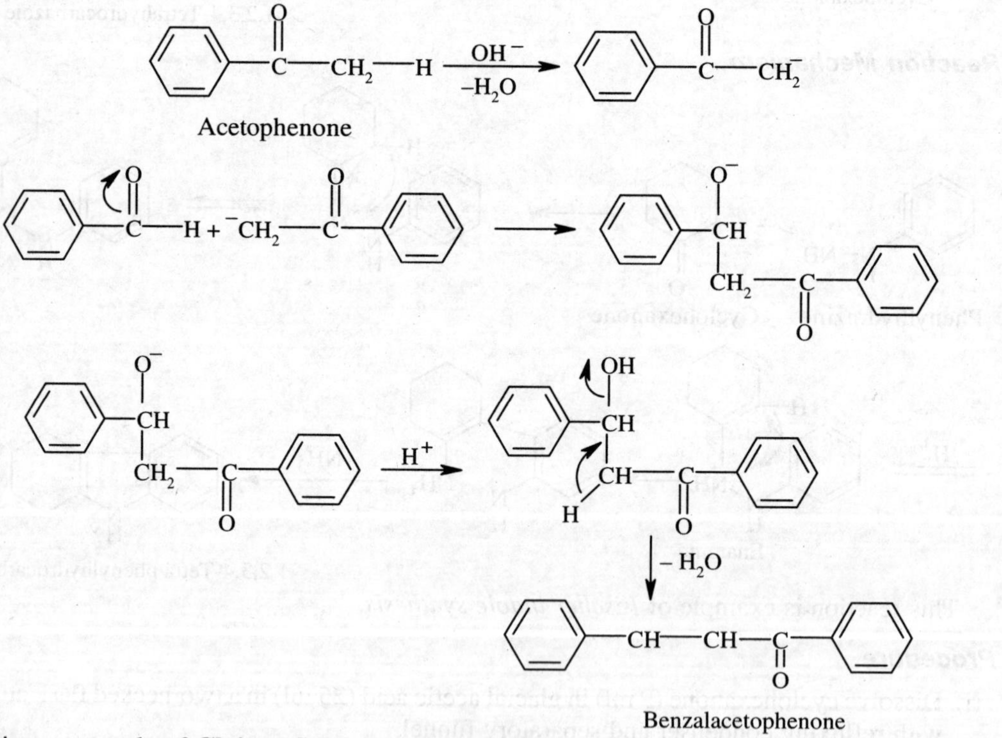

Acetophenone

Benzalacetophenone

It is an example of **Claisen-Schmidt condensation**.

Procedure

(i) Dissolve sodium hydroxide (0.5 g) in a mixture of water (50 ml) and ethanol (30 ml) in a flask.

(ii) Immerse the flask in the crushed ice bath and then add benzaldehyde (10 ml) slowly at a 10°C temperature.

(iii) Take out the flask and stir vigorously until the mixture becomes highly viscous at room temperature.

(iv) Keep the flask in a ice bath for 10 minutes.

(v) Filter the product with the help of cold water, wash with cold water until the washing are neutral to litmus and crystallize from ethanol, m.p. 57–58°C.

17. Preparation of 3-methyl-1-phenyl pyrazole-5-one

Requirements

Ethyl acetoacetate	1.2 ml
Phenylhydrazine	0.9 ml
Acetic acid	3.5 ml

Chemical Reaction

$$CH_3COCH_2COOC_2H_5 + C_6H_5NHNH_2 \longrightarrow$$

Ethyl acetoacetate

3-Methyl-1-phenyl pyrazole-5-one

$$+ \; C_2H_5OH + H_2$$

Reaction Mechanism

3-Methyl-1-phenyl pyrazole-5-one

Procedure

(i) Mix ethyl acetoacetate (1.2 ml) and phenylhydrazine (0.9 ml) and add acetic acid (3.5 ml) in a test tube.

(ii) Plug the test tube and heat the test tube for 30 minutes.

(iii) Cool the content and add ether (6 ml).

(iv) Filter the solids and wash with ether, dry it and recrystallize, m.p 128°C.

18. Preparation of *p*-acetylaminophenol or acetaminophen (paracetamol)

Requirements

p-Aminophenol	11 g
Acetic anhydride	15 ml

Chemical Reaction

$$(CH_3CO)_2O$$

p-Aminophenol   *p*-Acetylaminophenol

Reaction Mechanism

p-Acetylaminophenol

Procedure

 (i) Place p-aminophenol (11 g) in a conical flask and add acetic anhydride (15 ml).
 (ii) Shake the mixture vigorously and warm on a water bath till almost clear solution is obtained.
(iii) Cool the flask in ice bath, filter the acetylated derivative, wash with cold water and recrystallize with hot water, m.p. 169°C.

19. Preparation of phenacetin from acetaminophen

Requirements

Acetaminophen	1 g
Anhydrous K_2CO_3	1.9 g
Methyl ethyl ketone	15 ml
Ethyl iodide	1.4 g

Chemical Reaction

The conversion of acetaminophen (p-HOC_6H_4–NH–$COCH_3$) into phenacetin (C_2H_5–O-p-C_6H_4–NH–$COCH_3$) is an example of the *Williamson ether synthesis* using a phenol as the alcohol. The net reaction is:

Acetaminophen   Phenacetin

Reaction Mechanism

The Williamson ether synthesis actually a two-step conversion to form an ether. Initially, the acetaminophen reacts with carbonate to form the corresponding phenoxide ion:

$$HO - C_6H_4 - NH - COCH_3 + CO_3^{-2} \longrightarrow {}^-O - C_6H_4 - NH - COCH_3 + HCO_3^-$$

The phenoxide ion then acts as the nucleophile in the S_N2 reaction with ethyl iodide to form phenacetin:

$$CH_3CH_2I + {}^-O - C_6H_4 - NH - COCH_3 \longrightarrow CH_3CH_2 - O - C_6H_4 - NH - COCH_3 + I^-$$

Procedure

1. Powder the acetaminophen (1 g) using a mortar and pestle.
2. Set up the reaction in the hood with 50 ml round bottom flask and water cooled condensers.
3. Add the acetaminophen, K_2CO_3, 12 ml of MEK (methyl ethyl ketone, b.p. 80°C), and the ethyl iodide in the flask.
4. Connect the condenser and heat under refluxing condition for 1 hour.
5. Cool the flask in an ice bath and filter the contents of the flask into the separatory funnel. Rinse some ether through the flask and filter to carry additional product into the separatory funnel.
6. Wash the organic phase with 20 ml of 5% aqueous NaOH to remove any unreacted acetaminophen. Dry the organic layer over anhydrous Na_2SO_4, filter into a 100 ml beaker and evaporate out the MEK on the steam bath in the hood*.
7. Record the weight. Recrystallize the crude phenacetin from water. Collect the crystals with a small Buchner funnel and let them air dry.
8. Record the final weight and melting point, 137°C. Calculate the % yield.

20. Preparation of α-Phenylthiourea

Requirements

Ammonium thiocyanate	17 g
Dry acetone	150 ml
Benzoyl chloride	28 g
Aniline	18.6 g

Chemical Reaction

$$NH_4SCN + C_6H_5COCl \longrightarrow C_6H_5CONCS + NH_4Cl$$

$$C_6H_5CONCS + C_6H_5NH_2 \longrightarrow C_6H_5CONHCSNHC_6H_5$$

$$C_6H_5CONHCSNHC_6H_5 \xrightarrow{\text{NaOH}} C_6H_5NHCSNH_2$$
$$\text{α-Phenylthiourea}$$

Reaction Mechanism

---

* This evaporation can be hastened by using a hot plate (in the hood) but the process must be carefully watched to avoid burning of the product. Just before the last of the MEK has evaporated, remove the flask from the hot plate and keep it to allow the vapour to go out.

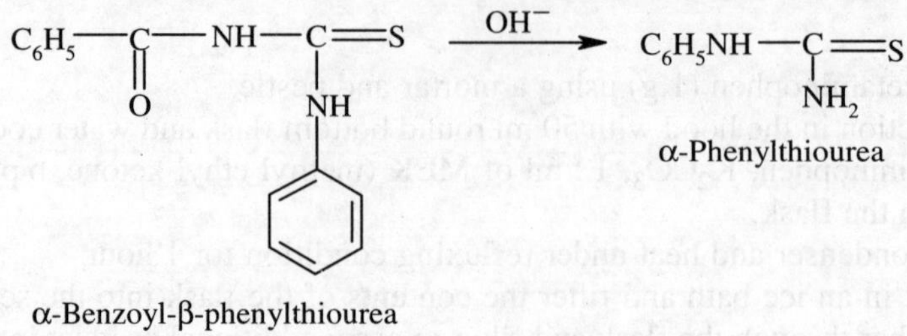

$$C_6H_5-\underset{\underset{O}{\|}}{C}-NH-\underset{\underset{NH}{\|}}{C}=S \xrightarrow{OH^-} C_6H_5NH-\underset{\underset{NH_2}{\|}}{C}=S$$

α-Phenylthiourea

α-Benzoyl-β-phenylthiourea

Procedure

1. Place ammonium thiocyanate (17 g) and dry acetone (75 ml) in R B flask fitted with reflux condenser.
2. Add slowly benzoyl chloride (28 g) to it with stirring.
3. After the addition, reflux the reaction mixture for 5 minutes.
4. Then, add a solution of aniline (18.6 g) dissolved in acetone (75 ml) at such a rate that the solution refluxes gently.
5. Pour the reaction mixture carefully in water (1 litre) with stirring and the filter the resulting precipitates of α-benzoyl-α-phenyl thiourea.
6. Dissolve the precipitate in 10% NaOH solution (250 ml).
7. After the removal of small amount of insoluble material, acidify the filtrate with concentrated HCl solution and then make slightly basic with ammonium hydroxide solution.
8. Allow to keep for a few minutes, filter the product and crystallize with ethanol, m.p. 153°C.

21. Preparation of glucosazone from glucose

Requirements

Glucose	4 g
Phenylhydrazine hydrochloride	10 g
Sodium acetate	10 g

Chemical Reaction

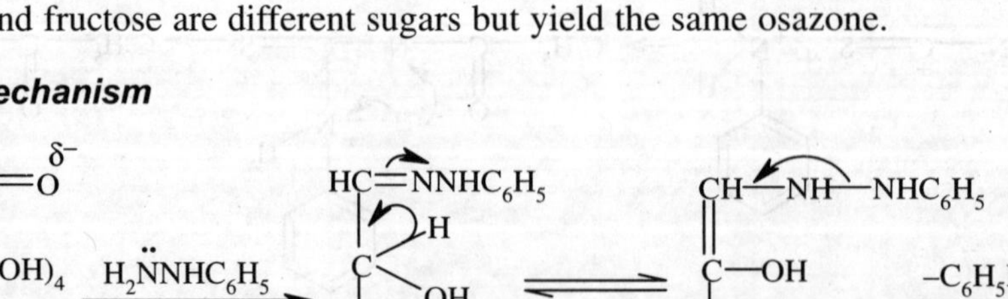

Glucose and fructose are different sugars but yield the same osazone.

Reaction Mechanism

$$\underset{\substack{\text{CH}=\text{NH} \\ \text{C}=\text{O} \\ (\text{CHOH})_3 \\ \text{CH}_2\text{OH}}}{} \xrightarrow[-\,\text{H}_2\text{O}]{\text{H}_2\text{NNHC}_6\text{H}_5} \underset{\substack{\text{CH}=\text{NH} \\ \text{C}=\text{NNHC}_6\text{H}_5 \\ (\text{CHOH})_3 \\ \text{CH}_2\text{OH}}}{} \xrightarrow[-\,\text{NH}_3]{\text{H}_2\text{NNHC}_6\text{H}_5} \underset{\substack{\text{CH}=\text{NNHC}_6\text{H}_5 \\ \text{C}=\text{NNHC}_6\text{H}_5 \\ (\text{CHOH})_3 \\ \text{CH}_2\text{OH} \\ \textbf{Glucosazone}}}{}$$

Procedure

(i) Place glucose (4 g), phenylhydrazine hydrochloride (10 g) and sodium acetate (10 g) in a beaker.

(ii) Add to it water (100 ml) and heat the content 30–45 minutes on water bath.

(iii) Cool the beaker in an ice bath, yellow crystals of glucosazone precipitate out.

(iv) Filter the crude product, wash with cold water and recrystallize it from ethanol, m.p. 205°C.

22. Preparation of phenolphthalein from phenol

Requirements

Phenol	25 g
Phthalic anhydride	12.5 g
Conc. H_2SO_4	8 ml

Chemical Reaction

Phthalic anhydride + 2 Phenol $\xrightarrow[-\,H_2O]{H_2SO_4}$ Phenolphthalein

Mechanism

Procedure

(i) Heat the phenol (25 g) and phthalic anhydride (12.5 g) in a round bottom flask on oil bath till the contents melt.

  (ii) At this stage, add concentrated sulphuric acid (8 ml) slowly and heat the reaction mixture on oil bath at 120°C for 6 hours or until the contents becomes semi solid and dark red in colour.

 (iii) Pour the reaction mixture in hot water (500 ml) and boil until the odour of phenol disappears.

 (iv) Filter the solid mass, wash with water and then dissolve in dilute NaOH solution (minimum quantity), filter off the any solid material and acidify the filtrate with dilute acetic acid and a few drops of hydrochloric acid.

  (v) Allow to keep for sometime, filter the yellow granules of Phenolphthalein and crystallize from ethanol, m.p. 256–258°C.

23. Preparation of urotropine (hexamethylenetetramine) from formaldehyde

Requirements

Formalin	8 ml
Ammonia solution	10 ml

Chemical Reaction

$$6HCHO + 4NH_3 \longrightarrow (CH_2)_6N_4 + 6H_2O$$
$$\text{Urotropine}$$

Mechanism

Urotropine

Procedure

  (i) Place formalin (40% solution of formaldehyde) in a porcelain dish and add to it liquid ammonia solution dropwise with stirring.

 (ii) Heat the porcelain dish on a water bath and evaporate the content with stirring.

 (iii) Remove the solid urotropine from the dish and crystallize it, m.p. 280°C.

24. Preparation of barbituric acid from urea

Barbituric acid or malonylurea has pyrimidine heterocyclic skeleton. It is an odourless powder soluble in water. Barbiturates are derivatives of barbituric acid. They can be used as hypnotics, sedatives, anticonvulsants and anesthetics, although they are probably most familiar as 'sleeping pills'. The different properties of the various barbiturates depend upon the side groups attached to the ring. Barbituric acid itself is not pharmacologically active. Using the *Knoevenagel condensation reaction*, barbituric acid can form a large variety of barbiturate drugs that behave as central nervous system depressants. The barbital (veronal) was the first to be used in medicine in 1903, and the second, phenobarbital was first marketed in 1912.

Barbituric acid
(malonyl urea)

Barbituric acid is prepared from condensation reaction of diethyl malonate with urea.

Reactions

Diethyl malonate + Urea $\xrightarrow[\text{C}_2\text{H}_5\text{OH}]{\text{Na}}$ Barbituric acid

Reaction mechanism

Barbituric acid

Chemicals required

Sodium metal	1.2 g
Absolute ethanol	50 ml
Diethyl malonate	8 g
Urea	3 g
HCl solution	5 ml

Procedure

1. Place 1.2 g of clean sodium metal into a dry 250 ml round-bottomed flask, fitted with a reflux condenser.
2. Add 25 ml of absolute ethanol slowly (portion-wise). If the reaction is unduly vigorous, immerse the flask momentarily in ice.
3. When all the sodium has reacted, add 8 g (7.6 ml) of diethyl malonate, followed by a solution of 3 g of dry urea in 25 ml of hot absolute ethanol (70°C). Shake the mixture well, and reflux it for 1 hour in an oil bath heated to 110°C. White solid separates out.
4. Add 45 ml of hot (50°C) water to the reaction mixture followed with concentrated hydrochloric acid, with stirring, until the solution is acidic. Filter the resulting mixture and leave clear solution in the refrigerator overnight.
5. Filter the solid on the Büchner funnel, wash it with cold water, drain well and then dry at 100°C for 2 hours. Weigh the product, calculate the yield of barbituric acid and measure the m.p. (lit. melts with decomposition at 245°C).

25. Preparation of phenyl azo-β-naphthol (an azo dye)

Requirements

Aniline	2 ml
Conc. HCl	6.5 ml
Sodium nitrite	1.6 g
β-Naphthol	3.2 g

Sodium hydroxide	2.0 g
Glacial acetic acid	12.0 ml
Ice	As per need
Distilled water	As per need

Chemical Reaction

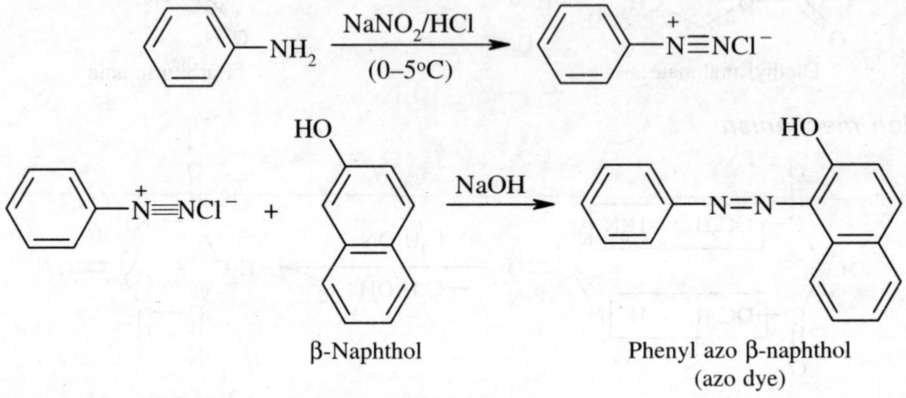

β-Naphthol   Phenyl azo β-naphthol
(azo dye)

Reaction Mechanism

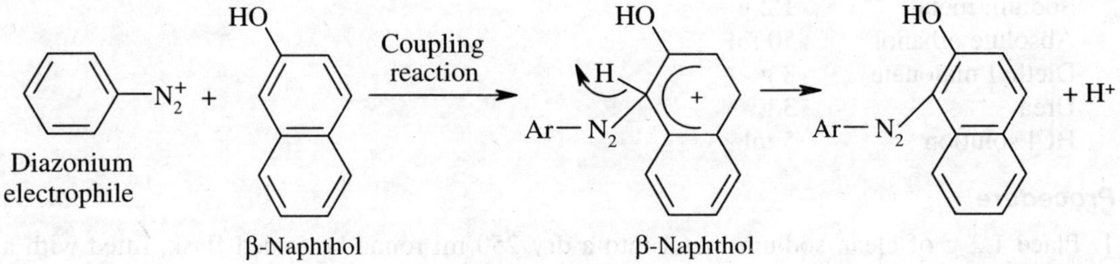

Diazonium
electrophile

β-Naphthol   β-Naphthol

Procedure

1. Place conc. hydrochloric acid (6.5 ml) in 100 ml beaker. Dilute it with equal quantity of water and dissolve aniline (2 ml) in it.
2. Cool the above mixture by placing the beaker in an ice bath maintained at 0–5°C temperature.
3. Diazotise the above mixture by slowly adding a solution of $NaNO_2$ (1.6 g) in water (10 ml) while maintaining the temperature below 5°C.
4. Dissolve β-naphthol (3.2 g) in 10% w/v NaOH solution (20 ml). Add crushed ice (25 g) to it.
5. Stir the β-naphthol solution well and add chilled diazonium chloride solution very slowly to it with constant stirring. An orange red dye of phenyl azo-β-naphthol is formed.
6. Allow the mixture to stand in the bath for 30 minutes with occasional shaking.
7. Filter the crystals and wash them well with cold water.
8. Recrystallize with glacial acetic acid.
9. Dry it and record the melting point, m.p. 132°C.

26. Preparation of dibenzalacetone (dibenzylidene acetone)

α-Hydrogen atom of aliphatic aldehydes and ketones is acidic in nature, therefore, in the presence of dilute alkali, such as aldehyde or ketone condenses with an aromatic aldehyde to give α,β-unsaturated aldehyde or ketone. This reaction is called *Claisen-Schmidt reaction*. For example, benzaldehyde undergoes condensation with acetone in the presence of aqueous sodium hydroxide (NaOH) to give dibenzalacetone.

Requirements

Ethanol	25 ml
NaOH	3.15 g
Benzaldehyde	3.2 ml
Acetone	2.5 ml
Ice	As per need
Ethylacetate	As per need

Chemical Reaction

Benzaldehyde — CHO + CH_3COCH_3 + OHC — (Acetone) $\xrightarrow{NaOH}$ — CH=CHCOCH=CH — Dibenzalacetone

Reaction mechanism

Please refer Claisen-Schmidt condensation (preparation 16).

Procedure

 (i) Prepare a solution sodium hydroxide (3.15 g) in a mixture of ethanol (25 ml) and distilled water (30 ml) taken in a 250 ml beaker. Cool the beaker in an ice bath maintained at a temperature of about 20 to 25°C.
 (ii) Prepare a mixture of benzaldehyde (3.2 ml) and acetone (2.5 ml) and add half of this mixture slowly in ice cooled NaOH solution prepared in step (i) with vigorously stirring. A fluffy precipitate is formed within 1–2 minutes. Stir the mixture gently for about fifteen minutes.
(iii) After 15 minutes, add remaining mixture of benzaldehyde and acetone and stir for 30 minutes more.
(iv) Filter the resulting pale yellow solid and then wash with cold water. Dry it and recrystallize it from ethanol or ethyl acetate.
 (v) Report the yield and the melting point of the compound, m.p. 110°C.

27. Preparations of cinnamic acid from benzaldehyde

Cinnamic acid is an unsaturated carboxylic acid with the formula $C_6H_5CH=CHCO_2H$. It is a white crystalline compound that is slightly soluble in water, and freely soluble in many organic solvents. Cinnamic acid is used in flavors, synthetic indigo, and certain pharmaceuticals. A major use is in the manufacturing of the methyl, ethyl, and benzyl esters for the perfume industry. Cinnamic acid is a precursor to the sweetener aspartame via enzyme-catalysed amination to phenylalanine.

Reaction

Cinnamic acid is prepared by **Perkin's reaction**. The benzaldehyde is heated with sodium acetate in presence of acetic anhydride. To get mono-benzylidene acetic anhydride. The later when heated with sodium carbonate solution undergoes hydrolysis to sodium cinnamate and acetate. The cinnamate is acidified to get free cinnamic acid.

$$C_6H_5CHO + HCH_2CO-O-OCCH_3 \rightarrow C_6H_5CH(OH)CH_2CO-OOCCH_3$$

$$C_5H_5CH(OH)CH_2CO\text{-}OOCCH_3 + Na_2CO_3 \rightarrow C_6H_5CH = CHCOONa + CH_3COONa + CO_2$$
Sodium cinnamate

Reaction mechanism

The **Perkin reaction** is an organic reaction developed by English chemist William Henry Perkin that is used to make cinnamic acids. The formation of cinnamic acid (α,β-unsaturated aromatic acid) by the reaction of an aromatic aldehyde with an acid anhydride, in the presence of an alkali salt of the acid, is knows as Perkin reaction. The active methylene moiety is generated by acetic anhydride. The alkali salt acts as a base catalyst. Reaction mechanism is as follows:

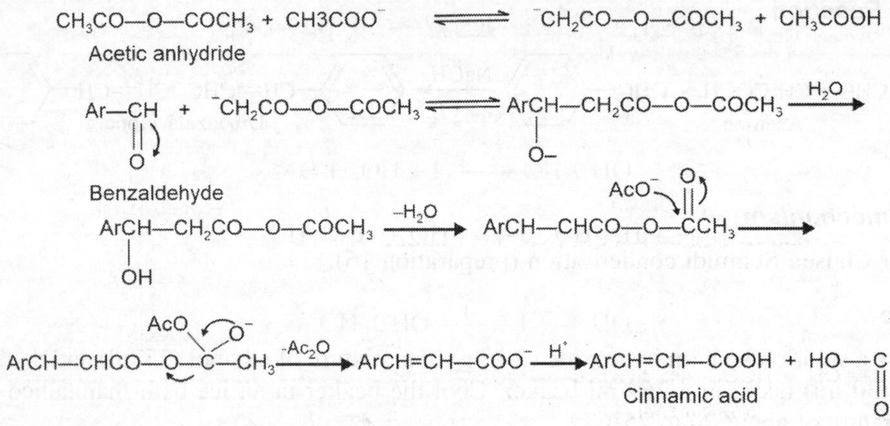

Requirements

Benzaldehyde	10 ml
Acetic anhydride	16 ml
Sodium acetate	5 g
Sodium carbonate solution	q.s.
Hydrochloric acid solution	q.s.
Rectified spirit	q.s.

Procedure

1. Place 10 ml of freshly distilled benzaldehyde (to ensure absence of benzoic acid), 16 ml of acetic anhydride and 5 g of sodium acetate in 50 ml of round bottom flask fitted with air condenser with anhydrous calcium chloride tube.
2. Heat the flask in an air or sand bath at 175–180°C temperature for 6 hours (the mixture boils vigorously and white precipitate may separate out in the liquid) (take the temperature by dipping the thermometer in the liquid).
3. Pour the hot liquid in 100 ml of water contained in round bottom flask of 500 ml capacity fitted for steam distillation.
4. Add with vigorous shaking saturated sodium carbonate solution drop-wise until solution becomes acidic (check by litmus paper—conversion of red litmus into blue color).
5. Now steam distilled the solution until unchanged benzaldehyde has been removed and the distillate is no longer turbid.
6. Cool the residual solution until the small quantity of insoluble oily impurity has formed a semi-solid sticky mass and the filter at the pump.

7. Acidify the clear filtrate by adding concentrated hydrochloric acid solution drop-wise with vigorous shaking until precipitation of cinnamic acid complete.
8. Cool if necessary in ice water and filter off the cinnamic acid.
9. Recrystallize from a mixture of 3 volumes of water and 1 volume of rectified spirit.
10. Determine its melting point, 133°C.

28. Preparation of *m*-nitrobenzoic acid

Requirements

Concentrated nitric acid	3 ml
Concentrated sulphuric acid	1 ml
Benzoic acid	1 g

Chemical Reaction

$$C_6H_5COOH + HNO_3 \longrightarrow$$

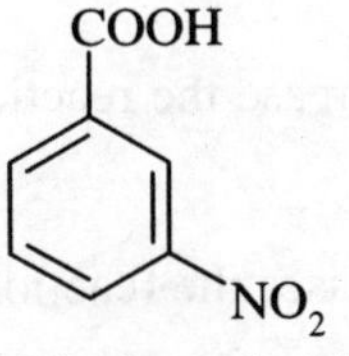

COOH

m-Nitrobenzoic acid

$$+ H_2O$$

Reaction Mechanism

$$HONO_2 + H_2SO_4 \rightleftharpoons H_2O + HSO_4^- + NO_2^+$$

Nitronium ion

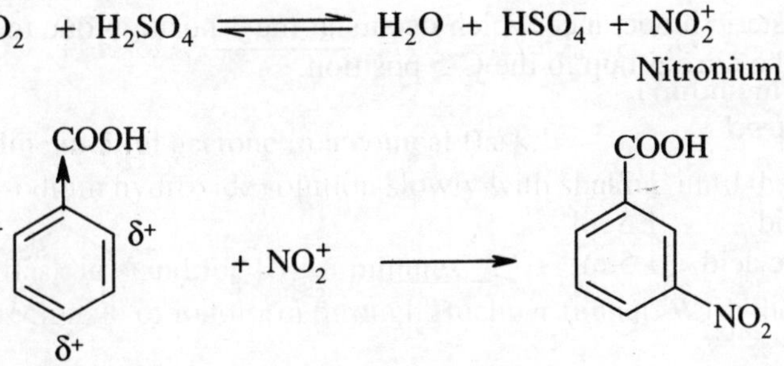

COOH

δ^+ δ^+

δ^+

$$+ NO_2^+ \longrightarrow$$

COOH

NO$_2$

COOH is a deactivating group and so it is meta directing.

Procedure

(i) Add the sulphuric acid to the nitric acid in a large test tube and heat to 90°C in a water bath.
(ii) Add the benzoic acid gradually with stirring/shaking to dissolve it.
(iii) Continue to heat the mixture at 90°C for ten minutes after all the benzoic acid has been added.
(iv) Cool down. The crystals of *m*-nitrobenzoic acid separates out.
(v) Filter it, wash with little cold water and recrystallize from hot water, m.p. 142°C.

29. Preparation of 5-nitrosalicylic acid from salicylic acid

5-Nitrosalicylic acid is available as yellow to orange-brown coloured powder and water soluble. 5-Nitrosalicylic acid is an important raw material and intermediate used in organic synthesis, pharmaceuticals, agrochemicals.

Reaction

5-Nitrosalicylic acid is synthesized by nitration reaction of salicylic acid.

Salicylic acid   5-Nitrosalicylic acid

Reaction mechanism

The nitration of salicylic acid is aromatic electrophilic substitution reaction. The nitronium (NO_2^+) ion is electrophilic reagent. At low temp, $0°C$, nitro group is added at the 5-position (favoured by both –OH and COOH substituents).

Activators

The phenolic OH group increase the reaction and ortho/para directing.

Deactivators

The carboxylic group decreases the reaction and meta directing.

1. Salicylic acid has a strong activator and a moderate deactivator (so there will be some cancelling affects, but salicylic acid is most likely more reactive than benzene).
2. Nitro group can be added at the 5 position (meta to carboxylic acid and para to hydroxyl group). It can also be added at the 3 position (ortho to the hydroxyl group)—this will not happen due to steric hinderance which occurs at the 3 position due to the hydroxyl group; thus directing the nitro group to the C-5 position.

Chemicals required

Salicylic acid	1.2 g
Conc. nitric acid	1.5 ml
Conc. sulphuric acid	1.5 ml

Procedure

1. Prepare an ice bath in 250 ml beaker.
2. Measure 3.0 ml of the mixed acid (1 : 1 sulphuric and nitric acids) into a 5 ml conical flask or in a test tube and cool in the ice bath.
3. Weigh 1.2 g of salicylic acid into a 50 ml round bottom flask. Attach an air condenser to the flask and then cool in ice bath.
4. Add slowly (drop-wise) the cold mixed acid to the salicylic acid. Stir/swirl flask after each addition to keep the temperature below 10°C (addition should be done slowly to control the exothermic reaction). This should take about 10–15 minutes to complete.
5. After addition is completed, remove the ice bath and allow the reaction to warm to room temperature. Continue to stir/swirl the flask.
6. After 5 minutes at room temperature, pour all the contents from the round bottom flask into a 50 ml beaker containing approx 5 g of crushed ice.
7. Using a glass rod thoroughly mix the ice and the solid product.
8. After the ice has completely melted, allow the mixture to stand at room temperature for 10 minutes.
9. Carefully decant the lighter water layer into another beaker.
10. Collect the remaining product by vacuum filtration.
11. Wash the solid product with cold water 2×2 ml.

12. Dry the product on a filter paper and recrystallize by dissolving in minimum amount of absolute ethanol, stir with a clean micro spatula using a twirling motion.
13. Once the solid is completely dissolved, add cold water drop-wise until product precipitates out.
14. Cool the mixture in an ice bath for 4–5 minutes.
15. Once crystallization is complete, filter using a Hirsch funnel and allow to air dry for 5 minutes, and determine melting point, 228–230°C.

30. Preparation of methyl salicylate (wintergreen oil)

Requirements

Salicylic acid	5 g
Methanol	10 ml
Sulphuric acid	0.5 ml
Ether	q.s.
5% $NaHCO_3$ solution	q.s.

Chemical Reaction

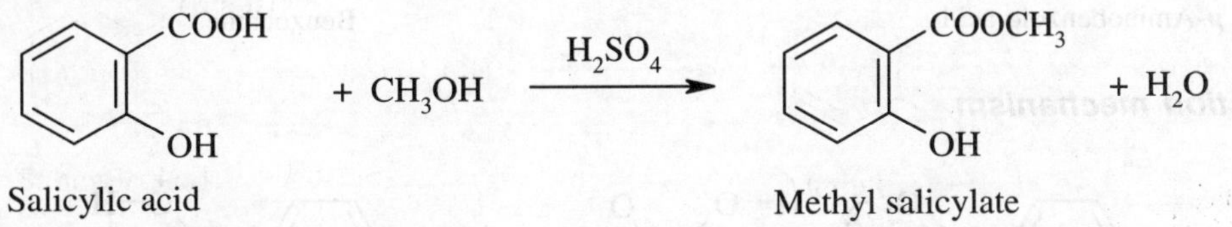

Salicylic acid   Methyl salicylate

Reaction mechanism

Salicylic acid

Methyl salicylate

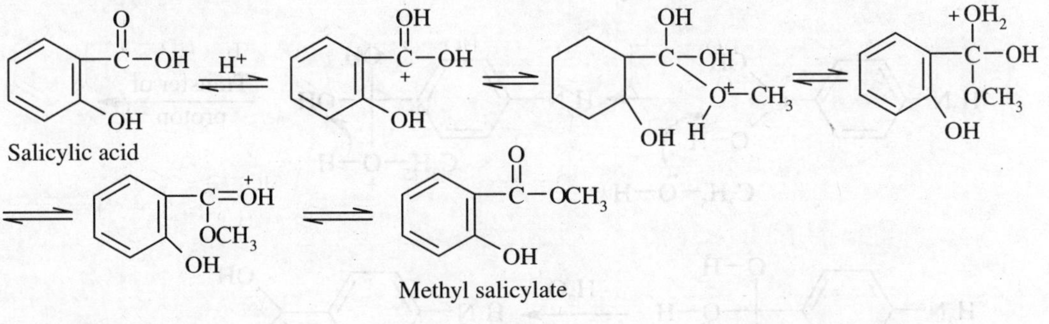

Procedure

1. Weigh out about 5.0 g salicylic acid, transfer it to a large dry test tube and add 10 ml of methanol to dissolve the salicylic acid completely.
2. Carefully add 0.5 ml of concentrated H_2SO_4 to the mixture (in the hood) and mix.
3. Place the mixture in the hot water bath for 20 minutes to complete the reaction.
4. After the completion of reaction, remove the test tube from the water bath and allow it to cool.
5. After it has cooled, smell the minty aroma of wintergreen.
6. Pour the mixture into cold water in a beaker and add 50 ml diethyl ether to it.
7. Transfer the content to a separating funnel and remove the aqueous layer.
8. To the organic layer, add 5 ml of 5% $NaHCO_3$ solution and mix. This will neutralize any remaining acid.

9. Transfer the ether layer to another dry flask and add anhydrous $CaCl_2$ or sodium sulphate until the product is dry.
10. Filter out the drying agent and evaporate off the ether.
11. Take the boiling point of methyl salicylate.
12. Calculate the yield density of methyl salicylate.

31. Preparation of Benzocaine

Requirements

p-Aminobenzoic acid	5 g
Absolute ethanol	40 ml
5% NaHCO$_3$ solution	0.5 ml

Chemical Reaction

p-Aminobenzoic acid   Benzocaine

Reaction mechanism

Benzocaine

Procedure

1. Dissolve 5.0 g of *p*-amino benzoic acid and 40.0 ml of absolute ethanol* in a round-bottom flask with a magnetic stirbar. Stir the mixture until the solid dissolved.
2. Cool the mixture in an ice bath and slowly add 1.0 ml of concentrated sulphuric acid (carefully). A large amount of precipitate will form when the sulphuric acid is added, but this solid will slowly dissolve during the reflux that follows. If precipitate persists, add 1–2 drops of sulphuric acid.
3. Boil gently under reflux for about 75 minutes. Take care not to overheat the flask and have too violent reflux rate.
4. After completion of reaction, allow the mixture to cool and transfer the content to a beaker containing 30 ml of water.
5. Add 5% sodium bicarbonate solution until gas is no longer evolved and the pH becomes around 8.
6. Filter the benzocaine precipitates using vacuum filtration and rinse the precipitates.
7. Allow the solid to dry at room temperature on a weighed piece of filter paper, weigh it, calculate the percentage yield, and determine its melting point. The melting point of pure benzocaine is 92°C. Recrystallization may be done from aqueous alcohol.

32. Preparation of 3,5-dimethylpyrazole from acetylacetone

Pyrazole is an organic compound with the formula $C_3H_3N_2H$. It is a heterocycle, characterized by a 5-membered ring of three carbon atoms and two adjacent nitrogen atoms. Notable drugs containing a pyrazole ring are celecoxib (Celebrex) (anti-inflammatory drug) and the anabolic steroid stanozolol (anabolic steroid).

Reaction

Substituted pyrazoles are prepared by condensation of 1,3-diketones with hydrazine. For example, acetylacetone and hydrazine gives 3,5-dimethylpyrazole.

Acetyl acetone   3,5-Dimethyl pyrazole

Reaction mechanism

On next page.

Chemicals required

Acetyl acetone	5 ml
Hydrazine hydrate	3 ml
Ethanol	25 ml
n-Hexane/petroleum ether b.p. 60–80°C	q.s.

---

* Benzocaine is prepared from *p*-aminobenzoic acid by *Fisher esterification*. DRY (absolute ethanol) is used rather than 95%. The 95% alcohol is wet and any water present will tend to prevent ester formation because water is the product of reacting carboxylic group with ethanol in presence of an acid (catalyst). To drive the reaction to completion the water is taken up by a dehydrating agent or can be distilled off into a Dean Stark trap...."

The enamine and imine formed make the heterocycle aromatic without having to carry out an oxidation step.

Procedure

1. Take 3 ml (~60 mmol) of hydrazine hydrate in a 250 ml flask.
2. To this, add 25 ml of ethanol with constant stirring.
3. Now place the flask in an ice cold water or ice-bath and wait for 10 minute.
4. Add slowly 5 ml (~50 mmol) of acetyl acetone drop-wise to the above solution at 15°C temperature with constant stirring.
   Note: The addition of acetyl acetone requires about ~20 minutes to complete.
5. Allow the reaction mixture to come to room temperature and then reflux for an hour (oil-bath temperature ~110ºC).
6. Then, remove the solvent to dryness on rotavapor and add few ml of *n*-hexane to dissolve the solid in lukewarm condition.
7. Place the flask in refrigerator to get crystalline solid. Collect the solid product by filtration. (You may use cold hexane to wash the product.)
8. Determine its melting point,107–108°C.

33. Preparation of phenothiazine from diphenyl amine

Phenothiazines are the largest chemical group, comprising more than 40 compounds (only the most relevant are listed below) grouped under three subtypes. Drugs in this group share the same three-ring structure with different side chains joined at the nitrogen atom of the middle ring. The activity of the group can be affected by substitutions at position 2 or 10. The phenothiazines are categorized into three subclasses based on substitutions at position 10: aliphatic, piperidine, and piperazine phenothiazines.

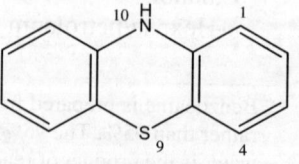

Phenothiazine

- **Aliphatic (a sedative neuroleptic)**
  - Chlorpromazine
  - Levomepromazine
  - Promazine
  - Triflupromazine
- **Piperidine (a less sedating preparation)**
  - Mesoridazine
  - Pericyazine
  - Pipotiazine
  - Thioridazine
- **Piperazine (a long-acting derivative for maintenance treatment)**
  - Perphenazine
  - Fluphenazine
  - Trifluoperazine.

Reaction

It is prepared by condensation reaction of diphenylamine with sulphur in presence of condensing reagent like anhydrous aluminum chloride, iodine, etc.

Diphenylamine   Phenothiazine

Chemicals required

Diphenylamine	22 g
Sulphur	8.2 g
Anhydrous aluminum chloride	3.2 g

Procedure

1. Melt together the 22 g of diphenylamine, 8.2 g of sulphur, and 3.2 g of anhydrous aluminum chloride by heating at 150°C temperature.
2. Maintain the reaction at 140–150°C temperature. There will be the rapid evolution of hydrogen sulphide; by lowering the temperature, a few degrees the reaction can be slackened.
3. When the reaction has moderated, raise the temperature to 160° C for a time. Cool down the melt, grind up and extract, first with water and then with dilute alcohol. The residue consists of almost pure phenothiazine.
4. Recrystallize from alcohol. Yield 93%, yellowish leaflets; m. p. 180°C.

34. Preparation of chlorobutanol from acetone and chloroform

Chlorobutanol, or trichloro-2-methyl-2-propanol, is a chemical preservative, sedative hypnotic and weak local anesthetic similar in nature to chloral hydrate. It has antibacterial and antifungal properties. Chlorobutanol is typically used at a concentration of 0.5% where it lends long-term stability to multi-ingredient formulations.

Chlorobutanol is colourless to white crystals with characteristic odour and taste. It is soluble in alcohol and glycerol; slightly soluble in water; readily soluble in ether, chloroform, and volatile oils. Its melting point is –97°C in anhydrous form and –78°C in hemihydrates form.

Chlorobutanol is formed by the simple nucleophilic addition of chloroform and acetone. The reaction is base driven by potassium or sodium hydroxide. The best result is obtained when powdered KOH is added to a mixture of acetone and chloroform, with the mole ratio $CHCl_3 : Me_2CO : KOH$ equal to $1 : 5 : 0.27$, and the reaction temperature being kept at $-5°C$ to $0°C$.

Reaction

Reaction mechanism

Reaction mechanism demonstrates the ability of chloroform to be deprotonated and act as a nucleophile; a powerful synthetic reagent in its own right.

Requirements

KOH	3.25 g
Dry acetone	50 g
Chloroform	100 g

Procedure

1. Add gradually 3.25 of finely powdered KOH to a mixture of 50 g of dry acetone and 100 g of chloroform over a period of 1 hour, maintained at below $0°C$ temperature.
2. Stir the mixture vigorously for 2 hour.
3. Filter the mass and wash with acetone. It may be difficult to filter due to fineness of solids.
4. Distill the combined filtrates and recover unchanged chloroform and acetone. Collect the fraction passing over $165°C$ and $172°C$ separately.
5. Pour down the distillate in ice cold water and filter off the solid.
6. Recrystallize from a mixture of alcohol and water.
7. Determine its melting point, $97°C$ (anhydrous).

Note: Chlorobutanol is extremely volatile even at room temperature and requires to be dried with great care.

35. Preparation of 2,5-diphenyl oxazole

Oxazole is the parent compound for a vast class of heterocyclic aromatic organic compounds. These are azoles with an oxygen and a nitrogen separated by one carbon. Oxazole is a weak base; its conjugate acid has a pK of 0.8, compared to 7 for imidazole.

The oxazole ring is present in numerous pharmacologically important compounds, including those used as antibiotics and antiproliferatives. The wide range of biological activities of oxazoles includes anti-inflammatory, analgesic, antibacterial, antifungal, hypoglycemic, antiproliferative, antituberculosis, muscle relaxant and HIV inhibitor activity.

Classical oxazole synthetic methods in organic chemistry are:

- Robinson–Gabriel synthesis by dehydration of 2-acylaminoketones
- Fischer oxazole synthesis from cyanohydrins and aldehydes
- Bredereck reaction with α-haloketones and formamide
- Van Leusen reaction with aldehydes and TosMIC

Wen-Chao Gao, Ruo-Lin Wang and Chi Zhang* reported the practical oxazole synthesis mediated by iodine from α-bromoketones and benzylamine derivatives (Org. Biomol. Chem., 2013, 11,7123).

Reaction

α-Bromoacetophenone   2,5-Diphenyloxazole

Reaction mechanism

Firstly, the S_N^2 reaction between α-bromoacetophenone and benzylamine proceed to produce the intermediate A, which could be oxidized to the keto imine B in the presence of iodine and K_2CO_3. After the removal of α-proton, the oxygen anion of enolate would attack the imine functionality to form the oxazoline D. Again, the iodine oxidation of D under basic conditions afforded the required oxazole (C).

Mechanism for I_2-mediated oxazole formation

Chemicals required

Iodine	1.2 g
α-Bromoacetophenone	0.5 g
Benzylamine	0.5 g
Potassium carbonate	1 g
DMF	10–15 ml
Ethyl acetate	50 ml
Saturated sodium thiosulphate solution	5 ml
Petroleum ether	q.s.

Procedure

1. Add iodine (1.2 g, 1.1 mmol) to the mixture of α-bromoacetophenone (0.5 mmol, 0.5 g), benzylamine (0.5 g, 0.6 mmol) and K_2CO_3 (1.0 g, 2 mmol) in 10–15 ml of DMF.
2. Stir the mixture at 80°C temperature.
3. After the completion of reaction as observed by TLC analysis, add EtOAc (about 30 ml) to dilute the reaction mixture, followed by the treatment of saturated $Na_2S_2O_3$ solution to quench the reaction.
4. Separate the organic layer, wash with water (3 × 10 ml), and dry over anhydrous Na_2SO_4.
5. After the removal of the solvent under vacuum, purify the residue by flash column chromatography/simple column chromatography with petroleum ether–EtOAc (10 : 1) to give the 2,5-diphenyloxazole.
6. Determine its melting point, 64–67°C.

36. Preparation of benztriazole from o-phenylenediamine

Benzotriazole (BTA) is a heterocyclic compound containing three nitrogen atoms, with the chemical formula $C_6H_5N_3$. This aromatic compound is colourless and polar and can be used in various fields. Benzotriazole has been known for its great versatility. It has already been used as a restrainer in photographic emulsions and as a reagent for the analytical determination of silver. More importantly, it has been extensively used as a corrosion inhibitor in the atmosphere and underwater.

Reaction

The BTA synthesis involves the reaction of o-phenylenediamine, sodium nitrite and acetic acid. The conversion proceeds via diazotization of one of the amino group.

o-Phenylenediamine   Benztriazole

Reaction mechanism

The first step in the reaction involves straightforward diazotization of one of the amino groups (exactly like what's done in the first part of the *Sandmeyer reaction*) to produce the *ortho*-amino diazonium ion. Instead of eliminating nitrogen as in the Sandmeyer case, the molecule loses a proton and then the diazomium ion internally captures the *ortho*-imino group to yield the triazole product.

o-Phenylenediamine   Benztriazole

Chemicals required

o-Phenylenediamine	10.8 g
Glacial acetic acid	11.5 ml
Sodium nitrite	7.5 g
Benzene	q.s.

Procedure

1. Dissolve 10.8 g o-phenylenediamine (0.1 mole) in a mixture of 11.5 ml (0.2 mole) of glacial acetic acid and 30 ml of water (slight warming is necessary).
2. Cool down to 10°C temperature and then add sodium nitrite solution (7.5 g dissolved in 15 ml of water (the reaction mixture may attain a temperature of 80–85°C temperature and color changes from deep red to pale brown).
3. Stir the mixture for 15 minutes and chill the mixture in ice water for 30 minutes.
4. Filter the products and wash with cold water.
5. Dry and crystallize from benzene.
6. Determine its melting point, 99–100°C.

37. Preparation of 2,4,5-triphenyl-1H-imidazole from benzil

2,4,5-triphenyl-1H-imidazole-1-yl derivatives are found to possess diverse activity like anti-inflammatory, antifungal and antibacterial activity.

2,4,5-Triphenylimidazole

Reactions

It is synthesized via **Radiszewski synthesis** from the reaction of benzil and benzaldehyde in presence of ammonium acetate.

Benzil   Benzaldehyde   2,4,5-Triphenylimidazole

Chemicals required

Benzil	5.2 g
Benzaldehyde	2.65 g
Ammonium acetate	10.0 g
Acetic acid	100 ml

Procedure

1. Dissolve 5.2 g of benzil (25 mmol), 2.65 g of benzaldehyde (25 mmol) and 10.0 g of ammonium acetate (130 mmol) in 100 ml acetic acid (100%) in 250 ml round bottom flask containing a magnetic stirrer bar.
2. Heat the mixture under refluxing in oil bath at 100°C temperature for 3–5 hours with stirring.
3. After this time, cool the mixture to room temperature and filter to remove precipitate which may be present.
4. Add 500 ml of water was added to filtrate and collected the precipitate by filtration with suction.
5. Neutralize the filtrate was neutralized with ammonium hydroxide and collect the second crop of solid.
6. Combine the two crop of solid and recrystallize from aqueous ethyl alcohol.
7. Determine its melting point, 292–295°C.

TWO STEPS PREPARATIONS

38. Preparation of p-nitroacetanilide from aniline

1st Step: Preparation of acetanilide from aniline

Requirements

Aniline	20 ml
Acetic anhydride	20 ml
Glacial acetic acid	20 ml

Chemical Reaction

$$\text{Aniline} + (CH_3CO)_2O \xrightarrow[\text{Reflux, 30 min.}]{CH_3COOH} \text{Acetanilide} + CH_3COOH$$

Procedure

(i) Place above three compounds in 250 ml conical flask and reflux the mixture for 30 minutes with frequent shaking.
(ii) Pour down the contents into ice cold water with constant stirring.
(iii) Filter the crude acetanilide, wash with cold water and recrystallize from boiling water along with small quantity of methylated spirit, m.p. 114°C.

2nd step: Preparation of p–nitroacetanilide from acetanilide

Requirements

Acetanilide	25 g
Glacial acetic acid	20 ml
Conc. H_2SO_4	50 ml
Conc. HNO_3	11 ml

Chemical Reaction

NHCOCH$_3$ (Acetanilide)	$\xrightarrow[\text{Conc. H}_2\text{SO}_4]{\text{Conc. HNO}_3}$	NHCOCH$_3$ / NO$_2$ (p-Nitroacetanilide (insoluble)) + NHCOCH$_2$ NO$_2$ (o-Nitroacetanilide)

Reaction Mechanism

$$HNO_3 + 2H_2SO_4 \longrightarrow NO_2^+ + 2HSO_4^- + H_3O^+$$
Nitronium ion

Procedure

(i) Dissolve dry acetanilide (25 g) in glacial acetic acid (30 ml) in a beaker and then introduce concentrated sulphuric acid (50 ml) slowly with constant stirring to obtain clear solution.

(ii) Place the beaker in a freezing mixture of ice and salt to cool the solution below 5°C.

(iii) Add a cold mixture of concentrated nitric acid (11 ml) and concentrated sulphuric acid (7 ml) dropwise with constant stirring to a reaction mixture while maintaining the temperature below 5°C.

(iv) After adding all the mixed acid, remove the beaker from the freezing mixture and keep it for 1 hour at room temperature with occasional shaking or crushed ice (50 g).

(v) Pour the reaction mixture into an ice cold water (30 ml) to obtain the crude product of p-nitroacetanilide.

(vi) Filter it on suction, wash with cold water till free from acid and recrystallize the pale yellow product from ethanol to get colourless crystalline solid, m.p. 214°C.

Note: o-Nitroacetanilide remains in the filtrate due to its more solubility in H$_2$O.

39. Preparation of *p*-bromoacetanilide from aniline

1st Step: Preparation of acetanilide from aniline

Requirements

Aniline	20 ml
Acetic anhydride	20 ml
Glacial acetic acid	20 ml

Chemical Reaction

Aniline + $(CH_3CO)_2O$ → $\xrightarrow[\text{Reflux, 30 min.}]{CH_3COOH}$ → Acetanilide + CH_3COOH

Procedure

 (i) Place above three compounds in 250 ml conical flask and reflux the mixture for 30 minutes with frequent shaking.
 (ii) Pour down the contents into ice-cold water with constant stirring.
 (iii) Filter the crude acetanilide, wash with cold water and recrystallize from boiling water along with small quantity of methylated spirit, m.p. 114°C.

2nd Step: Preparation of p-bromoacetanilide from acetanilide

Requirements

Acetanilide	13.5 g
Glacial acetic acid	70 ml
Bromine	5.5 ml
Sodium bisulphite	Sufficient quantity

Chemical Reaction

Acetanilide $\xrightarrow{Br_2}$ *p*-Bromoacetanilide (insoluble) + *o*-Bromoacetanilide

Reaction Mechanism

For preparation of acetanilide from aniline, see Preparation No. 38.

$Br_2 \longrightarrow Br^+ + Br^-$

p-Bromoacetanilide (insoluble)

Procedure

(i) Dissolve acetanilide (13.5 g) in glacial acetic acid (45 ml) in 250 ml conical flask.

(ii) Add dropwise by burette, bromine (5.5 ml) dissolved in glacial acetic acid (25 ml) with constant shaking. (*Precaution:* Reaction should be carried out in fuming cupboard).

(iii) Allow to stand the orange coloured reaction mixture at room temperature for half an hour and then pour the contents into cold water.

(iv) Stir well and add sufficient sodium bisulphite to discharge orange colour (which is due to slight excess bromine solution). Filter the crude product, wash with cold water and recrystallize with dilute ethanol to obtain white crystalline compound, m.p. 167°C.

Note: *o*-Bromoacetanilide remains in the solution during crystallization due to its high solubility.

40. Preparation of *p*-bromobenzanilide from aniline

1st Step: Preparation of benzanilide

Requirements

Aniline	5 ml
Benzoyl chloride	7 ml
10% sodium hydroxide	45 ml

Chemical Reaction

Aniline $+ C_6H_5COCl \xrightarrow{NaOH}$ Benzanilide $+ HCl$

Procedure

(i) Place aniline (5 ml) 10% sodium hydroxide solution (45 ml) in 250 ml conical flask and then add slowly benzoyl chloride (7 ml) with vigorous shaking.

(ii) Cork the flask and shake for further 15 minutes or till the odour of benzoyl chloride disappears.

(iii) Dilute the reaction mixture with cold water (100 ml).

(iv) Filter the crude benzanilide with suction on a Buchner funnel, wash with cold water and recrystallize from hot ethanol, m.p. 162°C.

2nd Step: Preparation of p-bromobenzanilide from benzanilide

Requirements

Benzanilide	2 g
Glacial acetic acid	30 ml
Bromine	2 ml

Chemical Reaction

Benzanilide $\xrightarrow{Br_2}$ *p*-Bromobenzanilide

Reaction Mechanism

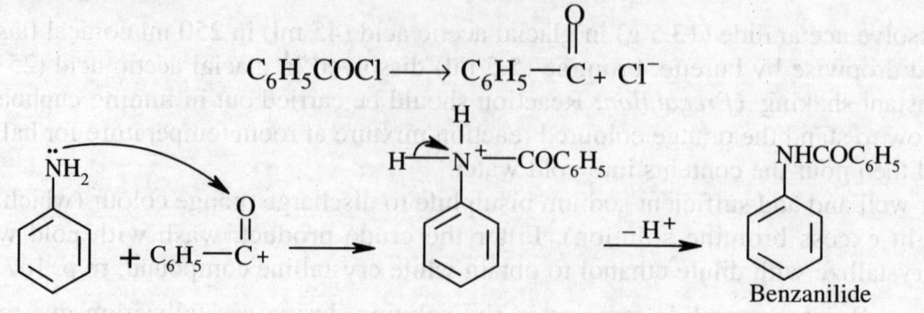

$$C_6H_5COCl \longrightarrow C_6H_5-\overset{\overset{\displaystyle O}{\|}}{C} + Cl^-$$

Benzanilide

$$Br_2 \rightarrow Br^+ + Br^-$$

p-Bromoacetanilide
(insoluble)

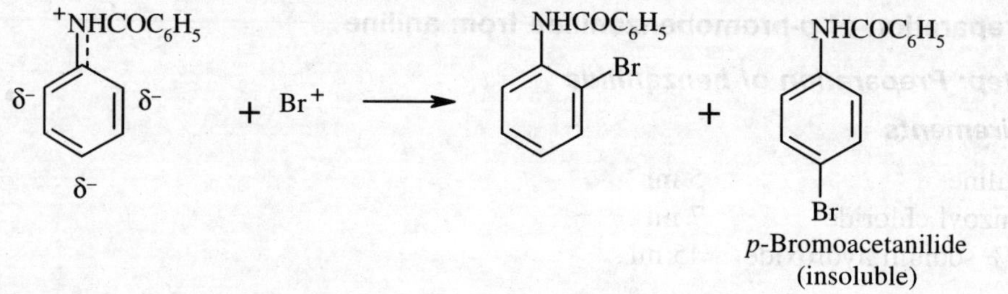

Procedure

Same as in p-bromoacetanilide replacing the acetanilide with benzanilide.

41. Preparation of methyl orange from aniline

Requirements

Aniline	20 ml
Sulphuric acid	40 ml

1st Step: Preparation of sulphanilic acid
Chemical reaction

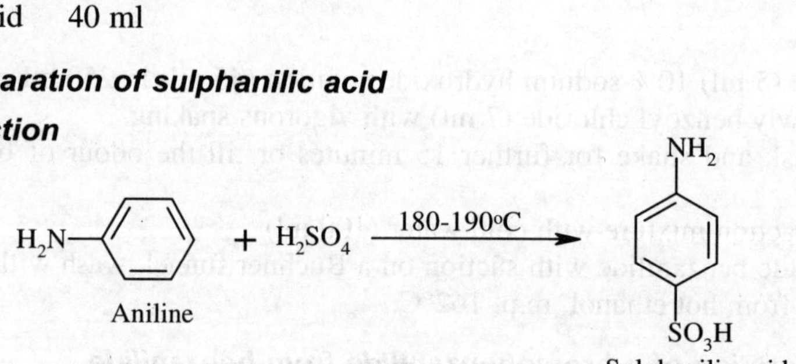

Aniline

Sulphanilic acid

Procedure

(i) Add concentrated sulphuric acid (40 ml) drop-wise with gentle shaking to aniline (20 ml) in a 250 ml conical flask. Keep the flask cool by occasionally immersing in cold water while adding sulphuric acid.

(ii) Heat the flask on oil bath at 180°–190°C for 5 hours (Precaution: Reaction should be carried out in fuming cupboard). Completion of the reaction can be checked by dissolving the reaction mixture (2 ml) in 2N sodium hydroxide (3 ml) without leaving the solution cloudy.

(iii) Cool the contents and pour them carefully into ice-cold water. Allow to stand for 10 minutes for complete separation of crystals.

(iv) Filter the crude sulphanilic acid on Buchner funnel, wash well with cold water and recrystallize from boiling distilled water to obtain shining white crystals, m.p. 300°C (decomposes).

2nd Step: Preparation of methyl orange from sulphanilic acid

Requirement

Sulphanilic acid	10.5 g
Anhydrous sodium carbonate	3 g
Sodium nitrite	3.5 g
Dimethyl aniline	6.5 ml
Sodium chloride	10 g
20% NaOH solution	35 ml
Conc. HCl solution	10.5 ml

Chemical Reaction

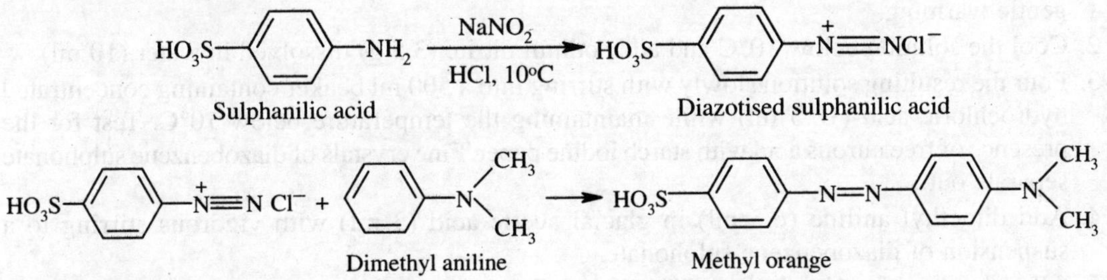

$$2H_2SO_4 \rightleftharpoons H_3O^+ + HSO_4^- + SO_3$$

Sulphanilic acid → Diazotised sulphanilic acid

Dimethyl aniline + → Methyl orange

Reaction Mechanism

Soluble in water

Insoluble in water

$$+ Na_2CO_3 \longrightarrow + CO_2 + H_2O$$

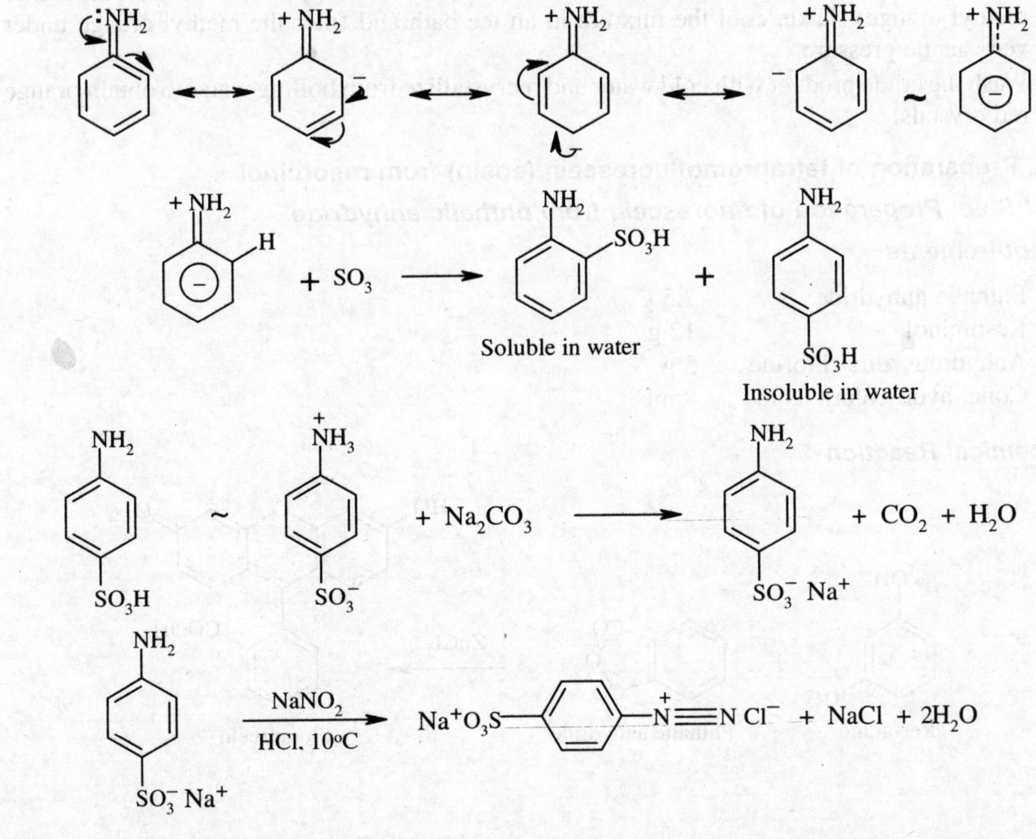

Methyl orange
(azo dye)

Procedure

1. Dissolve sulphanilic acid (10.5 g) and sodium carbonate (3 g) in water (about 100 ml) by gentle warming.

2. Cool the solution below 10°C and add sodium nitrite (3.5 g) dissolved in water (10 ml).

3. Pour the resulting solution slowly with stirring into a 500 ml beaker containing concentrated hydrochloric acid (10.5 ml) while maintaining the temperature below 10°C. Test for the presence of free nitrous acid with starch iodine paper. Fine crystals of diazobenzene sulphonate separate out.

4. Add dimethyl aniline (6.5 ml) in glacial acetic acid (3 ml) with vigorous stirring to a suspension of diazobenzene sulphonate.

5. Allow to stand for 10 minutes, the red methyl orange will be gradually separated out.

6. Add 20% sodium hydroxide solution (35 ml) with stirring to separate out the sodium salt of methyl orange.

7. Warm the solution to about 80°C and add sodium chloride (10 g) (helps in the separation of methyl orange) shake, cool the mixture in an ice bath and filter the methyl orange under very gentle pressure.

8. Wash the crude product with cold water and recrystallize from boiling water to obtain orange red crystals.

42. Preparation of tetrabromofluorescein (eosin) from resorcinol

1st Step: Preparation of fluorescein from phthalic anhydride

Requirements

Phthalic anhydride	7.5 g
Resorcinol	12 g
Anhydrous zinc chloride	5 g
Conc. hydrochloric acid	8 ml

Chemical Reaction

Resorcinol   Phthalic anhydride   Fluorescein

Method 1

Taking anhydrous zinc chloride and HCl.

Procedure

1. Grind phthalic anhydride (7.5 g) and resorcinol (12 g) in a mortar and then transfer to 500 ml round bottom flask.
2. Heat the contents to 180°C on an oil bath.
3. While oil bath is being heated, weigh rapidly anhydrous zinc chloride (5 g). Powder it and then transfer in a stopper bottle.
4. Add anhydrous zinc chloride in small portion from the stoppered bottle to the flask while stirring the mixture (zinc chloride should not be exposed to the air).
5. Continue heating at 180–190°C while stirring at interval of 2–3 minutes until it solidifies completely (about 1 hour is required).
6. Allow the oil bath to cool at about 90°C, add water (about 150 ml) and concentrated hydrochloride acid (5 ml) to the reaction mixture. Again raise the temperature of oil bath to boil the solution to obtain fluorescein with frequent stirring.
7. Continue boiling until the reaction mixture has disintegrated and all the zinc salt is dissolved.
8. Filter the insoluble residue of fluorescein on suction pump, grind it with water. Filter.
9. For purification, dissolve the crude fluorescein in dilute NaOH solution, filter if necessary and precipitate with dilute hydrochloride acid, re-filter, wash and dry it.

Method 2

Taking conc. H_2SO_4 instead of anhydrous zinc chloride and conc. HCl.

Procedure

1. Take 0.2 g of phthalic anhydride, 0.3 g of resorcinol in a dry conical flask. Add 6 drops of 4N H_2SO_4 and heat on a preheated oil-bath to a temperature between 180° and 200°C for half an hour avoiding overheating. Cool the reaction mixture for 5 minutes.
2. When the temperature is about 80°C, add 10 ml of acetone and stir vigorously for 5–10 minutes. The solution should turn yellow as the crude fluorescein dissolves. If the entire product did not dissolve, repeat the process with an additional 5 ml of acetone.
3. Combine the acetone layer in 50 ml beaker and evaporate off the acetone.
4. Dissolve the residue in 30 ml of diethyl ether and 1.5 ml of water.
5. Stir for several minutes, separate the layers using separatory funnel adding 15 ml of water. Separate the ethereal layer.
6. Dry the ether layer over anhydrous sodium sulphate.
7. Filter it and evaporate off the ether to get fluorescein.

2nd Step: Preparation of tetrabromofluorescein (eosin) from fluorescein

Requirements

Fluorescein	5 g
Glacial acetic acid	20 ml
Acetous bromine solution	3.8 ml in 15 ml of glacial acetic acid
Saturated sodium bisulphite solution	sufficient quantity

Procedure

(i) Dissolve powdered fluorescein (5 g) in rectified spirit (20 ml).
(ii) Cool the flask and add bromine solution drop-wise preferably with the help of dropping funnel to about 15 minutes with stirring.

Chemical Reaction

Fluorescein   Eosin (tetrabromofluorescein)

Reaction Mechanism

Fluorescein

(iii) When half the bromine solution has been introduced and the fluorescein has been converted into dibromo derivative, all the solid material disappears temporarily since dibromo derivative soluble in alcohol. On further addition of bromine, tetrabromo (slightly soluble in alcohol) separates out. Allow the reaction mixture to stand for 20 minutes.

(iv) Pour the content into cold water (300 ml) with stirring. If colour of bromine persists, add a few drops of dilute sodium bisulphite solution.

(v) Filter the crude eosin on suction pump, wash with water and dry it at 100°C.

43. Preparation of benzilic acid from benzoin

1st Step: Preparation of benzil from benzoin

Requirements

Benzoin	1 g
Glacial acetic acid	5 ml
Conc. nitric acid	2.5 ml

Chemical Reaction

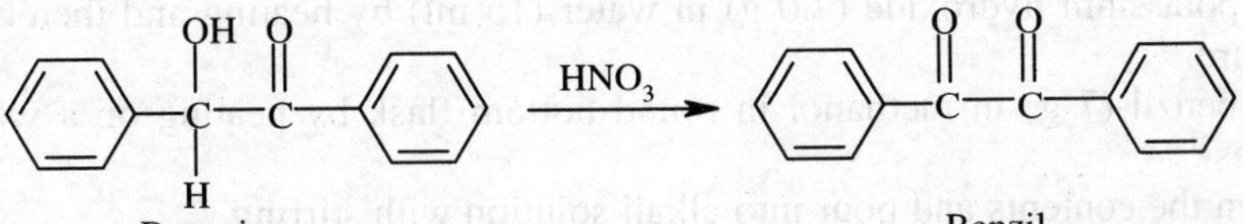

Benzoin → Benzil (via HNO_3)

Procedure

(i) Heat a mixture of benzoin (1 g), glacial acetic acid (5 ml) and conc. nitric acid (2.5 ml) in a test tube on boiling water bath for 1 hour.

(ii) Then, pour down the contents into ice cold water (50 ml) with continuous shaking.

(iii) Filter the product, wash the solid with cold water, and recrystallize from methanol, m.p. 92°C.

2nd Step: Preparation of benzilic acid

Requirements

Benzil	7 g
Potassium hydroxide	7 g
Methanol	25 ml
Conc. HCl	Sufficient quantity

Reaction

$$C_6H_5COCOC_6H_5 \xrightarrow{KOH} (C_6H_5)_2\overset{\displaystyle OH}{C}-COOK \xrightarrow{H^+} (C_6H_5)_2\overset{\displaystyle OH}{C}-COOH$$

Benzil ——— Benzilic acid

Reaction Mechanism

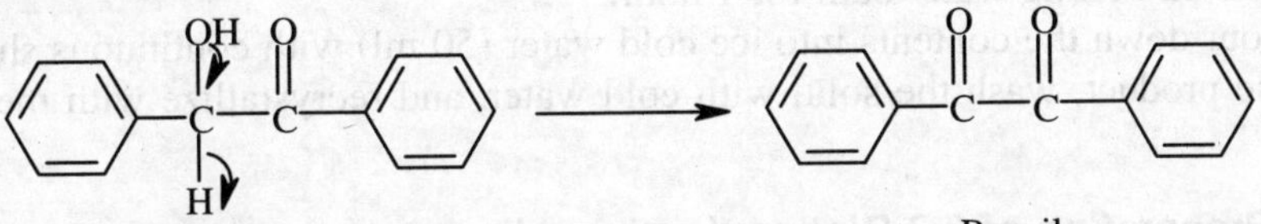

Benzoin → Benzil

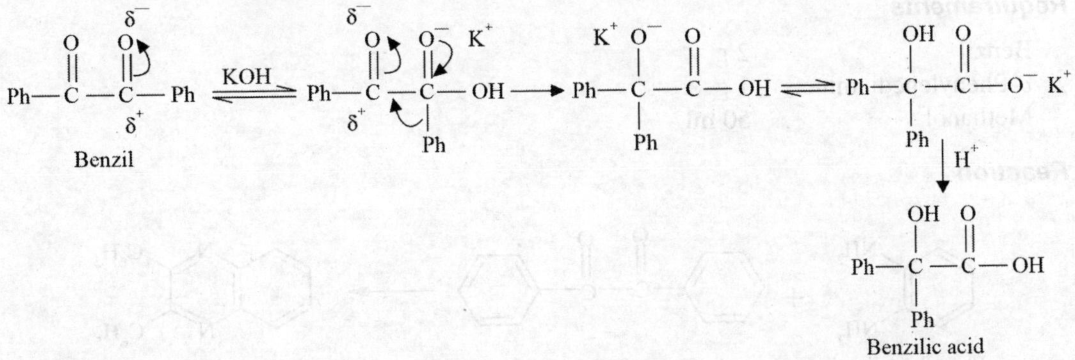

Benzil → Benzilic acid

Migration of phenyl group takes place. This rearrangement is known as *benzillic acid rearrangement*.

Procedure

1. Dissolve potassium hydroxide (7.0 g) in water (15 ml) by heating and then cool to room temperature.
2. Dissolve benzil (7 g) in methanol in round bottom flask by heating on a water bath for 15 minutes.
3. Cool down the contents and pour into alkali solution with stirring.
4. Reflux the content on a waterbath till blue colour disappears.
5. Cool in ice, collect the colourless needles of potassium benzillate.
6. Dissolve the solid in minimum quantity of hot water and acidify with hydrochloric acid.
7. Collect the solid benzillic acid and crystallize from ethanol.

44. Preparation of 2,3-diphenyl quinoxaline from benzoin

1st Step: Preparation of benzil from benzoin
Requirements

Benzoin	1 g
Glacial acetic acid	5 ml
Conc. nitric acid	2.5 ml

Chemical Reaction

Benzoin $\xrightarrow{HNO_3}$ Benzil

Procedure

(i) Heat a mixture of benzoin (1 g), glacial acetic acid (5 ml) and conc. nitric acid (2.5 ml) in a test tube on boiling water bath for 1 hour.
(ii) Then, pour down the contents into ice cold water (50 ml) with continuous shaking.
(iii) Filter the product, wash the solid with cold water, and recrystallize with methanol, m.p. 92°C.

2nd Step: Preparation of 2,3-Diphenyl quinoxaline
Requirements

Benzil	2 g
o-Phenylenediamine	1 g
Methanol	50 ml

Reaction

o-Phenylenediamine + Benzil ⟶ 2,3-Diphenylquinoxaline

Reaction Mechanism

2,3-Diphenylquinoxaline

Procedure

(i) Heat benzil (2 g) and *o*-phenylenediamine (1 g) in an dry flask.

(ii) Heat the flask on a water bath for 15 minutes.

(iii) Cool down the contents and dissolve the resulting solid in hot methanol (50 ml) and let the solution remain undisturbed for 5 minutes.

(iv) Filter the separated crystals as soon as possible and recrystallize with methanol to get brown needles of 2,3-diphenylquinoxaline, m.p. 110°C.

45. Preparation of 5,5-diphenylhydantoin from benzoin

1st Step: Preparation of benzil from benzoin

Requirements

Benzoin	1 g
Glacial acetic acid	5 ml
Conc. nitric acid	2.5 ml

Chemical Reaction

Procedure

(i) Heat a mixture of benzoin (1 g), glacial acetic acid (5 ml) and conc. nitric acid (2.5 ml) in a test tube on boiling water bath for 1 hour.

(ii) Then, pour down the contents into ice cold water (50 ml) with continuous shaking.

(iii) Filter the product, wash the solid with cold water, and recrystallize with methanol, m.p. 92°C.

2nd Step: Preparation of 5,5-diphenylhydantoin from benzil

Requirements

Benzil	10 g
Urea	6 g
30% aqueous sodium hydroxide	30 ml

Chemical Reaction

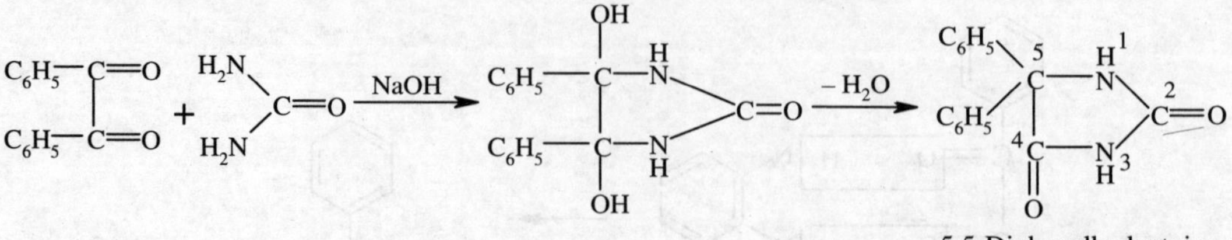

5,5-Diphenylhydantoin

Reaction Mechanism

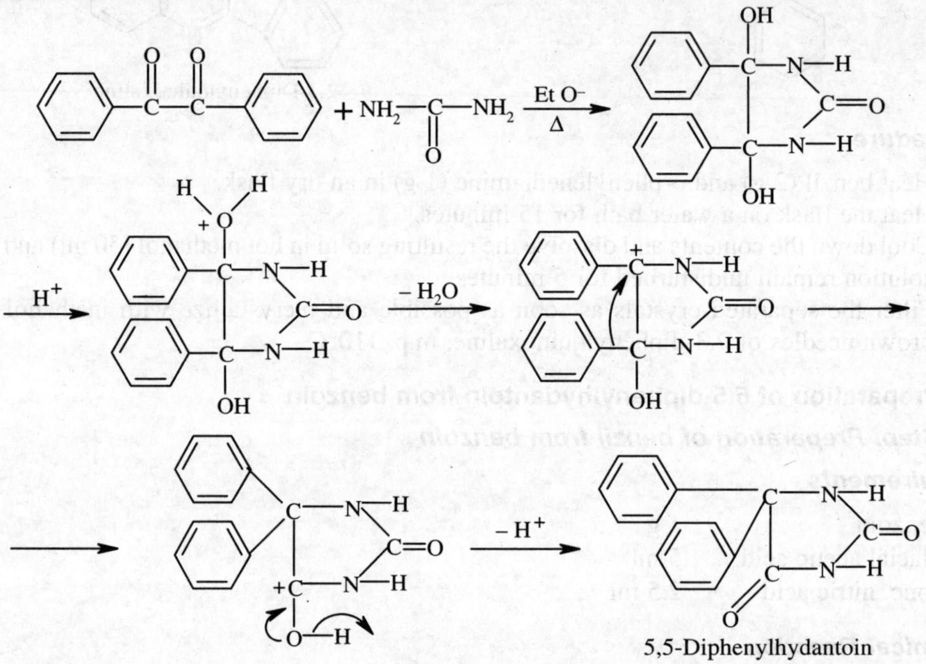

5,5-Diphenylhydantoin

Base catalyzed reaction between benzil and urea is used for the synthesis of hydantoin. The reaction proceeds via intramolecular cyclization to form intermediate which on acidification yields hydantoin as a result of 1,2-diphenyl shift.

Procedure

(i) Take benzil (10 g) and urea (6 g) in 30% aqueous sodium hydroxide solution (30 ml).

(ii) Add ethanol (100 ml) and heat the contents on a water bath for 2 hours.

(iii) Pour down the contents into ice cold water.

(iv) Filter, add concentrated hydrochloric acid to filtrate to make strongly acidic and then cool down the content.

(v) Filter the product and crystallize it from ethanol, m.p. 295–296°C.

46. Preparation of 4-benzylidene-2-phenyl oxazole-5-one from glycine

1st Step: Preparation of benzoyl glycine from glycine

Requirements

Glycine	1 g
Sodium hydroxide (10%)	10 ml
Benzoyl chloride	1.5 ml

Chemical Reaction

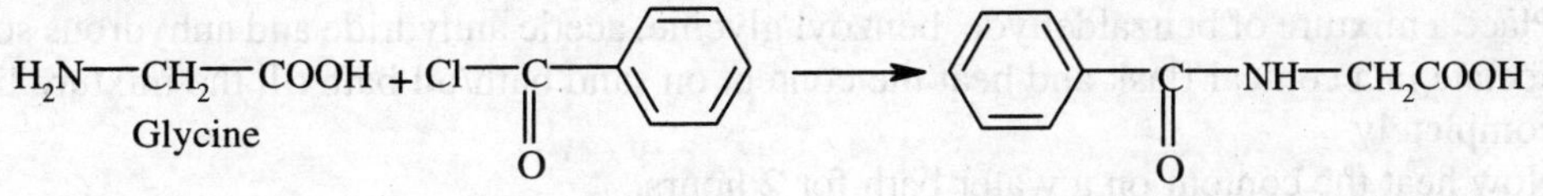
H₂N—CH₂—COOH + Cl—C(=O)—C₆H₅ → C₆H₅—C(=O)—NH—CH₂COOH
Glycine

Benzoyl glycine (hippuric acid)

Procedure

(i) Dissolve glycine (1 g) in 10% aqueous sodium hydroxide solution (10 ml) in a flask and add benzoyl chloride (1.5 ml) to it.

(ii) Plug the mouth of flask with cotton plug and shake vigorously until smell of benzoyl chloride can no longer be deleted.

(iii) Then, add 1–2 drops of conc. hydrochloric acid to make the mixture acidic.

(iv) Filter the product, wash with water and recrystallize, m.p. 192°C.

2nd Step: Preparation of 4-benzylidene-2-phenyl oxazole-5-one from benzoyl glycine (hippuric acid)

Requirements

Benzoyl glycine	1 g
Benzaldehyde	0.7 ml
Acetic anhydride	11.8 ml
Anhydrous sod. acetate	0.6 g

Chemical Reaction

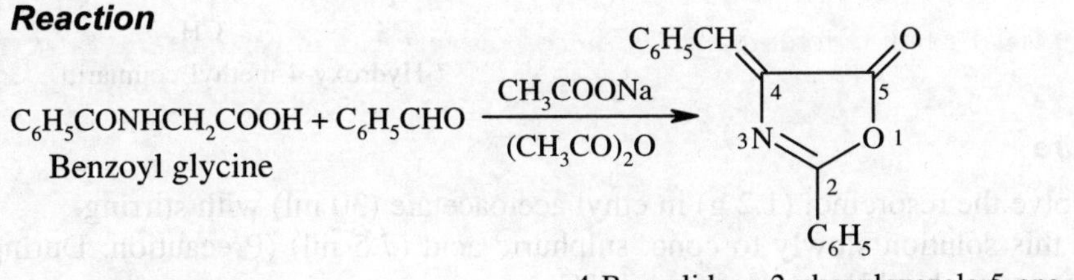
C₆H₅CONHCH₂COOH + C₆H₅CHO
Benzoyl glycine
CH₃COONa
(CH₃CO)₂O
C₆H₅CH
O
4
5
3N
O 1
2
C₆H₅

4-Benzylidene-2-phenyloxazole-5-one

Reaction Mechanism

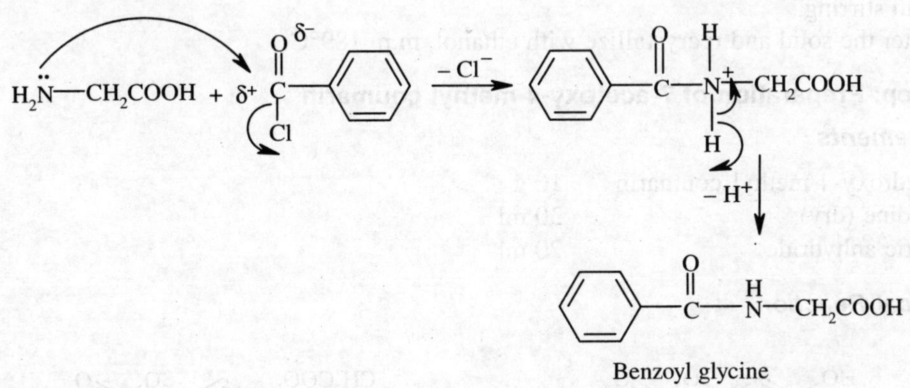
H₂N—CH₂COOH + δ+ C(=O δ−)(Cl)—C₆H₅
– Cl⁻
C₆H₅—C(=O)—N⁺(H)(H)—CH₂COOH
– H⁺
C₆H₅—C(=O)—N(H)—CH₂COOH

Benzoyl glycine

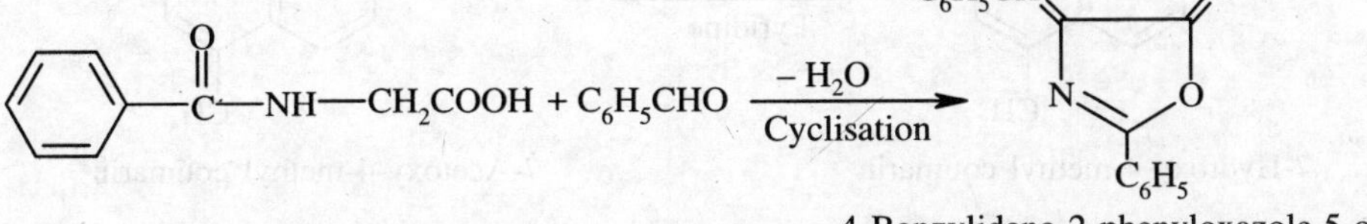
C₆H₅—C(=O)—NH—CH₂COOH + C₆H₅CHO
– H₂O
Cyclisation
C₆H₅CH
O
N
O
C₆H₅

4-Benzylidene-2-phenyloxazole-5-one

Procedure

(i) Place a mixture of benzaldehyde, benzoyl glycine, acetic anhydride and anhydrous sodium acetate in a conical flask and heat the content on sand bath/oil bath till the mixture liquify completely.

(ii) Now heat the content on a water bath for 2 hours.

(iii) Cool and then add 25 ml of ethanol slowly to the flask.

(iv) Filter the solids, wash with hot water and dry, m.p. 170°C.

47. Preparation of 7-acetoxy-4-methyl coumarin from resorcinol

1st Step: Preparation of 7-hydroxy-4-methyl coumarin

Requirements

Resorcinol	1.2 g
Ethyl acetoacetate	30 ml
Conc. sulphuric acid	7.5 ml

Chemical Reaction

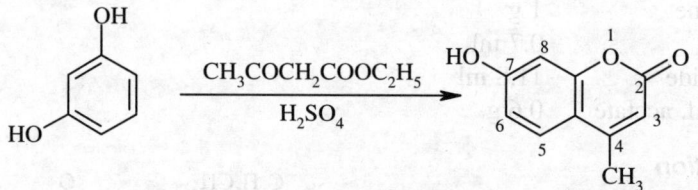

7-Hydroxy-4-methyl coumarin

Procedure

(i) Dissolve the resorcinol (1.2 g) in ethyl acetoacetate (30 ml) with stirring.

(ii) Add this solution slowly to conc. sulphuric acid (7.5 ml) (Precaution: During addition, temperature should not rise above 10°C).

(iii) Continue the stirring for 30 minutes. Pour the content into crushed ice, kept in a beaker with stirring.

(iv) Filter the solid and recrystallize with ethanol, m.p. 189°C.

2nd Step: Preparation of 7-acetoxy-4-methyl coumarin

Requirements

7-hydroxy-4-methyl coumarin	10 g
Pyridine (dry)	30 ml
Acetic anhydride	20 ml

Chemical Reaction

7-Hydroxy-4-methyl coumarin $\xrightarrow[\text{Pyridine}]{(CH_3CO)_2O}$ 7-Acetoxy-4-methyl coumarin

Reaction Mechanism

1st step

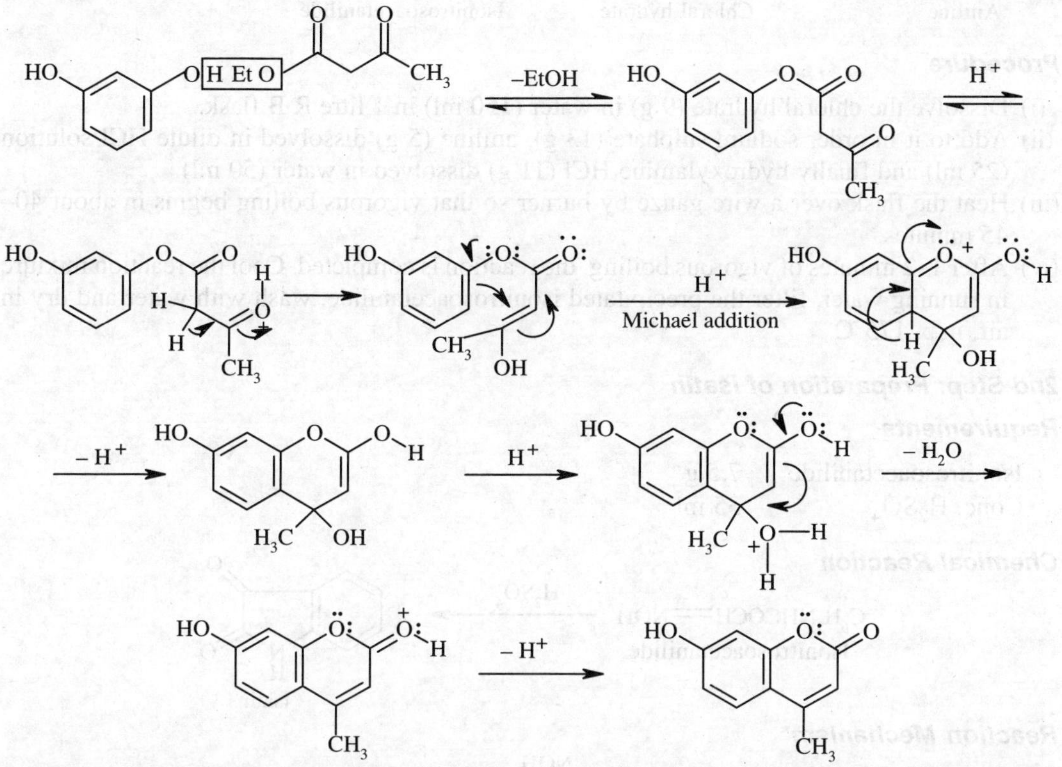

The condensation of resorcinol with β-keto ester is known as *Pachmann condensation*. The product on Michael addition gives the coumarin skeleton. The reaction proceeds by the formation of β-hydroxy ester.

2nd step

Please refer acetylation of salicylic acid (Aspirin).

Procedure

(i) Dissolve 7-hydroxy-4-methyl coumarin (10 g) in dry pyridine (30 ml) and to it add acetic anhydride (20 ml) to it.

(ii) Heat the content on a water bath for 45 minutes.

(iii) Pour the reaction mixture into ice cold water with continuous stirring.

(iv) Filter the solids and crystallize from ethanol, m.p. 122°C.

48. Preparation of isatin from chloral hydrate

1st Step: Preparation of isonitrosoacetanilide

Requirements

Chloral hydrate	9 g
Sodium sulphate	13 g
Hydroxylamine HCl	11 g
Aniline	5 g
Conc. HCl	Sufficient quantity

Chemical Reaction

$$C_6H_5NH_2 + NH_2OH + CCl_3CH(OH)_2 \longrightarrow C_6H_5NHCOCH=NOH + 3HCl + H_2O$$

Aniline   Chloral hydrate   Isonitrosoacetanilide

Procedure

(i) Dissolve the chloral hydrate (9 g) in water (150 ml) in 1 litre R B flask.

(ii) Add to it in order sodium sulphate (13 g), aniline (5 g) dissolved in dilute HCl solution (25 ml) and finally hydroxylamine HCl (11 g) dissolved in water (50 ml).

(iii) Heat the flask over a wire gauze by burner so that vigorous boiling begins in about 40–45 minutes.

(iv) After 1–2 minutes of vigorous boiling, the reaction is completed. Cool the reaction mixture in running water, filter the precipitated isonitrosoacetanilide, wash with water and dry in air, m.p. 175°C.

2nd Step: Preparation of isatin

Requirements

Isonitrosoacetanilide	7.5 g
Conc. H_2SO_4	35 ml

Chemical Reaction

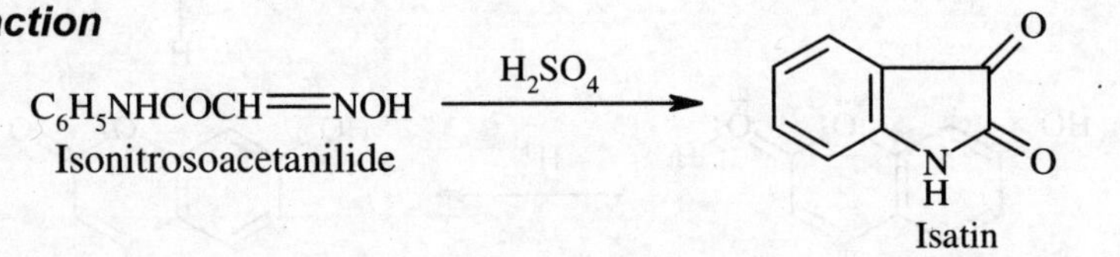

$$C_6H_5NHCOCH=NOH \xrightarrow{H_2SO_4}$$

Isonitrosoacetanilide   Isatin

Reaction Mechanism*

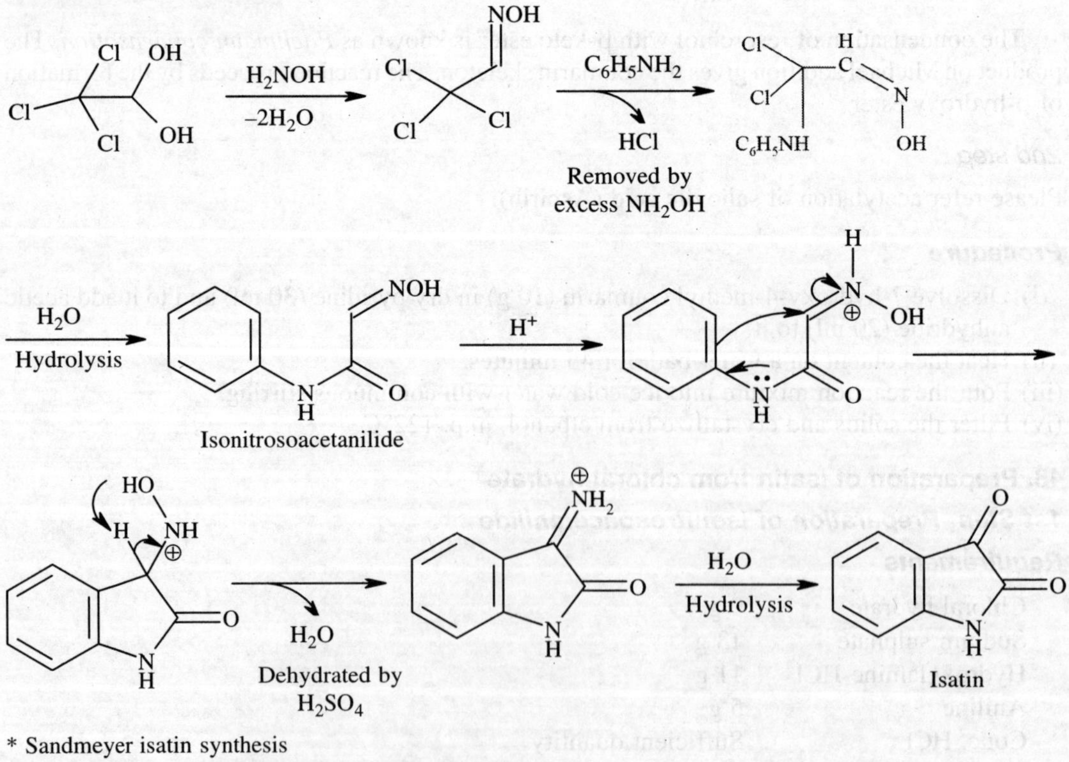

Removed by excess NH_2OH

Isonitrosoacetanilide

Dehydrated by H_2SO_4 Isatin

* Sandmeyer isatin synthesis

Procedure

(i) Warm the concentrated sulphuric acid (35 ml) to 50° temperature and add to it isonitroso-acetanilide (7.5 g) in a R B flask fitted with a mechanical stirrer at such a rate as to keep the temperature between 60° to 70°C but not higher. (**Note:** At higher temperature, charring occurs). External cooling may be provided to facilitate the reaction.

(ii) After the addition of isonitrosoacetanilide, heat the mixture at 80°C for about 10 minutes.

(iii) Then cool down the content at room temperature and pour into ice cold water.

(iv) Keep it for half an hour. Filter isatin which is precipitated out.

(v) Wash with cold water and recrystallized from glacial acetic acid, m.p. 189–192°.

49. Preparation of *p*-bromoaniline from acetanilide

1st Step: Preparation of p-bromoacetanilide

Requirements

Acetanilide	13.5 g
Glacial acetic acid	70 ml
Bromine solution	5.5 ml
Sodium bisulphite	Sufficient quantity

Chemical Reaction

Acetanilide $\xrightarrow{Br_2}$ *p*-Bromoacetanilide (insoluble) + *o*-Bromoacetanilide

Procedure

(i) Dissolve acetanilide (13.5 g) in glacial acetic acid (45 ml) in 250 ml conical flask.

(ii) Add drop-wise by burette, bromine (5.5 ml) dissolved in glacial acetic acid (25 ml) with constant shaking. (Precaution: Reaction should be carried out in fuming cupboard).

(iii) Allow to stand the orange coloured reaction mixture at room temperature for half an hour and then pour the contents into cold water.

(iv) Stir well and add sufficient sodium bisulphite to discharge orange colour which is due to slight brown colour of bromine.

(v) Filter the crude product, wash with cold water and recrystallize with dilute ethanol to obtain white crystalline compound, m.p. 167°C·

Note: *o*-Bromoacetanilide remains in the alcoholic solution during crystallization due to its high solubility.

2nd Step: Preparation of p-Bromoaniline

Requirements

p-Bromoacetanilide	5 g
Conc. HCl	7 ml
Ethanol	10 ml
5% NaOH solution	Sufficient quantity

Chemical Reaction

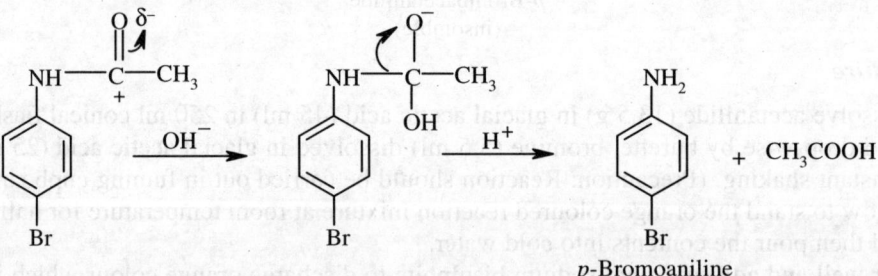

NHCOCH₃ ... p-Bromoacetanilide → NH₂ ... p-Bromoaniline + CH₃COOH

Reaction Mechanism

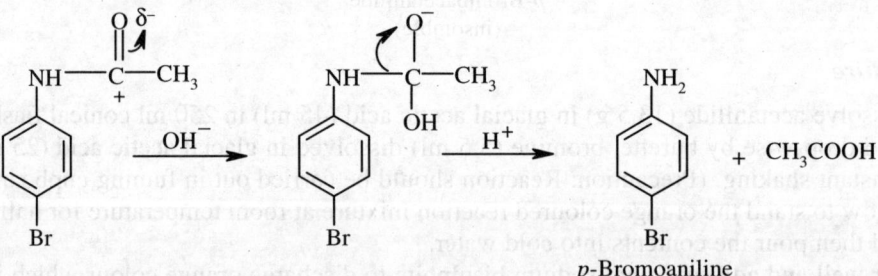

Procedure

(i) Dissolve p-bromoacetanilide (5.0 g) in ethanol (10 ml) by boiling in a flask attached with reflux condensor.

(ii) Add hydrochloric acid (7 ml) in installment to this boiling solution.

(iii) Continue heating under reflux for 1 hour.

(iv) Cool and add water (100 ml) and distil off the ethanol and ethyl acetate by heating on water bath.

(v) Cool the residual solution in a ice bath and add to it sufficient 5% sodium hydroxide solution till alkalinity with vigorous stirring. The p-bromoaniline separates first which then solidifies.

(vi) Filter it, wash with cold water and crystallize from dilute ethanol, m.p. 66°C.

50. Preparation of 2-phenyl indole from acetophenone

1st Step: Preparation of acetophenone phenylhydrazone from acetophenone

Requirements

Acetophenone	6.0 g
Phenylhydrazine	5.4 g
Ethanol	20 ml
Glacial acetic acid	q.s.

Chemical Reaction

Acetophenone   Acetophenone phenylhydrazone

Procedure

(i) Place acetophenone (6.0 g) in 100 ml beaker.

(ii) Add a solution of phenylhydrazine (5.4 g) dissolved in ethanol (20 ml) and 2–3 drops of glacial acetic acid.

(iii) Warm the mixture at 100°C for 20 minutes.

(iv) Filter the cold reaction mixture, wash it with dilute HCl solution, followed by cold ethanol. Recrystallize the crude product from ethanol, m.p. 100°C.

2nd Step: Preparation of 2-phenyl indole from acetophenone phenylhydrazone

Requirements

Crude phenylhydrazone	3.0 g
Polyphosphoric acid	20.0 g

Chemical Reaction

Reaction Mechanism

2–Phenyl indole

Procedure

(i) Transfer crude phenylhydrazone (3.0 g) to a 100 ml beaker containing polyphosphoric acid (20.0 g).

(ii) Heat on a boiling water bath, stir with a thermometer and maintain the temperature of reaction mixture at 100–120°C for 10 minutes.

(iii) Add 50 ml of cold water and stir well to ensure complete solution of polyphosphoric acid.

(iv) Filter with suction, wash with water and finally with little ethanol, m.p. 187°C.

51. Preparation of antipyrine

Step 1: Preparation of pyrazolones

Requirements

Ethyl acetoacetate	5.2 g (5.1 ml)
Phenylhydrazine	4.3 g (4 ml)
Ether	As per need

Chemical reaction

$$CH_3COCH_2 \quad + \quad H_2N \xrightarrow{\Delta}$$
$$COOC_2H_5 \qquad NHC_6H_5$$

Ethylacetoacetate   Phenylhydrazine

3-Methyl-1-phenyl-2-pyrazolin-5-one

Procedure

(i) Heat a mixture of ethyl acetoacetate (5.2 g) and phenylhydrazine (4.0 ml) at 110–120°C (oil bath) for 4 hours.

(ii) Cool the reaction mixture and add the ether.

(iii) Stir the mixture to give a solid product.

(iv) Filter, wash with ether and crystallize from ethanol to get yellow crystallise compound of 3-methyl-1-phenyl-2-pyrazolin-5-ene, m.p. 126–127°C.

Step 2: Preparation of 2,3-dimethyl-1-phenyl-3-pyrazolin-5-one (antipyrine)

Requirements

3-Methyl-1-phenyl-2-pyrazolin-5-one	21.75 g
Dimethyl sulphate	14 ml
NaOH solution	10 g (in 10 ml)
Methanol	20 ml

Chemical Reaction

$$\xrightarrow[\text{NaOH}]{(CH_3)_2SO_4}$$

3-Methyl-1-phenyl-2-pyrazolin-5-one

(2,3-Dimethyl-1-phenyl-3-pyrazolin-5-one)
Antipyrine

Chemical Mechanism

Procedure

(i) Dissolve 3-methyl-1-phenyl-2-pyrazolin-5-one (21.75 g) in a mixture of methanol (20 ml) and sodium hydroxide solution (10 g) in 10 ml of water.

(ii) To it, add dimethyl sulphate (14 ml) drop-wise with stirring and continue the stirring for another 30 minutes and then heat on a boiling water bath for 1 hour.

(iii) Evaporate off the methanol and add hot water to the residual solution.

(iv) Filter and extract the filtrate with benzene (3 × 50 ml).

(v) Evaporate off the benzene and crystallize the product as white solid, m.p. 113°C.

▌THREE STEPS PREPARATIONS

52. Preparation of acridone from anthranilic acid

Anthranilic acid is diazotized and then converted into o-chlorobenzoic acid (Sandmeyer reaction) (1st step). In 2nd step, o-chlorobenzoic acid is condensed with aniline to get N-phenylanthranilic acid and in the final step, N-phenylanthranilic acid is cyclised to form acridone.

1st step: Preparation of o-chlorobenzoic acid

Requirements

Anthranilic acid	7.0 g
Sodium nitrite	3.5 g
Conc. HCl solution	50 ml
Sodium chloride	12 g
Copper sulphate	13 g
Copper turnings	7 g
Urea	q.s.

Chemical Reaction

Anthranilic acid   Diazonium salt   o-Chlorobenzoic acid

Procedure

1. To prepare cuprous chloride solution, dissolve copper sulphate (13 g) and sodium chloride (12 g) in water (40 ml) in 500 ml round bottom flask.

2. Boil the solution and then add concentrated HCl solution (40 ml) followed by copper turnings (7.0 g).

3. Heat the solution under reflux until becomes colourless. Keep the solution in ice bath.

4. Place a solution of anthranilic acid (7 g) in a concentrated HCl solution (10 ml) and water (50 ml) in a beaker.

5. Cool this solution to below 5°C temperature and then diazotize it by slowly adding a cold solution of sodium nitrite (3.5 g) in water (20 ml). Check the presence of excess of free nitrous acid by placing a drop of it on starch iodide paper. If paper becomes dark blue, decompose the excess nitrous acid by adding solid urea.
6. Pour this cold diazonium solution slowly with shaking into cold solution of cuprous chloride prepared as above with shaking. The diazotised salt decompose to liberate nitrogen and frothing occurs.
7. Allow the contents to stay for 3–4 hours at room temperature and then transfer it to a beaker leaving the copper turnings in the flask.
8. Filter the precipitated acid and wash with cold water.
9. Dissolve the crude acid in hot water containing 2–3 ml of ethanol, add charcoal (1 g) and boil.
10. Filter the solution in hot condition, concentrate the filtrate and cool in a ice bath to get pure *o*-chlorobenzoic acid, m.p. 141°C.

2nd Step: Preparation of N–Phenyl anthranilic acid

Requirements

o-Chlorobenzoic acid	7.5 g
Aniline	30 ml
Anhydrous potassium carbonate	7.5 g
Cuprous oxide	0.2 g
Activated charcoal	3–4 g
Conc. hydrochloric acid solution	6 ml

Chemical Reaction

o-Chlorobenzoic acid   N-Phenylanthranilic acid

Procedure

(i) Place *o*-chlorobenzoic acid (7.5 g), aniline (30 ml), anhydrous potassium carbonate (7.5 g) and cuprous oxide (0.2 g) in R B flask fitted with air condenser.
(ii) Place the flask in a oil bath and reflux for about 2–3 hours at such a rate that water vapours escape from the top of the air condenser.
(iii) Allow to cool and subject to steam distillation to remove unreacted aniline.
(iv) To the brown residue, add charcoal (3–4 g), boil for about 15 minutes and filter while hot.
(v) To the filtrate, add concentrated hydrochloric acid (6 ml) to precipitate N-phenyl anthranilic acid.
(vi) Allow to cool, filter the acid, wash with cold water and crystallize from aqueous ethanol or acetic acid–water mixture, 183–184°C.

3rd Step: Preparation of acridone

Requirements

N-phenyl anthranilic acid	5 g
Conc. H_2SO_4 solution	35 ml
5% Sodium carbonate solution	200 ml

Chemical Reaction

N-Phenyl anthranilic acid   Acridone

Procedure

(i) Heat N-phenyl anthranilic acid (5 g) and concentrated H_2SO_4 solution (35 ml) in R B flask on water bath for 3–4 hours till green fluorescence is observed.

(ii) Cool the solution to room temperature and then in ice bath. Add ice cold water (50 ml) slowly with vigorous shaking and cooling the flask.

(iii) Filter the crystal of acridone and stir the precipitate with 5% sodium carbonate solution (200 ml) to dissolve the unreacted N-phenyl anthranilic acid.

(iv) Filter, wash the acridone with water and crystallize from glacial acetic acid. m.p. 351–352°C.

Reaction Mechanism

(i) HOOC—   [0°C]   HOOC—   Aryl free radical $\xrightarrow[\text{[0°C–60°C]}]{\text{CuCl}}$ HOOC—   + CuCl$_2$ o-Chlorobenzoic acid

(ii) HOOC   →   HOOC$^+$ $\xrightarrow{C_5H_5NH_2}$ HOOC $\xrightarrow{-H^+}$ HOC   N–Phenyl anthranilic acid

(iii) $\xrightarrow[\text{Cyclisation}]{H_2SO_4}$ Acridone

53. Preparation of succinanil from succinic anhydride

Succinic anhydride is prepared from dehydration of succinic acid with acetic anhydride or acetyl chloride. Succinic anhydride react with aniline to form succinanilic acid which on cyclisation gives succinanil.

1st Step: Preparation of succinic anhydride

Requirements

Succinic acid	12 g
Acetic anhydride	20 ml
Ether	20 ml

Chemical Reaction

$$\text{HOOCCH}_2\text{--CH}_2\text{COOH} + (\text{CH}_3\text{CO})_2\text{O} \longrightarrow (\text{CH}_2\text{CO})_2\text{O} + 2\text{CH}_3\text{COOH}$$

Succinic acid   Succinic anhydride

Procedure

 (i) Place succinic acid (12 g) and acetic anhydride (20 ml) in a flask.
 (ii) Plug it tightly with cotton plug and heat it on water bath till clear solution is obtained.
(iii) Cool the reaction mixture at room temperature first and then in ice bath.
(iv) Filter the crystals of succinic anhydride and wash with ether, m.p. 119–120°C.

Note: Succinic anhydride can also be prepared by dehydrating succinic acid with acetyl chloride or acetic anhydride.

2nd Step: Preparation of succinanilic acid

Requirements

Succinic acid	1.0 g
Aniline	0.9 ml
Benzene	35 ml

Chemical Reaction

$$(\text{CH}_2\text{CO})_2\text{O} + \text{C}_6\text{H}_5\text{NH}_2 \longrightarrow$$

$$\begin{array}{l}\text{CH}_2\text{COOH} \\ | \\ \text{CH}_2\text{CO.NH.C}_6\text{H}_5\end{array}$$

Succinic anhydride   Succinanilic acid

Procedure

 (i) Dissolve succinic anhydride (1 g) in benzene (30 ml) with heating on a boiling water bath.
 (ii) Add all at once a solution of aniline (0.9 ml) in benzene (5 ml) to it. The separation of product occur immediately.
(iii) Cool the mixture, filter the solids and wash with benzene. Recrystallize it, m.p. 178°C.

3rd Step: Preparation of succinanil from succinanilic acid

Requirements

Succinanilic acid	0.4 g
Acetyl chloride	1 ml

Chemical reaction

$$\begin{array}{l}\text{CH}_2\text{COOH} \\ | \\ \text{CH}_2\text{CO.NH.C}_6\text{H}_5\end{array} + \text{CH}_3\text{COCl} \longrightarrow \begin{array}{l}\text{CH}_2\text{CO} \\ \diagdown \\ \diagup \\ \text{CH}_2\text{CO}\end{array}\!\!\text{N}\!\!-\!\!\bigcirc + \text{HCl}$$

Succinanilic acid   Succinanil

Reaction Mechanism

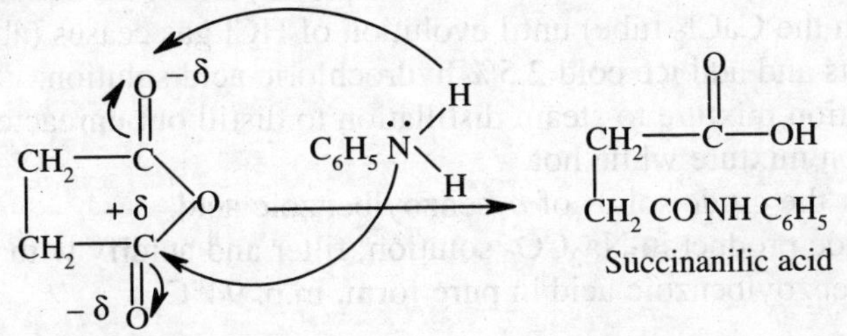

Succinanilic acid

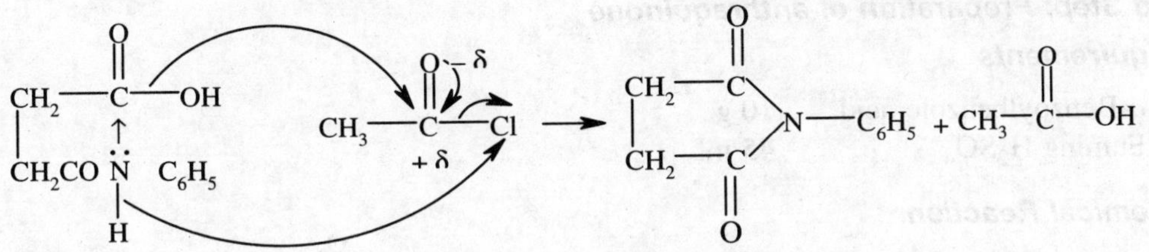

Succinanil

Procedure

(i) Transfer succinanilic acid (0.4 g), cover it with acetyl chloride (1 ml) and heat on a water bath for 15 minutes.

(ii) Cool the reaction mixture, filter the solid and wash with ether and recrystallize, m.p. 154°C.

54. Preparation of anthrone from phthalic anhydride

Phthalic anhydride on **Friedal-Craft reaction** with benzene form *o*-benzoyl benzoic acid. In second step, the acid is cyclised to yield anthraquinone which on reduction gives anthrone.

1st Step: Preparation of o-benzoyl benzoic acid

Requirements

Phthalic anhydride	10 g
Benzene	40 ml
Anhydrous $AlCl_3$	20 g
Na_2CO_3	6 g
Conc. HCl	25 ml

Chemical Reaction

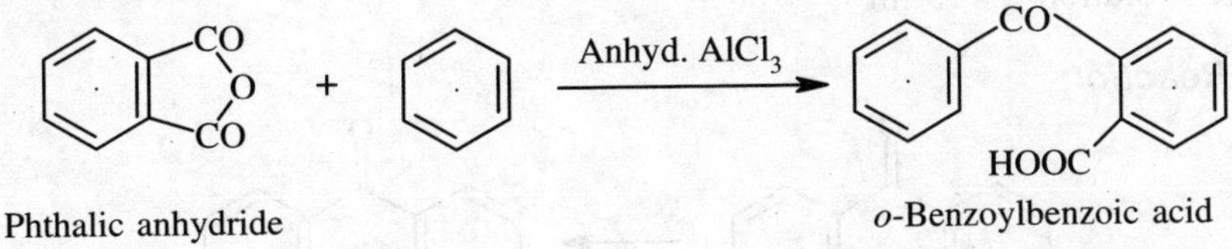

Phthalic anhydride   *o*-Benzoylbenzoic acid

Procedure

1. Suspend anhydrous aluminium chloride (10 g) in benzene in R B flask with a provision for reflux condenser and guard tube.

2. To this, add phthalic anhydride in portion of about 0.5 g with constant shaking. If the reaction does not start on addition of first installment of phthalic anhydride, heat the flask slowly on water bath for a few minutes and if the reaction becomes violent cool the flask in a ice bath. (Start of reaction can be observed by evolution of HCl gas or bubbling in the reaction mixture).

3. When the addition of phthalic anhydride is completed, reflux the contents under anhydrous condition (attach the $CaCl_2$ tube) until evolution of HCl gas ceases (about 3 hours).
4. Cool the contents and add ice cold 2.5% hydrochloric acid solution.
5. Subject the reaction mixture to steam distillation to distill out unreacted benzene.
6. Filter the reaction mixture while hot.
7. Cool it and filter the crude solids of o-benzoylbenzoic acid.
8. Dissolve the crude product in Na_2CO_3 solution, filter and acidify with hydrochloric acid to separate out o-benzoylbenzoic acid in pure form, m.p. 94°C.

2nd Step: Preparation of anthraquinone

Requirements

o-Benzoylbenzoic acid	10 g
Fuming H_2SO_4	45 ml

Chemical Reaction

o-Benzoylbenzoic acid $\xrightarrow{H_2SO_4}$ Anthraquinone

Procedure

(i) Heat the o-benzoylbenzoic acid (10 g) and fuming sulphuric acid (45 ml) on a water bath for 2 hours in fuming cupboard.
(ii) Cool the reaction mixture and pour it into crushed ice taken in a beaker with stirring when anthraquinone separates out.
(iii) Filter the solid, wash with water, little ammonium hydroxide solution and again with water.
(iv) Dry it and crystallize with hot acetic acid, m.p. 286°C.

3rd Step: Preparation of anthrone

Requirements

Anthraquinone	5 g
Granulated tin	5 g
Glacial acetic acid	35 ml
Conc. HCl solution	15 ml

Chemical Reaction

Anthraquinone → Anthrone

Procedure

(i) Heat anthraquinone (5 g), granulated tin (5 g) and glacial acetic acid (35 ml) for 15–30 minutes.

(ii) Allow to cool and then add slowly, almost drop by drop, HCl solution (15 ml) to it. If anthraquinone does not dissolves, add more granulated tin and hydrochloric acid.

(iii) Filter and dilute the filtrate with water (5–10 ml).

(iv) Cool the filtrate in ice bath when crystals of anthrone separate out.

(v) Filter it and crystallize from a mixture of benzene and petroleum ether, m.p. 155°C.

Reaction Mechanism

$$H^+ + [AlCl_4]^- \rightarrow HCl \uparrow + AlCl_3$$

Anthraquinone

55. Preparation of acetanilide from benzene

In the first step benzene undergoes **Friedal Craft reaction** to form acetophenone. The carbonyl group reacts with hydroxyamine to form the oxime in the second step. In the final step oxime forms the acetanilide (Beckmann rearrangement).

1st Step: Preparation of acetophenone from benzene

Requirements

Benzene	50 ml
Anhydrous AlCl$_3$	20 g
Acetyl chloride	14 ml

Chemical Reaction

$$C_6H_6 + CH_3COCl \xrightarrow{\text{Anhyd. AlCl}_3} C_6H_5COCH_3 + HCl$$

Procedure

1. Place anhydrous aluminium chloride (20 g) and benzene (50 ml) in three neck flask fitted with a reflux condenser and dropping funnel while its third neck is stoppered. Attach the CaCl$_2$ tube to the reflux condenser.

2. Cool it in water bath.

3. Add acetyl chloride slowly to it with continuous shaking through the dropping funnel.

4. After the complete addition, heat the flask on a water bath for 1 hour at 60°C temperature.
5. Cool the reaction mixture and pour it into cold water when a dark coloured oil starts floating on the surface.
6. Cork the flask and shake it vigorously. If any solid separates at this stage add little concentrated HCl to dissolve it.
7. Transfer the mixture to a separating funnel and discard the lower aqueous layer.
8. Wash the benzene layer first with dilute NaOH solution and then with water several times.
9. Finally dry the benzene layer over anhydrous calcium chloride. Transfer the content in distillation assembly and continue the distillation on an air bath and collect acetophenone between 195°C and 202°C (b.p. 201°C).

2nd Step: Preparation of acetophenone oxime

Requirements

Acetophenone	6 g
Hydroxylamine HCl	4 g
Sodium hydroxide	7 g
Conc. HCl solution	20 ml
Rectified spirit	15 ml

Chemical Reaction

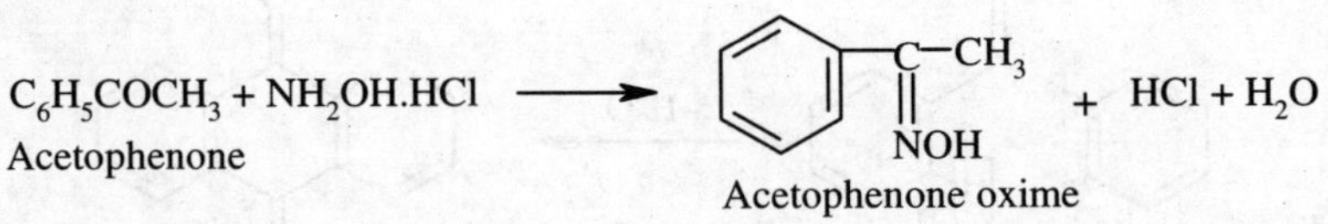

$$C_6H_5COCH_3 + NH_2OH.HCl \longrightarrow$$

Acetophenone

$$+ \; HCl + H_2O$$

Acetophenone oxime

Procedure

 (i) Take acetophenone (6 g), hydroxylamine hydrochloride (4 g), rectified spirit (15 ml) and water (2–3 ml) in a R B flask.
 (ii) To this mixture, add sodium hydroxide (7 g) in a portion of 0.5 g only.
 (iii) Heat the reaction mixture under refluxing condition for 2–3 hours.
 (iv) Cool and pour the content into a 20% hydrochloric acid solution (100 ml) to separate out acetophenone oxime.
 (v) Filter the oxime or alternatively extract with ether and evaporate off the ether to get oxime, crystallize from ethanol or petroleum ether.

3rd Step: Preparation of acetanilide from acetophenone oxime

Requirements

Acetophenone	4 g
Phosphorus pentachloride	6 g
Dry ether	100 ml

Chemical Reaction

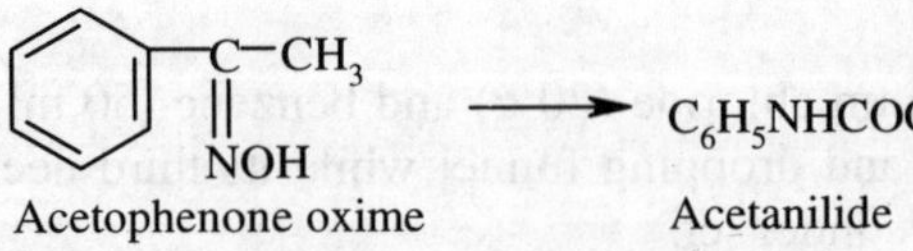

Acetophenone oxime $C_6H_5NHCOCH_3$

                           Acetanilide

Reaction Mechanism

$$CH_3COCl + AlCl_3 \rightarrow [CH_3CO]^+ \, [AlCl_4]^- \leftrightarrow [CH_3CO]^+ + [AlCl_4]^-$$

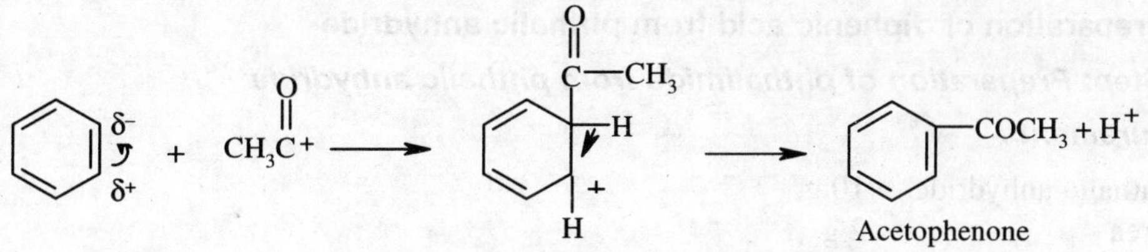

Acetophenone

$$H^+ + AlCl_4^- \rightarrow HCl + AlCl_3$$

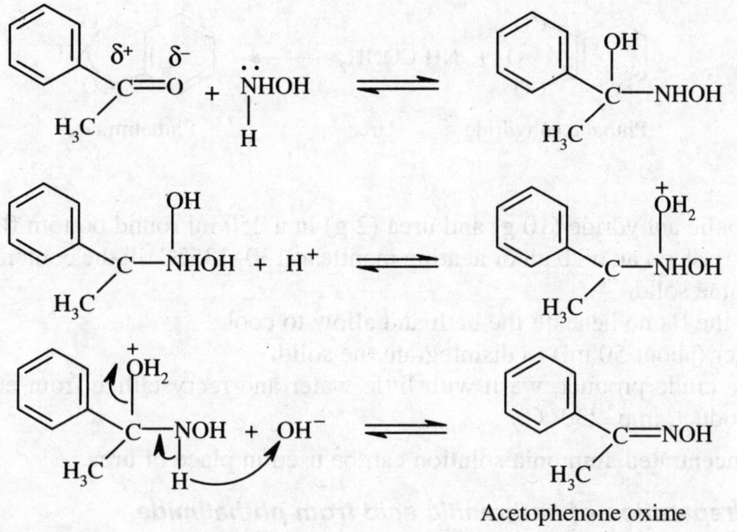

Acetophenone oxime

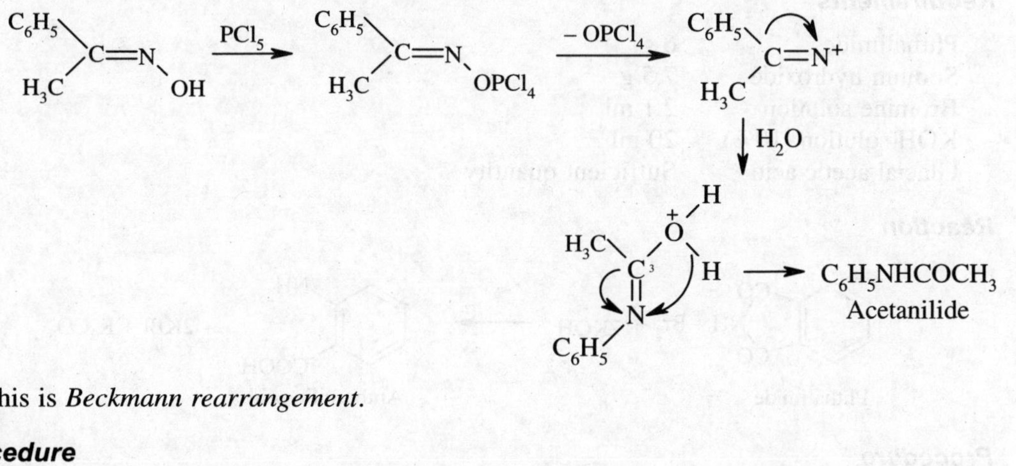

C_6H_5NHCOCH_3
Acetanilide

This is *Beckmann rearrangement*.

Procedure

 (i) Dissolve the acetophenone oxime (4 g) in dry ether (100 ml) in R B flask and then add PCl$_5$ (6 g) with shaking.
 (ii) Allow to stay for about 30 minutes and distill off the ether.
 (iii) To the residue, add water (50 ml), boil the reaction mixture, filter hot and allow the filtrate to cool.
 (iv) Filter the separated crystals of acetanilide, wash with water and crystallize from hot water, m.p. 114°C.

56. Preparation of diphenic acid from phthalic anhydride

1st Step: Preparation of phthalimide from phthalic anhydride

Requirements

Phthalic anhydride	10 g
Urea	2 g

Chemical Reaction

Phthalic anhydride   Urea   Phthalimide

Procedure

(i) Mix phthalic anhydride (10 g) and urea (2 g) in a 250 ml round bottom flask.

(ii) Heat the flask on an oil bath or heating mantle at 130–135°C till the contents melt, froth up and become solid.

(iii) Remove the flame beneath the bath and allow to cool.

(iv) Add water (about 50 ml) to disintegrate the solid.

(v) Filter the crude product, wash with little water and recrystallize from ethanol to obtain white product, m.p. 230°·C.

Note: Concentrated ammonia solution can be used in place of urea.

2nd Step: Preparation of anthranilic acid from phthalimide

Requirements

Phthalimide	6 g
Sodium hydroxide	7.5 g
Bromine solution	2.1 ml
KOH solution (10%)	20 ml
Glacial acetic acid	Sufficient quantity

Reaction

Phthalimide   Anthranilic acid

Procedure

(i) Dissolve sodium hydroxide (7.5 g) in water (about 40 ml) and cool in ice bath to about 0°C temperature and then add bromine solution (2.1 ml) to it.

(ii) To this solution, add phthalimide (6 g) and 10% KOH solution, then heat the solution for 5–10 minutes till phthalimide dissolves.

(iii) Filter the solution and neutralize the solution with glacial acetic acid.

(iv) Filter the solid crystals of anthranilic acid, wash with water and recrystallize, m.p. 146°C.

3rd Step: Preparation of diphenic acid * from anthranilic acid

Requirements

Anthranilic acid	2 g
Sodium chloride	0.25 g
Sodium nitrite	1.2 g
Conc. HCl solution	20 ml
Copper sulphate	5 g
Ammonia solution	8.5 ml
Hydroxylamine HCl	1.5 g

Chemical Reaction

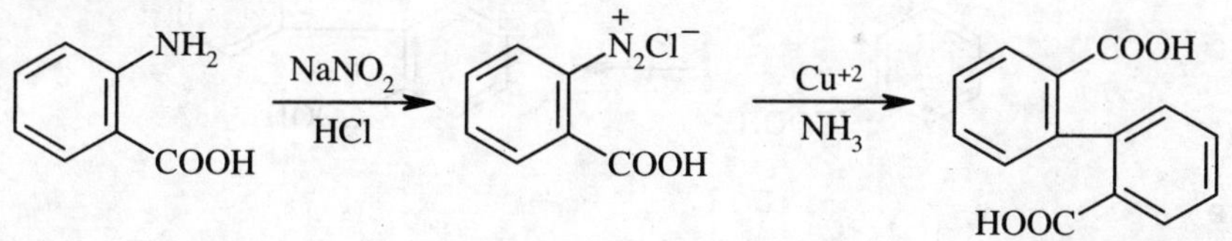

Anthranilic acid (with NH$_2$ and COOH) $\xrightarrow[\text{HCl}]{\text{NaNO}_2}$ diazonium salt ($N_2^+Cl^-$ and COOH) $\xrightarrow[\text{NH}_3]{\text{Cu}^{+2}}$ Diphenic acid (biphenyl with two COOH / HOOC groups)

Diphenic acid

Reaction Mechanism

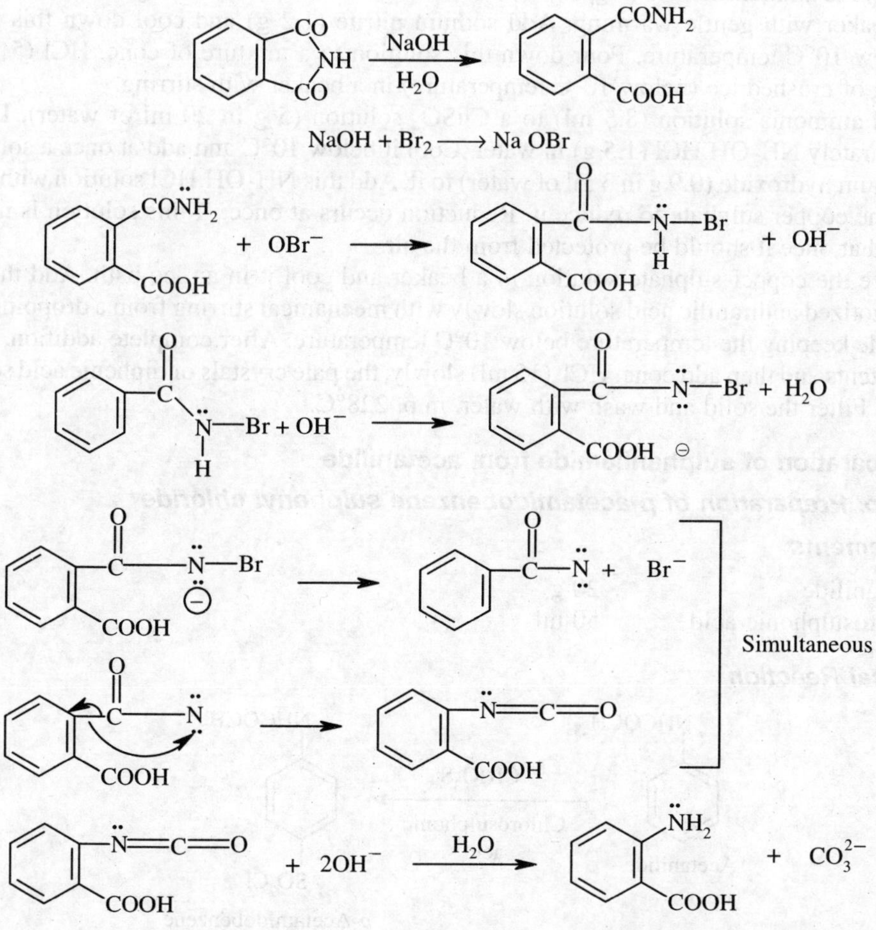

Phthalimide-type (CO—NH—CO) $\xrightarrow[\text{H}_2\text{O}]{\text{NaOH}}$ structure with CONH$_2$ and COOH

$$NaOH + Br_2 \longrightarrow Na\,OBr$$

Structure with CONH$_2$ and COOH $+\ OBr^- \longrightarrow$ structure with $C(=O)$—N—Br, H and COOH $+\ OH^-$

Structure $C(=O)$—$N(H)$—Br + COOH $+\ OH^- \longrightarrow$ structure $C(=O)$—N—Br + COOH$^-$ $+\ H_2O$

Structure $C(=O)$—N^-—Br + COOH $\longrightarrow$ $C(=O)$—N + Br^- (with COOH)

Structure $C(=O)$—N (with COOH) $\longrightarrow$ $N=C=O$ (with COOH)   Simultaneous

$N=C=O$ (with COOH) $+\ 2OH^- \xrightarrow{\text{H}_2\text{O}}$ NH_2 (with COOH) $+\ CO_3^{2-}$

Anthranilic acid

---

* Organic Synthesis, Coll. Vol. I, p. 222 (1941), Vol. 7, p. 30 (1927).

Procedure

Adopt the following sequence to prepare the biphenic acid.

(i) Dissolve anthranilic acid (2 g) in a solution of sodium carbonate (0.2 g) in water (20 ml) in a beaker with gentle warming. Add sodium nitrite (1.2 g) and cool down this mixture below 10°C temperature. Pour down this solution to a mixture of conc. HCl (5 ml) and 12 g of crushed ice (below 10°C temperature) in a beaker with stirring.

(ii) Add ammonia solution (8.5 ml) to a CuSO$_4$ solution (5 g in 20 ml of water). Dissolve separately NH$_2$OH.HCl (1.5 g) in water. Cool it below 10°C and add at once a solution of sodium hydroxide (0.9 g in 3 ml of water) to it. Add this NH$_2$OH.HCl solution with stirring to the copper sulphate to reduce it. Reduction occurs at once. If this solution is not to be used at once it should be protected from the air.

(iii) Place the copper sulphate solution in a beaker and cool it in an ice bath. Add the above diazotized anthranilic acid solution slowly with mechanical stirring from a dropping funnel while keeping the temperature below 10°C temperature. After complete addition, boil the contents and then add conc. HCl (15 ml) slowly, the pale crystals of diphenic acid separates out. Filter the solid and wash with water, m.p. 228°C.

57. Preparation of sulphanilamide from acetanilide

1st Step: Preparation of p-acetamidobenzene sulphonyl chloride

Requirements

Acetanilide	20 g
Chlorosulphonic acid	50 ml

Chemical Reaction

p-Acetamidobenzene
sulphonyl chloride

Procedure

1. Take dry acetanilide (20 g) in 500 ml two mouth round bottom flask, fitted with dropping funnel and a reflux condenser.
2. Attach a gas trap device to the top of the condenser (Fig. 15.1).
3. Place chlorosulphonic acid (50 ml) in a dropping funnel and fix a calcium chloride guard tube to it.
4. Add chlorosulphonic acid in small portions to the acetanilide with occasional shaking to ensure thorough mixing.
5. Heat the mixture for 1 hour in order to complete the reaction.
6. Allow to cool and pour the oily mixture into ice cold water.
7. Filter the crude product on suction pump, wash with cold water and press well to obtain the dry product of *p*-acetamidobenzene chloride.

Note: Chlorosulphuric acid must be handled with great care, it is very corrosive to the skin and to clothing and reacts with water with violence.

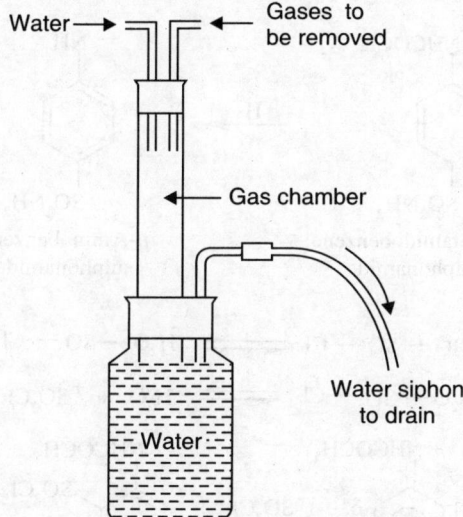

Fig. 15.1: HCl gas trap device

2nd Step: Preparation of p-acetamidosulphonamide

Requirements

p-Acetamidobenzene sulphonyl chloride	21 g
Strong ammonia solution	70 ml
Sulphuric acid	q.s.

Chemical Reaction

NHCOCH$_3$ $\xrightarrow{\text{NH}_4\text{OH}}$ NHCOCH$_3$

SO$_2$Cl   SO$_2$NH$_2$

p-Acetamidobenzene
sulphonamide

Procedure

(i) Add a mixture of strong ammonia solution (70 ml) and water (70 ml) to a crude *p*-acetamidobenzene sulphonyl chloride (21 g) in a 500 ml flask.

(ii) Heat the contents with occasional shaking for about 15 minutes to just below the boiling point.

(iii) Cool the suspension in ice and then add dilute sulphuric acid until the mixture is just acidic to Congo red paper.

(iv) Filter the crude *p*-acetamidobenzene sulphonamide, wash it with cold water and dry in air.

3rd Step: Preparation of p-aminobenzene sulphonamide (sulphanilamide)

Requirements

p-Acetamidosulphonamide	15 g
Conc. HCl solution	10 ml
Sodium bicarbonate	q.s.

Chemical Reaction

| *p*-Acetamidobenzene sulphonamide | *p*-Aminobenzene sulphonamide |

Reaction mechanism

p-Aminobenzene sulphonamide

Procedure

 (i) Add the crude *p*-acetamidobenzene sulphonamide (15 g) to a mixture of concentrated acid (10 ml) and water (30 ml).
 (ii) Boil the mixture gently under reflux for 30–45 minutes. The solution when cooled to room temperature, should not deposit the solid amide; if a solid separates, heat further for a short period.
(iii) Heat the solution to obtain with decolourizing carbon (2 g) for 15 minutes, filter and to the filtrate, cautiously add sufficient sodium bicarbonate in portions with stirring until the solution becomes neutral.
(iv) Filter the crude product and then recrystallize the crude product from water or from ethanol to obtain pure product, m.p. 163–164°C.

58. Preparation of tolbutamide from toluene

Tolbutamide, N-(*p*-methylbenzenesulphonyl)-N′-butylurea, is an oral antihyperglycemic agent used for the treatment of non-insulin-dependent diabetes mellitus (NIDDM). It is structurally similar to acetohexamide, chlorpropamide and tolazamide and belongs to the sulphonylurea class of insulin secretagogues, which act by stimulating β cells of the pancreas to release insulin. Sulphonylureas increase both basal insulin secretion and meal-stimulated insulin release.

Tolbutamide

Tolbutamide is a white, or partially white, crystalline powder. It has a slightly bitter taste and is odourless.

Tolbutamide is synthesized in three/four steps.

Chemical reactions

Step 1: Synthesis of p-toluene sulphonyl chloride from toluene

Chemicals required

Toluene	130 g
Conc. sulphuric acid solution	450 g

Phosphorus pentachloride	q.s.
Iodine	q.s.
Lime water	q.s.

Procedure

1. Heat 130 g pure toluene with 450 g conc. sulphuric acid in a cast iron pot fitted with a soluble agitator. Add a few crystals of iodine, and allow the temperature to rise to 100°C.
2. The sulphonation becomes complete in about 6 hours. Transfer the reaction mixture in a large basin, dilute with water. Add lime water gradually to neutralize the excess acid.
3. Filter out the calcium sulphate and any ferric hydroxide and wash with hot water.
4. Add sodium carbonate to the filtrate until just alkaline to phenolphthalein, and remove the calcium carbonate by filtration.
5. Evaporate the filtrate almost to dryness, when the sodium salts of o-toluenesulphonyl and p-toluene sulphonyl acids separate out. The total yield of o-toluene sulphonyl and p-toluene sulphonyl acids are 95% (340 g). o-Sodium tosylate crystallizes with $2H_2O$ as plates. p-Sodium tosylate crystallizes with $4H_2O$ as plates or prisms. In order to obtain o-toluene sulphonyl chloride and p-toluene suphonyl chloride, treat the mixture prepared above gradually with an equal weight of ground phosphorus pentachloride.
6. When the reaction becomes complete, add cold water, keep the reaction mixture in a freezing mixture. The p-toluene suphonyl chloride* separates as a solid (m.p. 69°C), purified by recrystallization from ethanol. The o-toluene suphonyl chloride is an oily liquid (m.p. 10°C), and is separated from the filtrate by means of a separatory funnel.

   * Note: Unstable. Highly reactive and hygroscopic. Hydrolyzes to hydrogen chloride and p-toluene sulphonic acid.

Step 2: Synthesis of p-toluene sulphonamide*

Chemicals required

| p-Toluene suphonyl chloride | 5 g |
| Ammonium carbonate | 10 g |

Procedure

1. Thoroughly mix 5 g of p-toluene sulphonyl chloride and 10 g of ammonium carbonate by grinding in mortar until a fine uniform powder is obtained.
2. Heat the mixture on a water bath (15–20 minutes) with continuous stirring to convert sulphonyl chloride into sulphonamide.
3. Crystallize the product from hot water.
4. Filter off the almost pure p-toluene sulphonamide as colourless crystal, m.p. 137°C.

Step 3: Synthesis of ethyl p-toluene sulphonyl carbamate*

Chemicals required

p-Toluene sulphonamide	49 g
Ethyl chloroformate	42 g
Anhydrous potassium carbonate	3 g
Dry acetone	300 ml
Acetic acid	q.s.

---

* Alok Singh Thakur, Ravita Deshmukh, Arvind Kumar Jha, P. Sudhir Kumar, Saudi Pharmaceutical Journal, 23 (5), 475–482 (2015).

* US patent, 3, 799, 760, Patented, Mar. 26, 1974.

Procedure

1. Mix corresponding sulphonamide (49 g, 20 mmol) with ethyl chloroformate (42 g, 26 mmol) and anhydrous potassium carbamate (3 g) in dry acetone (300–400 ml) and reflux for 18–20 hours.
2. Remove acetone by distillation under reduced pressure and keep the solution for overnight and then add in water (200–250 ml).
3. Neutralize with acetic acid.
4. Filter the solid product and wash with distilled water.
5. Dry it and recrystallize from ethyl alcohol, m.p. 79–81°C.

Step 4: Synthesis of tolbutamide

Chemicals required

Ethyl *p*-toluene sulphonyl carbamate	2.4 g
Butyl amine	1.0 g

Procedure

1. Dissolve the specified carbamate derivative in hot toluene (30 ml).
2. In the above solution, add the butylamine slowly and reflux for 3–4 hours.
3. On cooling the refluxed solution, precipitation of desired product occurs. Filter and dry it, m.p. 126–128°C.

Alternate method

It consists of conversion of the sulphonamide prepared in Step 2 to a salt of the desired sulphonyl urea derivative through reaction with the butyl isocyanate in the presence of a base. This reaction is preferably performed in dry acetone using anhydrous potassium carbamate as the base. The potassium salts of the desired sulphonyl urea derivatives are, with a few exceptions, insoluble in anhydrous acetone and are thus recovered by distillation.

Step 5: Synthesis of tolbutamide

Chemicals required

p-Toluene sulphonamide	0.85 g
Butyl isocyanate	0.49 g (0.55 ml)

Procedure

1. Mill the mixture of 0.50 mmol of sulphonamide and 0.50 mmol of K_2CO_3 (1 equiv) at a frequency of 30 Hz for 1 hour.
2. Then add 0.50 mmol butyl isocyanate (1 equiv) and subsequently mill for another 2 hours at 30 Hz.
3. Add 20 ml of deionized water and dilute HCl to the crude mixture. Set off pH of the resultant suspension to pH 3 using pH paper and left to stir for 15 minutes.
4. Filter the product isolated via vacuum filtration and dry in air.

59. Synthesis of 3-hydroxycoumarin

Step 1: Synthesis of hippuric acid (benzoyl glycine)

Requirements

Glycine	7.5 g
Benzoyl chloride	12.4 ml
10% Sodium hydroxide solution	100 ml

Chemical Reaction

Procedure

(i) Dissolve glycine (7.5 g) in 10% NaOH solution (100 ml).

(ii) Add benzoyl chloride (12.4 ml) in two lots with shaking. Shake the mixture vigorously until all the benzoyl chloride has reacted.

(iii) Add crushed ice, acidify with concentrated HCl to congo red, filter the solid and wash with cold water.

(iv) Heat the solid product with CCl_4 to dissolve unreacted benzoic acid.

(v) Filter it and crystallize with hot water.

(vi) Record its melting point, m.p. 187°C.

Step 2: Synthesis of 2-phenyl-4-(2'-acetoxybenzal) oxazolone

Requirements

Salicyldehyde	22 ml
Hippuric acid	42.0 g
Fused sodium acetate	15 g
Acetic anhydride	60 ml
Ethanol	q.s.

Chemical Reaction

2-Phenyl-4-(2'-acetoxybenzal) oxazolone

Procedure

(i) Heat salicyldehyde (22 ml), hippuric acid (42 g) and fused sodium acetate (15 g) with acetic anhydride (60 ml) on a water bath for 30–45 minutes under anhydrous conditions in R.B. flask. A bright yellow crystalline solid that formed redissolves on further heating.

(ii) Add alcohol (20 ml) to the reaction mixture and cool.

(iii) Filter the separated azalactone, wash with alcohol and then with hot water till the washings are colourless.

(iv) Crystallize from ethanol and use the product for the Step 3.

Step 3: Synthesis of 3-Hydroxycoumarin

Requirements

Oxazolone	40 g
NaOH	20 g
SO_2 gas	As per need
Conc. HCl solution	60 ml

Chemical Reaction

2-Phenyl-4-(2'-acetoxy benzal)
Oxazolone

3-Hydroxycoumarin

Reaction mechanism

Procedure

(i) Reflux the above oxazolone (40 g) with NaOH solution (20 g/100 ml) till no more ammonia evolved.

(ii) Dilute the resulting solution with water (100 ml) and saturate with SO_2 gas with cooling.

(iii) Keep the reaction mixture for 12 hours in an ice chest and filter the separated benzoic acid.

(iv) Heat the clear filtrate for 3 hours on water bath with conc. HCl solution (60 ml).

(v) Cool down the content, filter the separated product and crystallize from alcohol, m.p. 151–152°C.

Extraction Procedures for Isolation of Particular Constituents

EXTRACTION PROCEDURES

1. Isolation of caffeine (1,3,7-trimethylxanthine)
2. Isolation of eugenol from cinnamon leaf oil
3. Isolation of eugenol from clove buds
4. Isolation of pectin from orange peels
5. Isolation of piperine from black peeper
6. Isolation of hesperidin from orange peel
7. Isolation of hippuric acid from urine
8. Isolation of cystine from human hair

1. Isolation of Caffeine (1,3,7-Trimethylxanthine)

Caffeine ($C_8H_{10}N_4O_2$) is the common name for trimethylxanthine (systematic name is 1,3,7-trimethylxanthine or 3,7-dihydro-1,3,7-trimethyl-1H-purine-2,6-dione).

Caffeine

The purified caffeine is an intensely bitter taste white powder. It is soluble in hot water, alcohol, acetone, chloroform, benzene and ether.

The isolation of caffeine from tea leaves presents the chemist with a major problem: caffeine does not occur alone in tea leaves, but is accompanied by other natural substances from which it must be separated. The major components of tea leaves are:

1. Cellulose: The major structural material of all plant cells. Since cellulose is virtually insoluble in water it presents no problems in the isolation procedure.
2. Caffeine: One of the major water soluble substances present in tea leaves. Caffeine comprises as much as 5% by weight of the leaf material in tea plants.
3. Tannins: High molecular weight, water soluble compounds that are responsible for the colour of tea. The term "tannin" does not refer to a single compound or even to substances having

similar chemical structure. Rather, "tannin" refers to a class of compounds that have certain properties in common. They contain phenol groups, are acidic and are used to convert animal skin to leather [tanning].

4. **Flavonoid pigments:** Water soluble coloured compounds that are widely distributed in plant life.
5. **Chlorophylls:** Water soluble green plant pigments that enable plants to convert carbon dioxide and water to carbohydrates and oxygen [photosynthesis].

Requirements

Tea leaves	100 g
Basic lead acetate solution	300 ml
Dilute H_2SO_4 solution	Sufficient quantity
Chloroform	150 ml
Decolourizing carbon	1 g

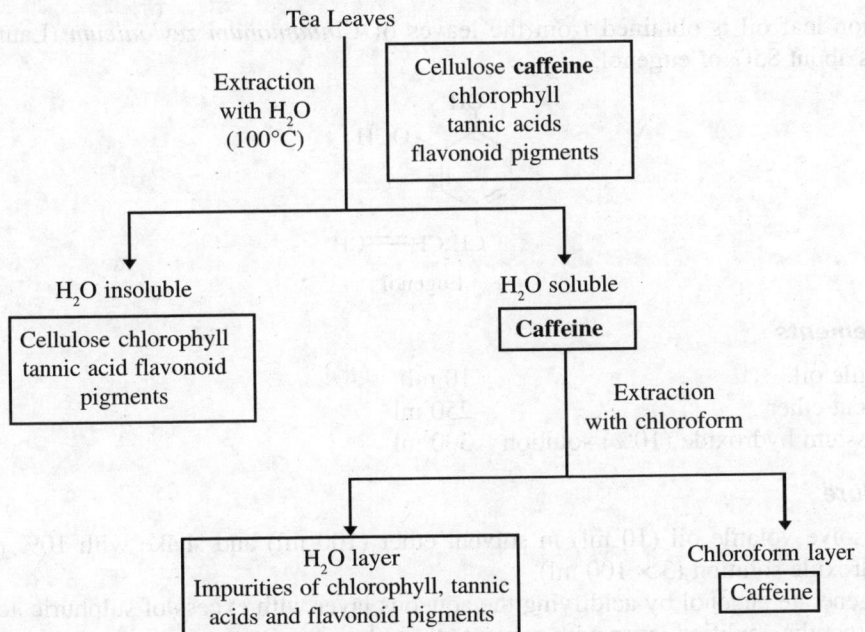

Experimental Procedure

1. Place 100 g of a powdered tea and 250 ml of water in a 600 ml beaker and boil gently for 30 minutes.
2. **Removal of tannins:** Strain the resulting hot extract through muslin. Carefully, add a solution of basic lead acetate [$Pb(C_2H_2O_2)_2$] solution to the filtrate until no more precipitate forms.
3. **Removal of unreacted lead acetate:** Heat the mixture of boiling to boiling and filter through a Buchner funnel and vacuum system. Heat the filtrate to boiling and add dilute sulphuric acid solution until precipitation occurs. Filter it.
4. **Removal of colouring impurities:** Add approximately 1 g of decolorizing charcoal to the filtrate, boil for a few minutes and then filter.
5. **Extraction of caffeine:** Cool the filtrate and transfer to a separatory funnel and shake out with three successive 10 ml portion of chloroform. Transfer the combined extracts to a small capacity flask.

6. Dry the combined $CHCl_3$ extracts with anhydrous sodium sulphate. Swirl for several minutes to allow enough time for the sodium sulphate to become hydrated with the water.
7. Filter the dry $CHCl_3$ solution into a dry pre-weighed 100 ml round-bottom flask. Wash the filter paper and drying agent with about 1 ml of $CHCl_3$.
8. Either remove the $CHCl_3$ by simple distillation or rotaevaporate off the solvent, until about 5 ml of liquid remains in the round-bottom flask. Do not allow the flask to go dry otherwise the caffeine may decompose.
9. Place the round-bottom flask on a steam bath and evaporate the contents to dryness at low-medium heat.
10. Weigh the flask to find the crude mass of caffeine.
11. Scrape out the residue, transfer to a small beaker and dissolve in a small amount of hot CH_3OH. Let stand overnight and filter off the caffeine crystals.
12. Record the weight of the caffeine, m.p. 235°C.

2. Isolation of Eugenol from Cinnamon Leaf Oil

Cinnamon leaf oil is obtained from the leaves of *Cinnamonum zeylanicum* (Lauraceae). It contains about 85% of eugenol.

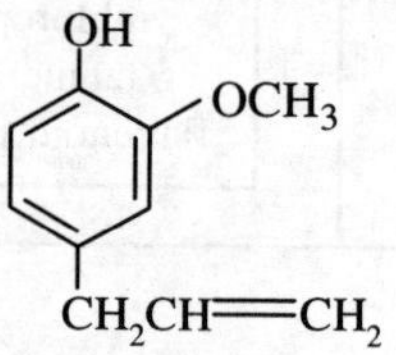

Eugenol

Requirements

Volatile oil	10 ml
Solvent ether	250 ml
Potassium hydroxide (10%) solution	300 ml

Procedure

 (i) Dissolve volatile oil (10 ml) in solvent ether (100 ml) and shake with 10% potassium hydroxide solution (3 × 100 ml).
 (ii) Regenerate eugenol by acidifying the aqueous layer with excess of sulphuric acid.
(iii) Extract the acidified layer with solvent ether (3 × 50 ml).
(iv) Distil off the solvent and dry the eugenol in a desiccator.

3. Isolation of Eugenol from Clove Buds

Eugenol is isolated from cloves. These flower buds are collected and dried to give the familiar spice used in cooking. The essential oil distilled from cloves (from *Eugenia caryophyllata*) is rich in **eugenol** (4-allyl-2-methoxyphenol; b.p. 250°C), which is a phenolic compound. **Caryophyllene** (sesquiterpene) is also present in relatively small amounts, along with other terpenes. Eugenol is responsible for giving cloves their distinctive aroma and taste. The structure of eugenol is shown below along with caryophyllene.

Requirements

Clove buds	5 g
Solvent ether	50 ml

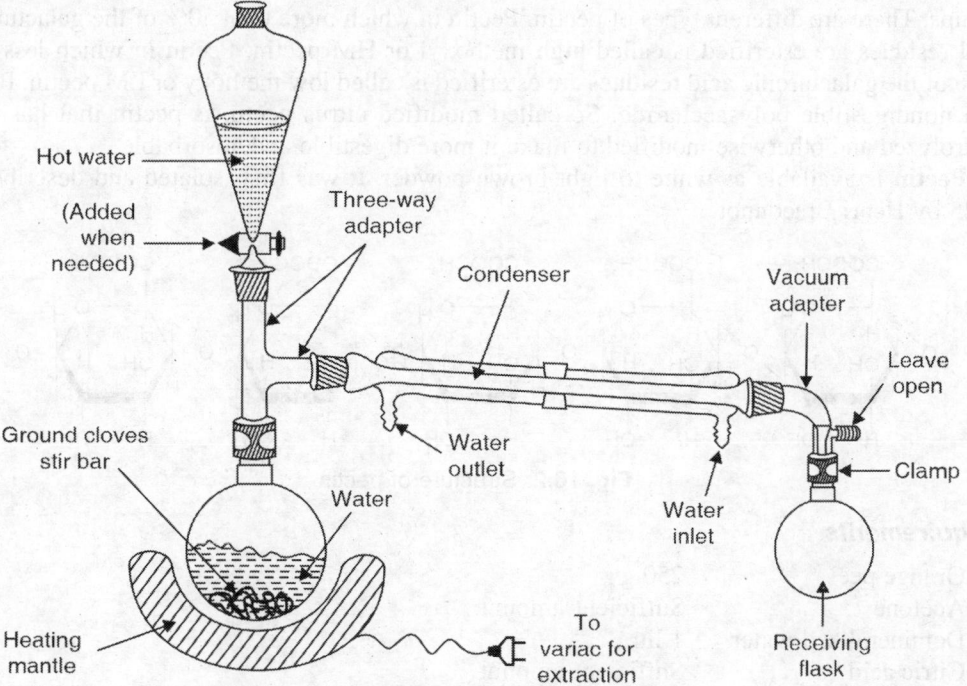

Caryophyllene

Eugenol

Experimental procedure

1. Grind up whole cloves with a mortar and pestle to a powder. Weigh out 5.0 g of this powder and place it in a 500 ml round-bottom flask along with 150 ml of water, and a magnetic stir bar.
2. Assemble the apparatus for steam distillation as shown in Fig. 16.1, and place a stir motor below the heating mantle. While stirring, heat the mixture using a Variac to control the rate of the distillation. A steady and even rate of distilling is better. During distillation, add small portions of water from the addition funnel to the distillation flask to maintain the original volume in the distillation flask.
3. The distillate that collects in the receiving flask will contain two immiscible liquids, a large amount of water and a small amount of your organic product. This will often make it look cloudy (which is a good sign).
4. Collect about 100 ml of distillate and then stop the distillation.
5. Now disassemble the apparatus and transfer the distillate into the empty separatory funnel.

Fig. 16.1: Distillation assembly for extraction

6. Now extract the distillation mixture successively with two 25 ml portions of ether. Combine the upper ether layers in a Erlenmeyer flask and dry the solution by adding anhydrous magnesium or sodium sulphate. Allow the solution to remain over the drying agent for roughly 10 minutes.

7. Filter the liquid into a beaker. Carefully evaporate the ether on a steam bath in the fume hood, using a wooden stick to prevent bumping. When only 1–2 ml of solution remains, transfer the liquid into large pre-weighed vial with a pipet. Now resume heating on a steam bath until only an oily residue remains in the vial, which is eugenol.

8. Dry the outside of the vial and weigh it to determine how much eugenol is isolated from the cloves. Calculate the weight percentage of eugenol isolated from the cloves according to this equation:

$$\text{Percentage of eugenol} = \frac{\text{Mass of eugenol isolated (in grams)}}{\text{Mass of cloves used (in grams)}} \times 100$$

It was shown that about 7.5% of an oil could be recovered from cloves by steam distillation.

4. Isolation of Pectin from Orange Peels

Pectin is classified as a soluble fiber. It is found in most of the plants, but is most concentrated in citrus fruits (oranges, lemons, grapefruits) and apples. Pectin is obtained by the aqueous extraction of citrus peels and apple pulp under mild acidic conditions. Pectin obtained from citrus peels is referred to as citrus pectin.

Chemically, pectin is a linear polysaccharide containing from about 300 to 1000 monosaccharide units (Fig. 16.2). D-Galacturonic acid is the principal monosaccharide unit of pectin. Some neutral sugars are also present in the substance. The D-galacturonic acid residues are linked together by α-1,4 glycosidic linkages. The molecular weight of pectin ranges from 50,000 to 150,000 daltons. The galacturonic acid residues in pectin may be esterified with methyl groups. There are different types of pectin. Pectin in which more than 50% of the galacturonic acid residues are esterified is called high methoxyl or HM pectin. Pectin in which less than 50% of the galacturonic acid residues are esterified is called low methoxy or LM pectin. Pectin is a nondigestible polysaccharide. So-called modified citrus pectin is pectin that has been hydrolyzed and otherwise modified to make it more digestible and absorbable.

Pectin is available as white to light brown powder. It was first isolated and described in 1825 by Henri Braconnot.

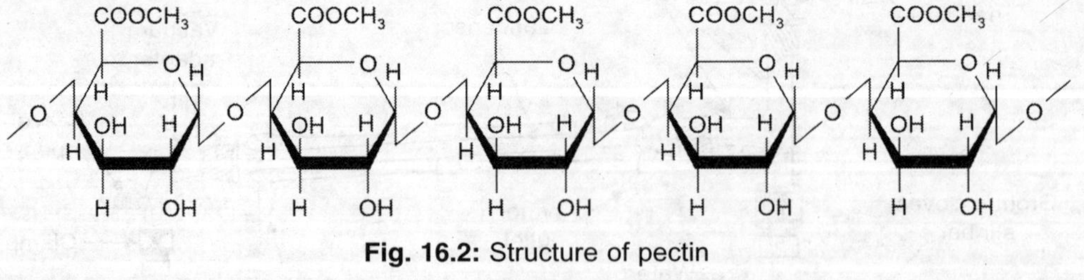

Fig. 16.2: Structure of pectin

Requirements

Orange peel	250 g
Acetone	Sufficient amount
Demineralized water	1 litre
Citric acid	Sufficient amount

Experimental procedure

Follow Flowchart 16.1 for its isolation.

Flowchart 16.1: Isolation of pectin

250 g of orange peel
  (i) Add 1 litre of distilled water
  (ii) Homogenise in a blender

Homogenate
  (i) Adjust the pH to 5 with citric acid or NaOH
  (ii) Heat at 90–95°C for 1 hr, stir
  (iii) Check pH every 15 minutes (maintain at 5.0)
  (iv) Replace water lost in last 20 minutes
  (v) Filter through cheese cloth

Precipitate   Filtrate
  (i) Collect in ice cream container
  (ii) Cool rapidly to 40°C (in ice bath)
  (iii) Add 95% ethanol acidified with 1M HCl (pH 0.7–1)
  (iv) Stir for 10 minutes
  (v) Filter through cheese cloth

Filtrate   Precipitate
  (i) Wash with 300 ml portion of 70% alcohol
  (ii) Test for chloride (with 0.1M AgNO₃)
  (iii) Wash with acetone dropwise
  (iv) Filter through cheese cloth

Filtrate   Precipitate
  (i) Test for NH₃ (with NaOH, heat)
  (ii) Wash with 60% ethanol, 65% ethanol, 95% ethanol and acetone
  (iii) Dry overnight

Pectin

Result: .... g

Calculate the pectin % in the rind.

5. Isolation of Piperine from Black Pepper

Piperine is the alkaloid responsible for the pungency of black pepper along with clavicine (an isomer of piperine). It has also been used in some forms of traditional medicine and as an insecticide.

Piperine is a solid substance essentially insoluble in water. It is a weak base that is tasteless at first, but leaves a burning aftertaste. Piperine belongs to the vanilloid family of compounds, a family that also includes capsaicin, the pungent substance in hot chili peppers. Piperine is the trans-trans stereoisomer of 1-piperoylpiperidine. It is also known as (*E, E*)-1-piperopylpiperidine and (*E, E*)-1-[5-(1,3-benzodioxol-5-yl)-1-cxo-2,4-pentdienyl] piperidine. It is represented by the following chemical structure:

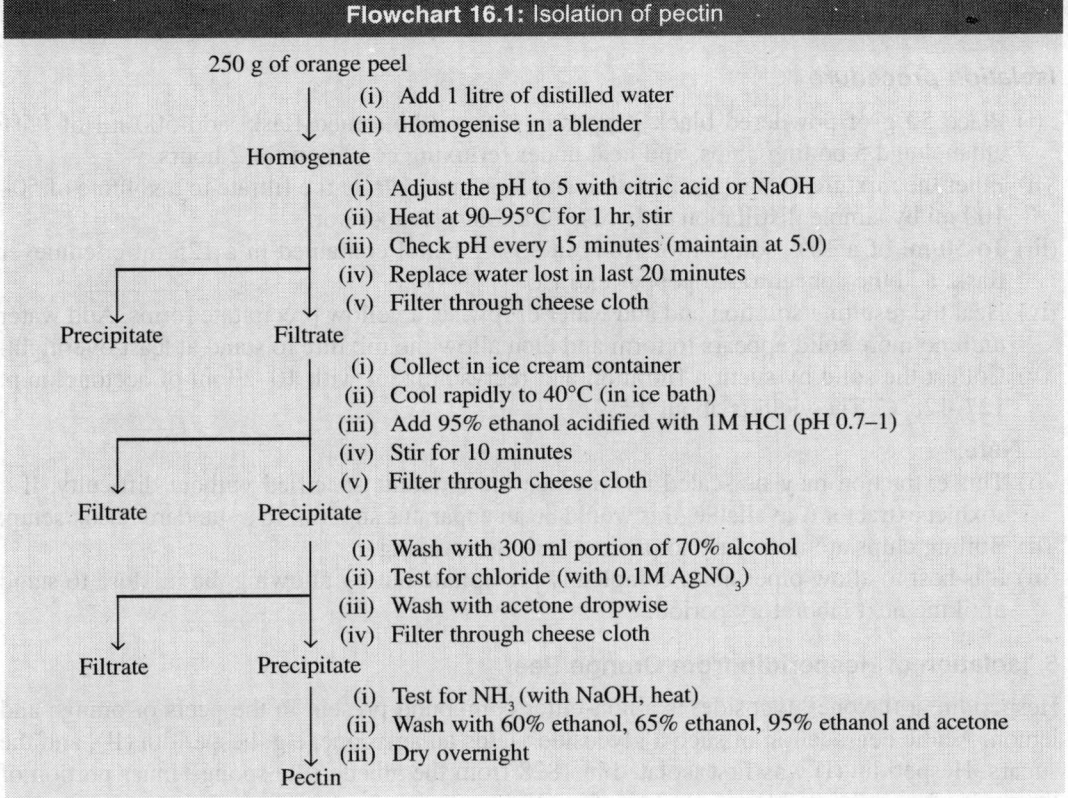

Piperine

Requirements

Black pepper	50 g
Ethanol (95%)	500 ml
Alcoholic KOH (10%)	50 ml

Isolation procedure

 (i) Place 50 g of powdered black pepper in a round-bottomed flask, add 500 ml of 95% ethanol and 5 boiling chips, and heat under refluxing condition for 2 hours.
 (ii) Filter the mixture by suction filtration and then concentrate the filtrate to a volume of 50–100 ml by simple distillation or by use of a rotary evaporator.
 (iii) To 50 ml of a 10% solution of KOH in 95% ethanol contained in a 125 ml erlenmeyer flask, add the concentrated pepper extract.
 (iv) Heat the resulting solution and add water dropwise, a yellow precipitate forms. Add water until no more solid appears to form and then allow the mixture to stand at least overnight.
 (v) Collect the solid by suction filtration and recrystallize it with 10–20 ml of acetone. m.p. 127–128°C. The yield is about 2.5%.

Note:

 (i) This extraction may be scaled up to twice the amounts specified without difficulty. If a soxhlet extractor is available, this would be an apparatus superior to a standard reflux setup.
 (ii) Boiling chips are necessary to prevent serious bumping.
 (iii) It is best to allow piperine to completely precipitate out by allowing the mixture to stand until the next laboratory period.

6. Isolation of Hesperidin from Orange Peel

Hesperidin, a flavone glycoside, is a non-bitter compound present in the peels of orange and lemon. Acidic degradation of such a glycoside yields an aglycone, e.g. hesperidin (II), and the sugars. Hesperidin (I) was first isolated in 1828 from the albedo (the spongy inner portion of the peel) of oranges, and has since been found in lemons and other citrus fruits.

Requirements

Orange peel	250 g
Petroleum ether	1 litre
Methanol	1 litre

Experimental procedure

(i) Place powdered dried orange peel (250 g) and petroleum ether (1 litre) in a round bottomed flask and heat at reflux for one hour.

(ii) While hot, filter the mixture through a Buchner funnel.

(iii) Allow the powder to dry at room temperature and re-extracted with refluxing methanol (1 litre) for 2 hours.

(iv) Filter the hot solution, and concentrate the filtrate under reduced pressure to get a syrup. This syrup is crystallized by the procedure given below.

Recrystallization of Hesperidin (I)

(i) Add the crude hesperidin to dimethylformamide (7 ml per g of syrup). Stir the mixture vigorously at room temperature for 15 minutes, and then filter to remove any insoluble material. To save some time and materials, do not try to recrystallize more than 7.5 g of the syrup.

(ii) In a fumehood, add the filtrate drop-wise with stirring to a boiling solution of water (20 ml per g of hesperidin) and acetic acid (0.5 ml per g of hesperidin).

(iii) Allow the mixture to cool to get hesperidin.

(iv) Collect the precipitated hesperidin by suction filtration and wash with a little cold water. Pure hesperidin has m.p. 252–254°C.

The compound gives a wine-red colour with alcoholic ferric chloride.

7. Isolation of Hippuric acid from urine

$$C_6H_5CO\text{–}NH\text{–}CH_2COOH$$
Hippuric acid

Requirements

Urine of herbivorous animal (cow, horse, etc.) 50 ml	
Calcium hydroxide solution	Sufficient quantity
Conc. HCl	Sufficient quantity

Procedure

(i) Add excess of calcium hydroxide solution to urine (50 ml) until the solution remain alkaline even on boiling.

(ii) Boil the solution when a thick white flocculent precipitate appears.

(iii) Filter it and concentrate the filtrate to about one fourth volume.

(iv) Cool it and add concentrated hydrochloric acid when colourless needles of hippuric acid separate out. Recrystallize it from hot water, m.p. 187°C.

8. Isolation of Cystine from human hair

Cystine may be obtained by the hydrolysis of a large number of proteins. However, the keratins are only common protein rich enough in cystine to serve as a source of this amino acid.

Human hair $\xrightarrow[\text{aq. HCl}]{\text{NaOH, NaOAc}}$

Cystine

Requirements

Human hair	250 g
Sodium hydroxide solution	Sufficient quantity
Conc. HCl solution	Sufficient quantity

Procedure

1. Add thoroughly clean and dry hair in portion of 50 g of hairs to concentrated hydrochloric acid (500 ml) in a round bottom flask.
2. Heat under refluxing condition for 5–6 hours until a drop of it no longer gives violet colour with alkaline copper sulphate solution (Biuret reaction). *This step is necessary to split peptide bonds.*
3. Partially neutralize the solution in hot condition with a sodium hydroxide solution and then add sufficient sodium acetate solution. The Congo red litmus paper test for mineral acid should then be entirely negative at this stage. Care must be taken not to make the solution alkaline with NaOH.
4. Allow the contents to rest overnight and filter it to get brown-coloured precipitate which in addition to cystine also contains some 'human' pigments and tyrosine.
5. Transfer the precipitate to beaker and add hydrochloric acid (about 150 ml). Boil and filter. Add a further hydrochloric acid (150 ml), boil and filter.
6. To the hot clear filtrate, add concentrated solution of sodium acetate until Congo red paper reaction is negative and then cool in ice bath when Cystine separates as colourless crystalline powder.
7. Filter the cystine and wash with hot distilled water (in portion) and dry.
8. Do not allow the filtrate to stand for a longer time, otherwise tyrosine may also crystallize out.

Calculate the % yield.

Note: *An alkaline reaction must always be avoided, as even dilute sodium carbonate decomposes cystine. For this reason some have preferred to omit the partial neutralization with NaOH and to employ sodium acetate only.*

Physical Methods for Analysis

VISCOSITY

Definition

Viscosity is the property which measures the resistance to flow offered by a fluid layer when another adjacent and parallel fluid layer tends to flow over the first layer.

If the distance between the adjacent layers is dx, the required difference of velocities between these layers is du and the area of each layer is A, then at given temperature the force, f, required for maintaining the selected velocity difference between the two layers, is related to the other factors by the following proportionality.

$$f \propto A.\frac{du}{dx} \text{ (at constant temperature)} \qquad \qquad ...(17.1)$$

$$f = \eta A.\frac{du}{dx} \qquad \qquad ...(17.2)$$

where η is the proportionality constant given by eq. 17.3, it has a characteristic value for a fluid at a specified temperature and also known as the *coefficient of viscosity*.

$$\eta = \frac{f}{A.\dfrac{du}{dx}} \qquad \qquad ...(17.3)$$

Coefficient of viscosity of a liquid at a given temperature is the force required per unit area of layers to maintain a unit difference of velocity between two parallel layers of the liquid one unit distance apart.

In the CGS system, the dimensions of η are $g\ cm^{-1}s^{-1}$ and expressed in units of dyne $s\ cm^{-2}$. The unit of coefficient of viscosity in CGS system is poise (g/cm.s). Since in practice, a poise is too large for many liquids, smaller units of centipose (1/100 poise) and millipose (1/1000 poise) are generally used.

The reciprocal of viscosity is called *fluidity* and is denoted by ϕ ($\phi = 1/\eta$).

Significance

Viscosity measurements are sometimes used for:

- Determining compositions of mixtures of two miscible liquids.
- Determining the temperature coefficient of viscosity of a given liquid. The viscosity of liquid decreases by 1–2% for each degree rise in temperature.
- Quality control purposes in the formulation and evaluation of emulsion, colloids, suspension, etc.

DETERMINATION OF VISCOSITY

A. OSTWALD VISCOMETER

Ostwald viscometer (named after Wilhelm Ostwald) consists of a fine capillary tube, a bulb B at its upper end and a U-tube and bulb tube A at the lower end (Fig. 17.1). There are two marks X and Y on the tube above and below the bulb B.

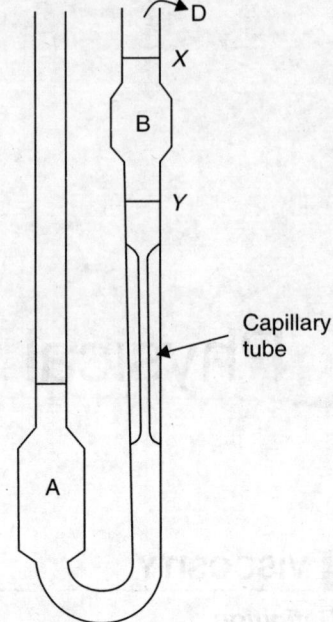

Fig. 17.1: Ostwald viscometer

Experiment 17.1. Determine the viscosity of glycerin by Ostwald Viscometer

Procedure

(i) For viscosity determinations, clean and dry the viscometer and set it vertically in the thermostatic condition in a tall cylinder full of water.

(ii) Suck the glycerin up into the bulb B through a rubber tube attached at D to a level some what above the mark X while maintaining the liquid in U-bend.

(iii) Allow the glycerin to flow through the capillary and note the time for the flow of liquid from X to Y. Record in the Table 17.1.

(iv) Repeat this process with water (standard) of which viscosity is known.

(v) Record the time and density of glycerin and water in Table 17.1.

Observation and calculation

S. No.	Time of flow (in second)	Density of liquid	Viscosity of glycerin
Glycerin			
1.	t_1	r_1	$\eta_1 = \dfrac{\rho_1 t_1}{\rho_2 t_2} \times n_2$
2.			
3.			
Standard liquid			
1.	t_2	r_2	
2.			
3.			

Table 17.1: Observation data

The viscosity of two liquids (glycerin and standard) can be correlated by the following equation:

$$\frac{\eta_1}{\eta_2} = \frac{\rho_1 t_1}{\rho_2 t_2} \qquad \qquad ...(17.4)$$

The η_1 and η_2 are the viscosities of glycerin and water (standard liquid respectively), ρ_1 and ρ_2 are the densities of the glycerin and standard, t_1 and t_2 are the respective times (flow times) in seconds. The viscosity and density of standard liquid is known as particular temperature. From this, viscosity of unknown liquid (glycerin) is calculated.

Eq. 17.4 is based on Poiseuille's law which is:

$$\eta = \frac{\pi r^4 t \Delta \rho}{8lv} \qquad \qquad ...(17.5)$$

where, v is the volume in ml of the liquid flowing in seconds through a narrow tube of radius r cm and length l cm under hydrostatic (driving) pressure ρ dynes per square centimeter and η is the viscosity.

For a given Ostwald viscometer, the radius, length and volume of the liquid are constant and may be combined into a single constant, K. Then, equation 17.5 may be written as:

$$\eta = Kt\rho \qquad \qquad ...(17.6)$$

Note: *Density of liquid is estimated by a specific gravity or pycnometer methods.*

$$Density\ of\ liquid = \frac{W_3 - W_1}{W_2 - W_1} \qquad \qquad ...(17.7)$$

where W_1 = weight of the empty specific gravity bottle; W_2 = *weight of bottle with water;* W_3 = *weight of bottle with test liquid (here it is glycerin)*

In the above determination, as viscosity is determined with reference to that of standard (usually water). Hence, it is termed relative viscosity.

Table 17.1a: Standard densities of liquids at room temperature (25°C)	
Liquid	**Density (g/ml)**
Water	0.9961
Benzene	0.8702
Toluene	0.8592
CCl_4	1.5806
Methyl alcohol	0.7848
Ethyl alcohol	0.8010
Ethyl acetate	0.897
Glycerin	1.2610

Table 17.1b: Standard viscosities of some liquids at room temperature (25°C)	
Liquid	**Viscosity (millipoise)**
Water	8.379
Benzene	5.816
Toluene	3.388
CCl_4	8.682
Methyl alcohol	5.354
Ethyl alcohol	11.900
Acetone	3.06

Experiment 17.2. Determine % composition (water and ethanol) of a given mixture by viscosity measurement

Procedure

(i) Prepare a different dilution of ethanol, e.g. 90 : 10, 80 : 20, 70 : 30 ...... with water and measure the time of flow (thus viscosity) of mixture of known composition as mentioned earlier.

(ii) Similarly, determine the time of flow of unknown composition of same ethanol and water system. Record in the Table 17.2.

Table 17.2: Observation data		
Percentage of components		**Time of flow (in second)**
Ethanol	**Water**	
1. 10	90	–
2. 20	80	–
3. 30	70	–
4. 40	60	–
5. 50	50	–
6. 60	40	–
7. 70	30	–
8. 80	20	–
9. 90	10	–
10. Unknown composition		–

(iii) Determine the viscosity of standard (known composition) and unknown composition with the help of Eq. 17.4.

(iv) Plot the graph between the % composition and viscosity or time of flow.

(v) Read out the composition of unknown mixture in a graph with the determination of the viscosity/time of flow.

SURFACE TENSION

Definition

Surface tension of a liquid is the force acting per centimeter along the surface of liquid at right angles to any line taken in the surface of the liquid in any direction.

It may also be considered as the force per cm which is required to prevent edge of surface of the liquid from being pulled in wards when liquid exists only on other side of the edge.

SI units for surface tension is newton per meter (Nm^{-1}) but CGS unit of dynes per cm is most commonly used.

The surface tension of a solid is a characteristic of surface properties and interfacial interactions, such as adsorption, wetting or adhesion.

Determination of Surface Tension

The surface tension of a liquid is generally determined by the following methods:

(i) Stalagmometer method

(ii) Capillary rise methods (Single and double capillary methods)

(iii) Torsion balance method

Only stalagmometer method, used in undergraduate laboratory, is discussed here.

(i) Stalagmometer method

Two following methods are adopted with the help of stalagmometer.

Drop Weight Method

The size of the drop falling off from the end of capillary tube depends on the surface tension of the liquid and size of the capillary which provides the outer line of attachment for the drop. The total surface tension force supporting the drop is $2\pi r\gamma$, where r is the circumference of the drop at the end of capillary tube.

Along this line, the liquid, glass and air meet and the force of surface tension operates. The drop falls when its weight force, w $(= mg)$, just exceeds the surface tension acting along the circumference.

$w = mg = 2\pi r\gamma$
w = Weight of the drop
m = Mass of liquid
γ = Surface tension
$2\pi r$ = External circumference of contact of the drop with capillary tip.

Thus, the drop weight method can be employed for comparing the surface tension of two liquids generally a liquid of which is to be determined and other liquid of which surface tension is known.

If we have two liquids such that,

$$w_1 = m_1 g = 2p\gamma_1 \qquad \qquad ...(17.8)$$

$$w_2 = m_2 g = 2p\gamma_2 \qquad \qquad ...(17.9)$$

then,
$$\frac{w_1}{w_2} = \frac{m_1}{m_2} = \frac{\gamma_1}{\gamma_2} \qquad \qquad ...(17.10)$$

where w_1 and w_2 are the weight of drops of two liquids, test and standard liquid (usually water); m_1 and m_2 are mass of the two liquids, test and standard; γ_1 and γ_2 are surface tension of the two liquids, test and standard.

From the Eq. 17.10, the surface tension of test liquid can be determined.

Drop number method

It is easier to count the number of drops formed by equal volumes of two liquid: unknown (surface tension of which is to be determined) and standard (surface tension of which is known). With two different liquids, masses of equal volumes are proportional to their densities. If n_1 and n_2 are the number of drops produced from the same volume v of two respective liquids, unknown (surface tension of which is to be determined) and it standard (surface tension of which is known), then:

Volume of a single drop of test liquid $= \dfrac{v}{n_1}$

Mass of its single drop $m_1 = \dfrac{v}{n_1} \times d_1$

where m_1 and d_1 are the mass and density of test liquid

$$2\pi r\gamma_1 = \frac{v}{n_1}.d_1.g \qquad \qquad ...(17.11)$$

where γ_1 is the surface tension of test liquid, and similarly, for the standard liquid,

$$2\pi r\gamma_2 = \frac{v}{n_2}.d_2.g \qquad \qquad ...(17.12)$$

where γ_1 and d_2 are the surface tension and density of standard liquid.

Dividing Eq. 17.11 by 17.12

$$\frac{\gamma_1}{\gamma_2} = \frac{n_2 d_1}{n_1 d_2} \qquad \qquad ...(17.13)$$

With the help of Eq. 17.13 the surface tension of test liquid can be determined.

Experiment 17.3: Determine the surface tension of acetone by stalagmometer by drops number method

Procedure

Stalagmometer (Fig. 17.2) is useful for comparing surface tensions. It consists of a capillary tube with a thick wall and a ground glass flattened end with sharp edges. This helps in giving large well formed drops. The function of capillary tube is to slow down the rate of the flow of liquid. On the stem of tube, two marks A and B are etched, one above and the other below the bulb.

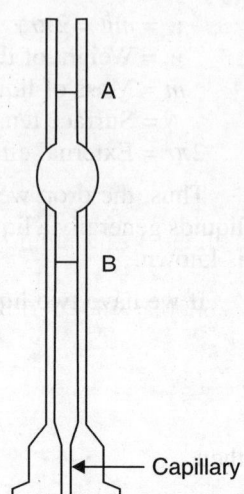

Fig. 17.2: Stalagmometer with a flat ground glass end

For determination of surface tension:

1. Clean the stalagmometer by chromic acid solution to remove the greasy material and then wash with distilled water.
2. Fix the stalagmometer to a stand firmly in a vertical position. Attach a small rubber tube having screw pinch coak on the upper end of the stalagmometer.
3. Dip the stalagmometer by immersing the lower end into distilled water (standard liquid of which surface tension is known) and suck the water above the mark 'A'. Close the pinch coak; insert the stalagmometer in the weighing bottle; lossen the pinch coak and count the number of drops, n_2 obtained from a volume of water between mark A and B. (In drop weight method, weight of this fixed volume is determined).
4. Remove the stalagmometer from the weighing bottle anb dry it.
5. Fill it with the test liquid of which surface tension is to be determined and repeat the same procedure as before and count the number of drops.
6. Determine the densities of both the liquid (standard d_2 and test liquid d_1) as given in Experiment 17.1.
7. Record the data in the Table 17.3.
8. Calculate the surface tension of unknown, γ_2, with the help of the Eq. 17.13 depending on the method.

Table 17.3: Determination of surface tension			
	No. of drops	**Density**	**Surface tension**
Unknown liquid	–	d_1	$\gamma_1 = \dfrac{\gamma_2(n_2 d_1)}{(n_1 d_2)}$
1.	–		
2.	–		
3.	–		
Standard liquid		d_2	γ_2 (known)
1.	–		
2.	–		
3.	–		

Table 17.3a: Standard surface tension of some liquids at room temperature (25°C)

Liquid	Surface tension (dynes/cm)
Water	71.50
Methyl alcohol	21.92
Ethyl alcohol	21.62
Benzene	27.83
Toluene	27.45
CCl$_4$	27.77
Acetone	22.65

Experiment 17.4. Determine the % composition of a mixture (benzene and acetone) by measurement of surface tension

Procedure

(i) Prepare a different dilution of benzene with acetone like 90 : 10, 80 : 20, 70 : 30, ..., 10 : 90 and count the number of drops during the flow of the solution from higher A to the lower mark B in a stalagmometer of each dilution.

(ii) Calculate the surface tension of each dilution as reported earlier. Record in Table 17.4.

(iii) Similarly, do the same with a mixture of unknown composition of the same system. Record the observations in Table 17.4.

(iv) Plot a standard graph between the % composition and number of drops formed/surface tension with standard liquid.

(v) From a standard graph, read out the % composition of unknown liquid.

Table 17.4: Observation data (Room temperature = ... °C)

S. No.	%age of components		No. of drops
	Benzene	Acetone	
1.	10	90	–
2.	20	80	–
3.	30	70	–
4.	40	60	–
5.	50	50	–
6.	60	40	–
7.	70	30	–
8.	80	20	–
9.	90	10	–
10.	Unknown	–	

PARTITION COEFFICIENT LAW

Definition

When a substance distributes itself between two immiscible liquid in equilibrium with each other, the ratio of concentration of substances in them is constant at a particular temperature, provided the molecular state of added substance is same in both the phases.

Consider the distribution of iodine between two immiscible like carbon disulphide and water or benzene and water. If varying amounts of iodine is added to them, concentrations of iodine in the two liquid phases remain constant at a constant temperature. Let C_1 be the concentration of iodine in carbon disulphide and C_2 in water layer, then

$$\frac{C_1}{C_2} = K \text{ (at constant temperature)} \qquad \qquad ...(17.14)$$

The constant K is known as the distribution coefficient or partition coefficient.

The partition coefficient is independent of the total quantity of the substance added or the quantity of solvents used or the units in which the concentration is expressed. The ratio of concentrations is not constant under all conditions. It is applicable only:

(i) When the concentrations of dissolved substance are low in both the solvents. If the concentration of the solute is high, C_1/C_2 may not remain independent of the amount of solute distributed. Hence, deviation is larger.

(ii) When the molecular state of the solute remains the same in two liquids. If the solute associates or dissociates in one or both the solvents, the law fails and C_1/C_2 may not remain constant.

(iii) When the miscibility of two solvents is not affected by addition of the solute.

(iv) When the temperature remains constant, the variation of K with temperature (T) is given by:

$$\frac{d \ln K}{dT} = \frac{2.303 d \log K}{dT} = \frac{\Delta H}{RT^2} \qquad \qquad ...(17.15)$$

where ΔH is the heat of transfer of the solute per mole from one solvent to the other.

Experiment 17.5: Determine the partition coefficient of succinic acid between ether and water

Succinic acid remains in normal molecular state in both water and ether. Hence, distribution law in the simplest form can be applied.

Procedure

(i) Make 4% w/v solution of succinic acid in water. Transfer 30, 40, and 50 ml of this solution in three stoppered flask (labelled them 1, 2, and 3) and add 20 ml and 10 ml of water respectively to flask 1 and 2 to make total 50 ml in each flask.

(ii) Now add 50 ml of ether to each bottle; shake vigorously and allow each flask to stay at constant thermostatic temperature for complete separation of ether and aqueous layer.

(iii) Separate out the ether layer (upper) and aqueous layer (lower) with the help of separating funnel.

(iv) Pipette out 10 ml of the ether layer (of flask no. 1); add 25 ml of water, 2–3 drops of phenolphthalein indicator and titrate with 0.05N sodium hydroxide solution till pink colour is obtained. Take three such readings. Similarly, repeat the procedure with the aqueous layer.

(v) Adopt the same procedure for upper and lower layers in flasks 2 and 3.

(vi) Record the observation data as per Table 17.5.

Observation and Calculation

Table 17.5: Observation data		
	Volume of 0.05N NaOH consumed	
	Ether layer (10 ml)	**Aqueous layer (10 ml)**
Flask 1	x ml	a ml
Flask 2	y ml	b ml
Flask 3	z ml	c ml

For ethereal layer (Flask no. 1):

$$\text{Succinic acid} = \text{NaOH}$$

$$10 \times N_1 = x \times 0.05N \quad \text{or} \quad N_1 = \frac{x \times 0.05N}{10} \qquad \qquad ...(17.16)$$

where N_1 is the normality of succinic acid in ether layer.

Strength or concentration of succinic acid/litre = N_1 × equivalent weight.

Concentration = $\dfrac{x}{10} \times 0.05N \times \dfrac{1}{2}$ mole/litre $\quad$ or $\quad \dfrac{x}{10} \times 0.05 \, N \times \dfrac{118}{2}$ mole/litre

$$= C_{ether} \text{ mole/litre}$$

Note: Gram equivalent weight of succinic acid is half of its gram molecular weight (mol. wt. 118).

For aqueous layer (Flask no. 1)

Concentration = $\dfrac{a}{10} \times 0.05N \times \dfrac{1}{2} mole/litre$ = $C_{aq.}$ mole/litre

Similarly, calculate concentration of succinic acid for flasks 2 and 3 and enter the values in the Table 17.6.

Table 17.6: Determination of K values		
	C $_{ether}$ $\quad$ **C** $_{aqueous}$	**K = C** $_{ether}$/**C** $_{aqueous}$
Flask 1		
Flask 2		
Flask 3		

The constant ether/aqueous values in all the three flasks will verify the partition coefficient law.

Experiment 17.6: Determine the partition coefficient of benzoic acid in benzene and water

Benzoic acid exist as double molecule in the benzene so distribution law in the simple form cannot be applied.

Procedure

(i) Make 8% w/v solution of benzoic acid in benzene. Take out 30, 40 and 50 ml in three separate stoppered flask (labelled as no. 1, 2, 3). Add 20 ml and 10 ml benzene to flask no. 1 and 2 respectively to make 50 ml in each flask.

(ii) Mix 50 ml of water in each flask with vigorous shaking and allow to stand for a few minutes for complete separation of layer.

(iii) Separate the water (lower) and benzene (upper) layer with the help of separating funnel.

(iv) Pipette out 10 ml from benzene layer, add 20 ml of water and titrate with 0.05N NaOH solution using phenolphthalein as indicator.

(v) Repeat the same procedure with aqueous layer. Calculate the normality and concentration of benzoic acid of each layer as given below.

(vi) Adopt the similar procedure with the other flasks 2 and 3.

(vii) Record the observation data as per Table 17.7.

Observation and Calculation

Table 17.7: Observation data

	Volume of 0.05N NaOH consumed	
	Ether layer (10 ml)	Aqueous layer (10 ml)
Flask 1	x ml	a ml
Flask 2	y ml	b ml
Flask 3	z ml	c ml

For benzene layer (Flask 1)

$$C_6H_5COOH = NaOH$$

$$10 \times N_1 = x \times 0.05N$$

$$N_1 = \frac{x \times 0.05}{10} \qquad \qquad ...(17.17)$$

where N_1 is the normality of benzoic acid in ether layer.

$$N_1 = \frac{x \times 0.05N}{10} \text{ or Concentration litre} = \frac{x \times 0.05 \times 122}{10}$$

Note: Gram equivalent weight of benzoic acid is same as molecular weight (Mol.wt.122)

Similarly, for aqueous layer, concentration $= \dfrac{a \times 0.05 \times 122}{10}$

In the same way, calculate the concentration of benzoic acid for flask 2 and 3 and record the value in the Table 17.8.

Table 17.8: Determination of K values

	$C_{benzene}$	$C_{aqueous}$	$K = \dfrac{\sqrt{C_{benzene}}}{C_{water}}$
Flask1			
Flask2			
Flask3			

The constant $K = \dfrac{\sqrt{C_{benzene}}}{C_{water}}$ values in all the three flasks will verify this law.

Note: As benzoic acid associates into double molecules in benzene, $C_{benzene}/C_{water}$ will not give constant value while $K = \dfrac{\sqrt{C_{benzene}}}{C_{water}}$ will give the constant value.

Experiment 17.7: Determine the partition coefficient of iodine in carbon tetrachloride and water

The molecular state of iodine in both the solvents, CCl_4 and water is the same as I_2 and hence, the partition coefficient is practically independent of concentration in dilute solutions. Hence, the distribution law may be applied.

Procedure

1. Prepare a saturated solution of iodine in CCl_4 at room temperature (about 5%) and filter it if necessary.
2. Place 20, 30, 40 ml of this solution in three stoppered flasks (no.1, 2, and 3). Add 20 and 10 ml of CCl_4 to flask no. 1 and 2, respectively.
3. Add 60 ml of water to each flask and shake vigorously.
4. After final shaking, put the flask in thermostate and wait till there is a complete separation of CCl_4 (lower) and aqueous layer (upper).
5. Separate the CCl_4 layer and aqueous layer with the help of separating funnel from flask no. 1.
6. Pipette out 20 ml from aqueous layer of flask no. 1 and titrate with 0.01N sodium thiosulphate solution using a starch mucilage as indicator (the solubility of iodine in water is very low).
7. Similarly repeat the procedure with CCl_4 layer. In the same manner, take the readings from flask no. 2 and 3.
8. Record the observation as shown in Table 17.9 and calculate the concentration of iodine.

Observation and Calculation

Table 17.9: Observation data		
Volume of 0.01N $Na_2S_2O_3$ solution consumed		
	CCl_4 layer (20 ml)	**Aqueous layer (20 ml)**
Flask 1	x ml	a ml
Flask 2	y ml	b ml
Flask 3	z ml	c ml

For carbon tetrachloride layer (Flask No. 1)

$$I_2 = Na_2S_2O_3$$

$$N_1V_1 = N_2V_2 \qquad \qquad \ldots(17.18)$$

where N_1 and N_2 are the normality of iodine and sodium thiosulphate, respectively; V_1 = volume of CCl_4 layer taken (here it is 20 ml); V_2 = volume of $Na_2S_2O_3$ solution consumed in the titration (here it is 'x' ml).

$$20 \times N_1 = x \times 0.01 \, N \text{ or } N_1 = \frac{x \times 0.01N}{20}$$

$$N_1 = \frac{x \times 0.01N}{20} \qquad \qquad \ldots(17.19)$$

$$\text{Concentration} = \frac{x \times 0.01N}{20} \times \frac{1}{2} \text{ gm eq/litre} = C_{CCl_4} \text{ mole/litre}$$

Note: Molecular weight of iodine is twice its equivalent weight which equals its atomic weight (which is 126.9).

$$\text{Concentration} = \frac{x \times 0.01\ N}{20} \times 126.9 \qquad \qquad ...(17.20)$$

For aqueous layer (Flask no. 1).

$$\text{Concentration} = \frac{x \times 0.01N}{20} \times \frac{1}{2} \text{ mole per litre} = C_{aq.} \text{ mole/litre}$$

9. Similarly, calculate the concentration of I_2 for flasks 2 and 3 and enter the values as per Table 17.9.
10. Calculate the partition coefficient (K) as shown in Table 17.10.

	C_{CCl4}	$C_{aqueous}$	$K = C_{CCl4}/C_{aqueous}$
Flask 1	x	a	–
Flask 2	y	b	–
Flask 3	z	c	–

Table 17.10: Determination of K value

The constant CCl_4/aqueous values in all the three flasks will verify the partition coefficient law.

APPLICATIONS OF PARTITION COEFFICIENT

1. Determination of solubilities

Partition coefficient is the ratio of concentration of a compound in the two phases of a mixture of two immiscible solvents at equilibrium. Hence, these coefficient are the measure of differential solubility of the compound between these two solvents. Normally, one of the solvent is water while the second one is hydrophobic. Hence, partition coefficient is measure of how hydrophobic (water hating) or hydrophilic (water loving) a chemical substance is:

$$\frac{C_1}{C_2} = \frac{S_1}{S_2} = K \qquad \qquad ...(17.21)$$

2. Determining association/dissociation of a solute in a liquid

In case the solute exists as single molecule in water as well as in hydrophobic solvent, then its concentration ratio in both the solvents remain constant K.

The inconsistent values indicates association/dissociation of solute in solvent.

3. In determining complex ions

This law has been successfully applied in determination of the formation of complex ions. For example, iodine and iodide ions form a complex ions I_3^- when a solution of iodine in carbon disulphide is shaken with water containing potassium iodide.

4. Process of extraction

(i) The solvent is selected on the basis of partition coefficient for extraction of desired constituent. The solvent should have high partition coefficient toward desired constituted and little or no miscibility with other constituents.

(ii) It is more economical to extract the desired material with the use of solvent in portions. For example, double or triple maceration is more efficient in comparison to simple maceration. In double or triple maceration is divided into two or three parts respectively. Similarly in desilverisation of lead by park's process, zinc used in extracting silver from lead is always taken in small quantities for each extraction and process is repeated several times.

5. Drug delivery system

Drugs which are newly developed must have some kind of delivery method. Most drugs have a partition coefficient which is 0 and 4 for oil and water phase potential. Drugs which has K near to 0 like to be solubilised in water. These drugs are administered directly into the blood-stream by injection. Drugs with K value mean to 4 like to be in oil. These drugs are absorbed through a patch or in ointment. Most of drugs have K value in between 0 to 4. These drugs are often delivered orally in the form of pill.

Experiment 17.8: Determine the partition coefficient of aspirin in chloroform and water

Aspirin is known as a salicylate and a non steroidal anti-inflammatory drug, used to reduce fever and relieve mild to moderate pain from conditions, such as muscle aches, toothaches, common cold, and headaches. Chemically, it is an acetyl derivative of salicylic acid, is a white, crystalline, weakly acidic substance, with a melting point of 136°C.

Aspirin

Procedure

1. Weigh about 1.0 g of the aspirin powder and transfer to a clean, dry 100 ml conical flask. Dissolve in approximately 50 ml chloroform.
2. Prepare at least 100 ml of a saturated sodium bicarbonate solution (about 10% w/v).
3. Add aspirin solution to a separating funnel and then add 50 ml portions of $NaHCO_3$. Your mentor will demonstrate the proper use of a separating flask. Shake the separating flask.
4. Allow to stand for 5 minutes. Collect the organic and aqueous layers in separate Erlenmeyer flasks. Note: Why will aspirin be extracted into the aqueous layer?
5. Set your organic layer aside. Slowly, add HCl solution to your aqueous layer while stirring until the pH is about 2. Cool the solution and filter off the solid by vacuum filtration. Wash your solid with cold distilled water and dry to constant mass.
6. Dry your organic layer with sodium sulphate and gravity filter into a pre-weighed round-bottom flask. Evaporate out the solvent on a water bath and determine the mass of solid you obtain.
7. Determine the partition coefficient (K) of aspirin:

K = Mass of aspirin (g) in chloroform layer/Mass of aspirin (g) in $NaHCO_3$ layer

Note: Aspirin can be also determined by titration with 0.5M NaOH solution (volumetric method). The obtained residue is titrated with standard (0.5M) NaOH solution by using phenol red as indicator.

Aspirin + NaOH $\longrightarrow$ Sodium salt + H_2O

Factor: Each ml of 0.5M NaOH solution = 0.090 g of aspirin.

Experiment 17.9: Determine the partition coefficient of caffeine in chloroform and water

Caffeine is a stimulant obtained from over 60 different types of plants worldwide. The scientific name for caffeine is 1,3,7-trimethylxanthine. Caffeine is a white, odourless and hygroscopic crystalline solid. Caffeine tastes bitter and the density is 1.23 g mL^{-1} and its melting point is 235°C and at higher temperatures, it decomposes. It is soluble in water.

Caffeine

Procedure

1. Weigh about 1.0 g of the caffeine powder and transfer to a clean, dry 100 ml conical flask. Dissolve in approximately 50 ml chloroform.
2. Prepare at least 100 ml of a hydrochloric acid solution (about 10% v/v).
3. Add caffeine solution to a separating funnel and then add 50 ml portions of hydrochloric acid solution. Your mentor will demonstrate the proper use of a separating flask. Shake the separating flask.
4. Allow to stand for 5 minutes. Collect the organic and aqueous layers in separate Erlenmeyer flasks.
5. Set your organic layer aside. Slowly, add dilute NaOH solution to your aqueous layer while stirring until the pH is about 9. Cool the solution and filter off the solid by vacuum filtration. Wash your solid with cold distilled water and dry to constant mass.
6. Dry your organic layer with sodium sulphate and gravity filter into a pre-weighed round-bottom flask. Evaporate out the solvent on a water bath and determine the mass of solid you obtain.
7. Determine the partition coefficient (K) of caffeine:

   K = Mass of caffeine (g) in chloroform layer/Mass of caffeine (g) in HCl layer

Note: Caffeine can also be estimated by iodometric method. Dissolve the caffeine in hot water and cool down. Add 10 ml of sulphuric acid and 25.00 ml standardized (0.05M) iodine solution to the mixture and swirl gently, brown-red precipitate will form. Filter the solution to remove out the precipitate. Titrate the filtrate against a standard (0.05M) sodium thiosulphate solution. Add a few drops of starch solution when the titrand becomes pale brown. Slowly run $Na_2S_2O_3$ until titrand become colourless from dark blue.

$$C_8H_{10}N_4O_2 \text{ (caffeine)} + 2\,I_2 + KI + H_2SO_4 \rightarrow C_8H_{10}N_4O_2.HI.I_4 + KHSO_4$$
$$I_2 + 2\,Na_2S_2O_3 \rightarrow 2NaI + Na_2S_4O_6$$

Determine the unreacted iodine volume from the volume of sodium thiosulphate. Then determine the iodine volume, reacted with caffeine.

Factor: Each ml of 0.05 I_2 solution = 0.00485 g of caffeine.

CRITICAL SOLUTION TEMPERATURE

When two liquids exhibit partial miscibility, a rise in temperature increases the miscibility of liquids. The temperature at, and above which, two partially miscible liquids become completely miscible is called the **critical solution temperature** or consolute temperature or consulate point for the liquid pair.

Consider an example of phenol and water system. Both phenol and water are only partially miscible at room temperature. Therefore, on shaking both the liquid together, two saturated solution of different compositions, one of phenol in water and other of water in phenol are obtained. Such solution of different composition in coexistance with one another are termed conjugate solution. The mutual solubility of phenol and water system increases with rise in temperature and therefore, the concentration of phenol in water as well as that of water in phenol goes on increasing with rise of temperature and ultimately at certain temperature, the conjugate solution change into homogeneous solution. This temperature is called **critical solution temperature**. This temperature for phenol–water system is found to be 68.1°C. The composition of the system is then 36.10% phenol and 63.90% water. Above this temperature, the two layers become miscible with each other in all proportion. The variation of mutual solubility of phenol and water is shown in Fig. 17.3.

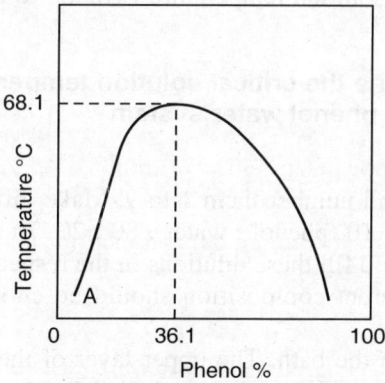

Fig. 17.3: Phenol–water system

Three other types of partially miscible liquid pairs are also encountered in practical field.

Type I: In this, the liquids become completely miscible at and below a certain temperature characteristic of the liquid pair, e.g. triethylamine and water (Fig. 17.4).

Type II: Here, the liquids become completely miscible both above a higher temperature and below a lower characteristic temperature, e.g. nicotine and water (Fig. 17.5).

Type III: In this, the state of complete miscibility of the liquids is reached neither by raising the temperature nor by lowering the temperature, e.g. ether and water.

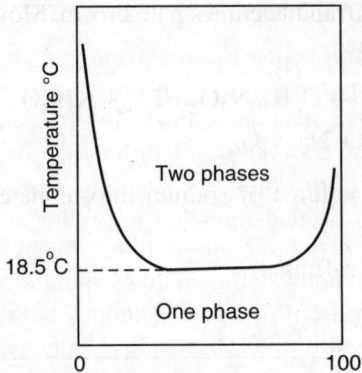

Fig. 17.4: Phase diagram for triethyl-amine in water system showing lower critical solution temperature

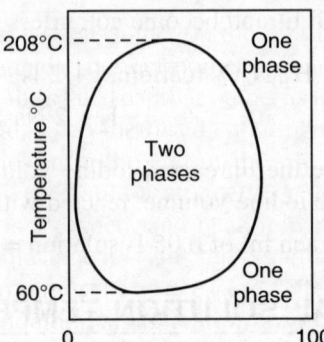

Fig. 17.5: Phase diagram for nicotine–water system showing upper and lower critical solution temperature

Thus, critical solution temperature is observed either by recording upper critical solution temperature by going in the direction of rising temperature or lower critical solution temperature by going in the direction of falling temperature.

Effect of impurities on critical solution temperature

Critical solution temperature is very sensitive to the presence of small amounts of impurities soluble in one or both components. This is the basis of crismer test for detection and estimation of water ion in alcohols.

If an impurity is soluble only in one of the components, its presence in the system raises the upper critical solution temperature and decrease the lower critical solution temperature. If the impurity be soluble in both the components, its presence lowers the upper critical solution temperature and raises the lower critical solution temperature.

The change in the critical solution temperature is found to be linearly proportional to the percentage of impurity.

Experiment 17.10: Determine the critical solution temperature and composition of the solution in the CST for phenol water system

Procedure

1. Take nine boiling tubes and number them 1 to 9. Make different compositions of phenol and water as follows: 90 : 10 (phenol : water), 80 : 20, 70 : 30, 60 : 40, 50 : 50, 40 : 60, 30 : 70, 20 : 80, 10 : 90, and fill these dilutions in the respective boiling tubes 1 to 9.
2. The volumes of the different composition should be enough to cover the bulb of the thermometer (Fig. 17.6).
3. Dip these boiling tubes in the bath. The upper layer of the volume of phenol and water mixture should be about 1cm or more below the level of bath liquid.
4. For recording of critical solution temperature, raise the bath temperature gradually while stirring the mixture and note the temperature (t_1) at which the last traces of cloudiness disappears.
5. Keep the clear solution and allow the bath temperature to decrease.
6. Record the temperature (t_2) at which cloudiness just reappears. The mean of the two temperature which should be nearly equal is the miscibility temperature. Repeat this operation thrice to get the concordant readings.
7. Calculate the CST of the phenol–water system (unknown) as shown in Table 17.11.

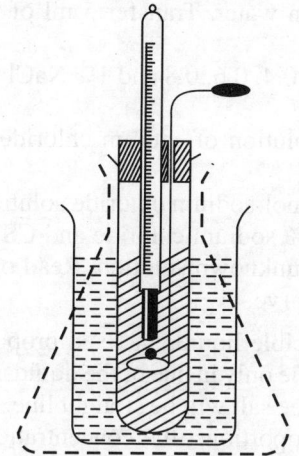

Fig. 17.6: Determination of CST

8. Find out the CST of composition of unknown solution of same system (phenol–water).
9. Plot a graph between per cent composition of phenol–water system of known composition and the critical solution temperature. Similarly determine the CST of unknown solution of same system.
10. Then read out the composition of unknown system in the standard graph.

Observation Data

Boiling tube	Vol. of phenol (ml)	Vol. of water (ml)	Temp. (°C)		Mean CST (t) $\dfrac{t_1 + t_2}{2}$
			t_1	t_2	
1.	90	10	–	–	
2.	80	20	–	–	
3.	70	30	–	–	
4.	60	40	–	–	
5.	50	50	–	–	
6.	40	60	–	–	
7.	30	70	–	–	
8.	20	80	–	–	
9.	10	90	–	–	

Table 17.11: Determination of mean CST

Experiment 17.11: Determine the concentration of aqueous sodium chloride with the help of critical solution temperature

Procedure

1. Prepare 1% NaCl solution.
2. Then, pipet out 1, 2, 4, 6 and 8 ml of this stock solution and transfer in a separate test tube or small capacity flask.
3. Add water 8, 6, 4 and 2 ml to each of the test tube to get 0.1, 0.2, 0.4, 0.6 and 0.8% NaCl solution.

4. Prepare 80% phenol solution in water. Transfer 5 ml of this stock solution in each of the 7 test tubes.
5. Then transfer 10 ml of 0.1, 0.2, 0.4, 0.6, 0.8 and 1% NaCl solution in each of six (1 to 6) test tube containing phenol.
6. Transfer 10 ml of unknown solution of sodium chloride and transfer in the 7th test tube containing phenol.
7. Find out the CST of all the phenol-sodium chloride solution of known concentration. Plot a calibration curve between the % sodium chloride and CST.
8. Similarly, find out the CST of unknown solution. Read out the % of NaCl in the unknown solution from the calibration curve.

The CST of two partially miscible liquids in fixed proportions increases linearly with the concentration of the impurity soluble only in one of the liquids. Thus, plot of the CST temperature of the liquids vs concentration of the salt will be straight line. Determining the CST of unknown NaCl with phenol in the same proportions, the concentration of the solution can be read off from the plot.

Observation

Table 17.12: Determination of CST (°C)

	80% phenol (ml)	% of NaCl solution	CST (0°C)
1.	5 ml	0.1	–
2.	5 ml	0.2	–
3.	5 ml	0.4	–
4.	5 ml	0.6	–
5.	5 ml	0.8	–
6.	5 ml	1.0	–
7.	5 ml	Unknown	–

POLARIMETRY

According to wave theory of light, an ordinary ray of light is considered to be vibrating in all plane at right angles to the direction of its propagation. If this ordinary light passes through a nicol prism, the emergent ray has its vibration only in one plane. The light having wave motion in only one plane is known as *plane polarized light.*

The plane along which vibrations are taking place is known as *plane of polarization.* The nicol prism used for this purpose is called the polarizer. Some substance in its pure state or in solution form has the ability to rotate the plane of polarization of a beam of polarized light. The property by virtue of which the plane of polarization of light is rotated is called *optical activity.* The substances possessing this property are called optically active substances. The substance which rotate the plane of polarized light toward the right (clockwise) is called *dextrorotatory* (+) and which rotate toward the left (anticlockwise) is called *levorotatory* (–). A mixture of these varieties in equal proportion is optically inactive and is called recemic mixture.

The presence and concentration of optically active substances can be determined by measuring the degree and direction in which plane of polarized light is rotated. The field devoted to the analysis of optically active compounds by measuring the rotation of plane of polarized light is called *polarimetry.* The magnitude of the rotation depend on the following factors:

(a) Nature of substance
(b) Length of liquid column through which light travels.
(c) Concentration of the solution
(d) Nature of the solvent
(e) Temperature of the solution
(f) Wavelength of light used.

The rotatory power of a given solution is generally expressed as specific rotation $[\alpha]^t_D$. It is the no. of degrees of rotation of the plane of polarised light produced by a liquid. If the active substance is used as such, then specific rotation is represented by Eq. 17.22.

$$[a]^t_D = \frac{\text{Observed angle of rotation}}{L \times d} \qquad ...(17.22)$$

where L = path length of light in decimeter; d = density of the liquid

If the substance is in solution, then concentration is taken into account and the Eq. 17.22 is rearranged accordingly as:

$$[a]^t_D = \frac{100 \times \text{Observed angle of rotation}}{L \times C} \qquad ...(17.23)$$

where C = concentration in g/100 ml.

It is essential to specify the solvent used to dissolve the substance as magnitude and even sign of the specific rotation may be markedly affected by the nature of the solvent. Specific rotation of a very dilute solution in a non-optically active solvent is always constant at constant temperature (t).

D refers to the D line of the sodium flame. When other light is used, the specific rotation is represented as $[\alpha]^t_l$ where l is the wavelenght of light.

Polarimeter

Polarimeter (Fig. 17.7) consists of light source, a polarizer, an analyzer attached to disk graduated in degrees and fraction of degrees, sample tube and half shadow device.

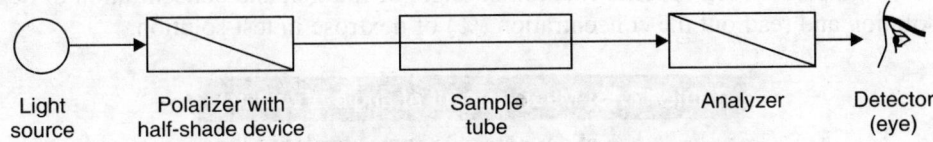

| Light source | Polarizer with half-shade device | Sample tube | Analyzer | Detector (eye) |

Fig. 17.7: Schematic representation of polarimeter

Sodium vapor lamp is used as light source.

Two different Nicol prisms are used as polarizer and analyzer in most of the polarimeter. Monochromatic light is plane polarized by the stationary polarizer and extent of rotation of this polarized light is related to rotation of the analyzer. The number of degrees of rotation of the analyzer is read on the graduated disk attached to it.

Sample tube is the container for the sample to be analysed and are placed between the polarizer and analyzer in the path of the plane polarised light.

Because it is easier for the human eye to match two adjacent areas to same degrees of brightness than to determine a point of maximum darkness or brightness, a third Nicol prism is placed behind the polarizer and rotated through a small angle to divide the field into halves of unequal brightness. An eyepiece is focussed on the field and by rotating the analyzer, the two halves may be brought to equal brightness (Fig. 17.8). This is called balance or zero point.

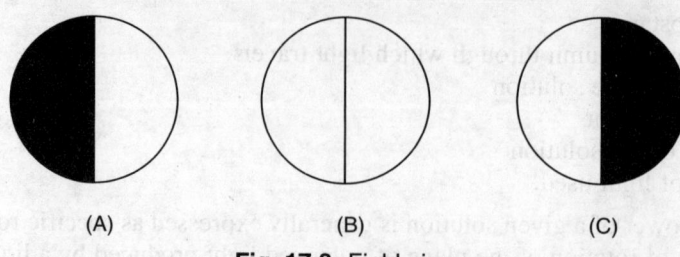

(A)   (B)   (C)

Fig. 17.8: Field view

When an optically active substance is placed in the path of plane polarized light, one half appears dark and other half appears bright. Rotation of analyzer returns the two halves to equal intensity of illumination. The number of degrees of rotation (either in left direction or right direction) as read on graduated disk measures the optical activity.

Application

Specific rotations are basis of identification and index of purity of volatile oils (peppermint, cinnamon), sugars (dextrose), vitamins (ascorbic acid), etc.

Experiment 17.12: Perform the quantitative estimation of dextrose by measuring specific rotation

Procedure

(i) Prepare a 5%, 10%, 15% dextrose solution and measure the angle of rotation.

(ii) Record in Table 17.13 as given below.

(iii) Similarly, measure the angle of rotation in unknown solution.

(iv) Calculate the specific rotation of each solution by the formula:

$$[\alpha]_D^t = \frac{100 \times \text{Observed angle of rotation}}{L \times C}$$

where C = concentration in g/100 ml; L = length of liquid column in decimeter.

(v) Plot a graph between specific rotation or angle of rotation and concentration of dextrose solution and read out the concentration (%) of dextrose in test solution.

Table 17.13: Measurement of angle of rotation

	% of dextrose	Angle of rotation
1.	Distilled water	—
2.	5	—
3.	10	—
4.	15	—
5.	Test solution	—

SOLUBILITY PRODUCT

Definition

Solubility product of a sparingly soluble salt at a given temperature may be defined as the product of the concentrations of its ions, each raised to the power of number of times the ion occurs in the chemical equation representing the dissociation of the electrolyte.

Certain electrolytes such as $BaSO_4$, and AgCl are sparingly soluble in water. Even in their saturated solutions, the concentration of the electrolyte is very low. So, whatever little of electrolytes, solid electrolyte is in equilibrium with the ions as:

$$\text{Undissolved electrolyte} \rightleftharpoons \text{Ions in solution}$$

For example, in aqueous solution of silver chloride

$$AgCl\ (s) \rightleftharpoons Ag^+\ (aq.) + Cl^-\ (aq.)$$

On applying law of chemical equilibrium,

$$K = \frac{[Ag^+][Cl^-]}{[AgCl]}$$

Since the solution is saturated and incontact with the solid so the concentration of silver chloride must be constant at given temperature. Hence:

$$K = \frac{[Ag^+][Cl^-]}{k}$$

$$K.k = K_{SP} = [Ag^+][Cl^-]$$

The product of K and AgCl (k) is replaced by new constant K_{SP}, known as solubility product. It is equal to the product of ionic concentration termed ionic product, for a saturated solution.

In general, for any sparingly soluble salt A_xB_y, which dissociates to set up the equilibrium:

$$A_xB_y \rightleftharpoons xA^{y+} + yB^{x-}$$

Solubility product constant may be expressed as:

$$K_{SP} = [A^{y+}]^x\ [B^{x-}]^y$$

A^{y+} and B^{x-} denote positive and negative ions respectively and x and y represent number of these ions in the formula of the electrolyte.

CALCULATION OF SOLUBILITY PRODUCT

Knowing the solubility of the salt, its solubility product K_{SP} can be calculated. For example, the solubility of barium sulphate at 25°C salt is 2.5×10^{-3} g per 1000 g of water. This weight must be divided by the mol.wt (233) to obtain molarity or molality in this dilute solution.

$$\frac{2.5 \times 10^{-3}}{233} = 1.1 \times 10^{-5}\ \text{litre}$$

Since barium sulphate is completely ionised, this is the concentration of each of its ion. Therefore,

$$K_{sp} = (1.1 \times 10^{-5})\ (1.1 \times 10^{-5}) = 1.2 \times 10^{-10}$$

At a given temperature, the more insoluble a salt, less is its solubility product. Since, in general, solubility is increased with the increase of temperature, its solubility product also likewise increases. For example, at 50°C the solubility product of barium sulphate is 2.0×10^{-10}.

APPLICATIONS OF SOLUBILITY PRODUCT

Calculations of Solubility

If solubility product of a sparingly soluble salt at a particular temperature is known, its solubility at that temperature can be calculated.

Predicting the precipitation of a salt

The concept of solubility product helps us to predict whether a salt will precipitate or not, on mixing the solutions containing its ions under particular concentration of the ions of the salt cannot exceed the value of solubility product. Thus, if ionic product exceeds solubility product, excess ions combine with each other to form precipitate of the salt.

∴   Precipitation occurs: If calculated ionic product $> K_{SP}$

        No precipitation: If calculated ionic product $< K_{SP}$

Precipitation of Soluble Salts

The principle of solubility product is also applied in the precipitation of soluble salts from their saturated solution, in pure state.

The salting out, phenomenon is used in the purification of sodium chloride. This is done by preparing saturated solution of impure sodium chloride in water:

$$NaCl\ (s) \rightleftharpoons Na^+ + Cl^-$$
$$\text{(In solution)}$$
$$K_{SP} = [Na^+]\ [Cl^-]$$

HCl gas is passed through this solution. The concentration of Cl^- ions, therefore increases considerably. The ionic product exceeds the solubility product of NaCl. Therefore, it precipitates out from the solution in pure state.

In inorganic qualitative analysis

The classification of basic redicals into different groups in the inorganic qualitative analysis is based upon the knowledge of solubility products of salts of these basic redicals.

Experiment 17.13: Determine the solubility product of $Ca(OH)_2$ at room temperature

Procedure

1. Prepare 0.025, 0.05 and 0.1N NaOH solution in separate flask and standardize them against 0.05N HCl solution.
2. Transfer the 100 ml of sodium hydroxide solution of each normality in separate flask and add about 2 g of $Ca(OH)_2$ into each flask.
3. Stopper them and shake for about 1 hour.
4. Filter the content of each flask. Reject a few initial ml of the solution and collect the remaining portion.
5. Titrate the 20 ml solution of each flask with 0.05N HCl solution by using phenolphthalein as indicator.
6. From titration result, calculate:
   (a) The concentration of OH^- ion (a) due to NaOH, (apply $N_1V_1 = N_2V_2$ formula and calculate the exact normality of NaOH, where N_1 and N_2 are the normality of NaOH and HCl solution V_1 and V_2 are the volume of NaOH and HCl solution.
   (b) Concentration of OH ion (b) after saturation with $Ca(OH)_2$, by similar procedure.
   (c) Excess OH^- ion ($b - a$) due to $Ca(OH)_2$
   (d) Concentration of Ca^{2+} ions from excess concentration OH^- ions.
7. Record the data in Table 17.14 as illustrated below and calculate the solubility product (K_{SP}).

Table 17.14: Determination of solubility product					
Normality of NaOH solution	Conc. of OH⁻ due to NaOH (*a*)	Conc. of OH⁻ due to NaOH and Ca(OH)₂ (*b*)	OH⁻ due to Ca(OH)₂ (*b – a*)	Conc. of Ca²⁺ = ½(OH⁻) = ½(*b – a*)	$K_{sp} = [OH^-]^2[Ca^{2+}]$
1.					
2.					
3.					

Note: Protect the solution from absorption of CO_2 gas from air.

CHEMICAL KINETICS

Chemical kinetics is the branch of chemistry which answer the question: "how fast do reactions go?" If Chemistry is involved in making new substances out of old substances (i.e. chemical reactions), then there are two basic questions that must be answered:

(i) Does the reaction want to go? This is the subject of chemical thermodynamics.

(ii) If the reaction wants to go, how fast will it go? This is the subject of chemical kinetics. Besides information about the speed at which reaction occurs, kinetics also shed light on reaction mechanism (how the reaction occurs).

Important factors which affect rates of reactions:

- Reactant concentration
- Temperature
- Action of catalysts
- Surface area
- Pressure of gaseous reactants or products.

Reaction Rates

Consider the reaction:

$$2NO(g) + O_2(g) \longrightarrow 2NO_2(g)$$

We can specify the rate of this reaction by telling the rate of change of the partial pressures of one of the gases. However, it is convenient to convert these pressures into concentrations, so we can specify the rate of this by telling the rate of change of the partial pressures of one of the gases. However, it is convenient these pressures to rate equations in terms of concentrations, where square brackets, means concentration in mol/L.

The rate of reaction can be written as:

$$\frac{d[NO_2]}{dt},$$

or as

$$-\frac{d[O_2]}{dt},$$

but these are not the same because each molecule of O_2 gives two molecules of NO_2. To arrive at an unambiguous definition of reaction rate we define the "reaction velocity", *v*, as:

$$v = \frac{1}{2}\frac{d[NO_2]}{dt} = -\frac{d[O_2]}{dt} = -\frac{1}{2}\frac{d[NO]}{dt} \qquad \ldots(17.24)$$

Table 17.15: Solubility products of some slightly soluble electrolytes in water

Substance	Solubility product (K_{SP})	Temperature (°C)
Aluminium hydroxide	7.7×10^{-13}	25
Barium carbonate	8.1×10^{-9}	25
Barium sulphate	1×10^{-10}	25
Calcium carbonate	9×10^{-9}	25
Calcium sulphate	6.1×10^{-5}	20
Ferric hydroxide	1×10^{-36}	18
Ferrous hydroxide	1.6×10^{-14}	18
Lead carbonate	3.3×10^{-14}	18
Lead sulphate	1.1×10^{-8}	18
Magnesium carbonate	2.6×10^{-5}	12
Pot.acid tartarate	3.8×10^{-4}	18
Silver iodide	1.5×10^{-16}	25
Zinc hydroxide	1.8×10^{-14}	18
Zinc sulphide	1.2×10^{-23}	18

This is unambiguous. The negative sign tells us that species is being consumed and the fractions take care of the stoichiometry. Anyone of the three derivatives can be used to define the rate of the reaction.

For a general reaction:

$$a\text{A} + b\text{B} \rightarrow c\text{C} + d\text{D} \qquad \qquad ...(17.25)$$

the reaction velocity can be written in a number of different but equivalent ways.

$$v = -\frac{1}{a}\frac{d[\text{A}]}{dt} = -\frac{1}{b}\frac{d[\text{B}]}{dt} = \frac{1}{c}\frac{d[\text{C}]}{dt} = \frac{1}{c}\frac{d[\text{D}]}{dt} \qquad ...(17.26)$$

As in our previous example, the negative signs account for material that is being consumed in the reaction and the positive signs account for material that is being formed in the reaction. The stoichiometry is preserved by dividing the rate of change of concentration of each substance by its stoichiometric coefficient.

Rate Laws

A rate law is an equation that tells us how fast the reaction proceeds and how the reaction rate depends on the concentrations of the chemical species involved. A rate law is an equation of the form:

$$v = f([\text{A}], [\text{B}], ... [\text{E}]) \qquad \qquad ...(17.27)$$

Equation 17.27 gives us a first order differential equation in t because the reaction velocity is related to a time-derivative of one of the concentrations (as in Eq. 17.28).

The rate law may contain substances which are not in the balanced reaction and may not contain some things that are in the balanced equation (even on the reactant side).

Usually, rate law takes the form:

$$v = k[\text{A}]^x [\text{B}]^y ... [\text{E}]^z \qquad \qquad ...(17.28)$$

where x, y, z are small whole numbers or simple fractions and k is called the "rate constant". The sum of $x + y + z + ...$ is called the "order" of the reaction.

COMMON TYPES OF RATE LAWS

First Order Reactions

In a first order reaction the rate is proportional to the concentration of one of the reactants. That is:

$$v = \text{rate} = k[B] \qquad \qquad ...(17.29)$$

where B is a reactant. If we have a reaction which is known to be first order in B, such as B + other reactants → products.

We would write the rate law as:

$$-\frac{d[B]}{dt} = k[B] \qquad \qquad ...(17.30)$$

The constant, k, in this rate equation is the first order rate constant.

Second Order Reactions

In a second order reaction the rate is proportional to concentration squared. For example, possible second order rate laws might be written as:

$$\text{Rate} = k\,[B]^2 \qquad \qquad ...(17.31)$$

or as if A and B are the two reactants,

$$\text{Rate} = k[A]\,[B] \qquad \qquad ...(17.32)$$

That is, the rate might be proportional to the square of the concentration of one of the reactants, or it might be proportional to the product of two different concentrations.

Third Order Reactions

There are several different ways to write a rate law for a third order reaction. One might have cases where:

$$\text{Rate} = k[A]^3 \qquad \qquad ...(17.33)$$

or

$$\text{Rate} = k[A]^2\,[B] \qquad \qquad ...(17.34)$$

or

$$\text{Rate} = k[A]\,[B]\,[C] \qquad \qquad ...(17.35)$$

and so on.

A, B, C are the reactants.

Experiment 17.14: Determine of rate constant for hydrolysis of ethyl acetate in presence of HCl at room temperature

The hydrolysis of methyl acetate in presence of an acid may be represented as:

$$CH_3COOCH_3 + H_2O \xrightarrow{\ H^+\ } CH_3COOH + CH_3OH$$

Reaction Mechanism

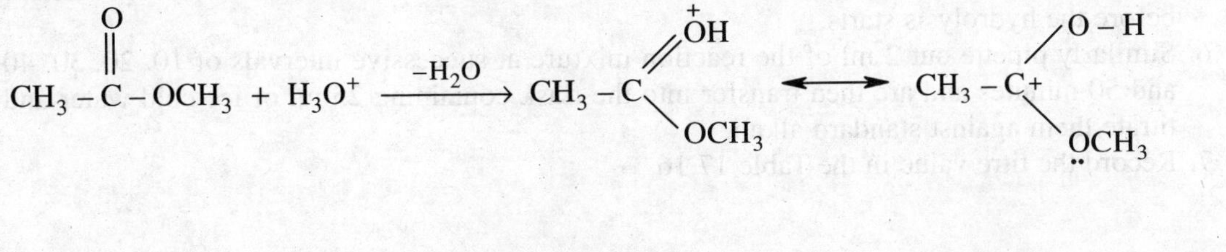

$$CH_3-\underset{+}{\overset{\overset{\displaystyle OH}{|}}{C}}-OCH_3 + H_2O \longrightarrow CH_3-\underset{\overset{|}{^+OH_2}}{\overset{\overset{\displaystyle OH}{|}}{C}}-OCH_3 \xrightarrow{\text{Transfer of proton}} CH_3-\underset{\overset{|}{OH}}{\overset{\overset{\displaystyle OH}{|}}{C}}-\underset{\overset{|}{H}}{\overset{+}{O}}CH_3$$

$$CH_3-\underset{\diagdown OH}{\overset{\diagup OH}{C+}} \quad + \ HOCH_3$$

$$\downarrow H_2O$$

$$CH_3-C\underset{\diagdown O-H}{\overset{\diagup\!\!\diagup O}{}} \quad + \ H_3O^+$$

The reaction is an example of pseudo unimolecular reaction. [The concentration of water is high and remain constant during the reaction. Concentration of H$^+$ ions also remain constant]. Thus, the rate of reaction is determined by one concentration (e.g. methyl acetate).

$$\frac{dx}{dt} = k\,[CH_3COOCH_3]$$

and so the following formulae for the first order reaction may be used.

$$k = \frac{2.303}{t} \times \log\frac{a}{a-x}$$

where a = initial concentration of ester; $a - x$ = concentration of ester which is hydrolyzed.

Procedure

1. Place 50 ml of 0.05 HCl solution in a clean 100 ml conical flask and about 10 ml of ethyl acetate in a test tube. Cork both of them and keep them in thermostate maintained at room temperature.
2. Maintain a stock of ice cold carbonate free water. Arrange five conical flask of 100 ml capacity and put 25 ml of ice cold water in each flask before titration of reaction mixture during the course of reaction.
3. Pipette out 2 ml of ethyl acetate from the test tube into the conical flask containing 50 ml of hydrochloric acid solution. Start the stopwatch when half the pipette has been discharged ($t = 0$).
4. Shake the mixture and at once take out 2 ml of the reaction mixture and immediately transfer it to one of the flask containing 25 ml of the ice cold water. The lowering of temperature slow down the reaction.
5. Titrate it quickly against 0.05N NaOH using phenolphthalein as indicator. This volume of v_o of the alkali very nearly corresponds to the concentration of HCl in the reaction mixture before the hydrolysis starts.
6. Similarly pipette out 2 ml of the reaction mixture at successive intervals of 10, 20, 30, 40 and 50 minutes and are then transfer into the flask containing 25 ml of ice cold water and titrate them against standard alkali.
7. Record the titre value in the Table 17.16.

Time (minutes)	Titre value (ml)	$a - x$ (ml)	$\log (a - x)$	k
	Table 17.16: Observation data			
0	v_0	–	–	–
10	v_{10}	$v_\infty - v_{10}$	–	–
20	v_{20}	$v_\infty - v_{20}$	–	–
30	v_{30}	$v_\infty - v_{30}$	–	–
40	v_{40}	$v_\infty - v_{40}$	–	–
50	v_{50}	$v_\infty - v_{50}$	–	–
∞	v_∞	–	–	–

8. Record the infinite (∞) time reading as follows:

Take out 10 ml of the reaction mixture in dry conical flask. Keep the flask on a water bath maintained at 50°C for an hour or so that the hydrolysis is completed. Now cool it at room temperature. Take out 2 ml of this mixture and do the same as done in step (4) and (5).

Observation and Calculation

Remarks

(i) The initial titre value or titre value at $t = 0$, v_o is proportional to the amount of HCl present in 2 ml of the reaction mixture at zero time when no acetic acid is yet formed.

(ii) v_∞ is proportional to the amount of acid present in 2 ml of the reaction mixture when the hydrolysis is completed (initial HCl + CH_3COOH formed).

(iii) $v_\infty - v_o$ is proportional to the concentration of acetic acid produced when the hydrolysis is completed and proportional to the amount of ester hydrolysed in 2 ml of the reaction mixture.

(iv) $v_\infty - v_o$ is proportional to the initial concentration of the ester ['a' in the formula]. Since we have a ratio of volumes in the integrated rate equation, the proportionality factor will cancel out and the $v_\infty - v_t$ values can be used in place of '$a - x$' in the formula.

(v) Substitute the titre values in the formula and calculate 'k' value for different values of 't':

$$k = \frac{2.303}{t} \times \log \frac{(v_\infty - v_o)}{(v_\infty - v_t)}$$

Experiment 17.15: Determine of rate constant for hydrolysis of ethyl acetate in presence of alkali

The reaction (saponification) of ethyl acetate by sodium hydroxide illustrates a biomolecular reaction and may be represented as:

$$CH_3COOC_2H_5 + NaOH \longrightarrow CH_3COONa + C_2H_5OH$$

The rate of reaction can be determined by the following equation:

$$\frac{dx}{dt} = k\,[CH_3COOC_2H_5]\,[NaOH]$$

As the reaction proceeds, NaOH is consumed, hence the progress of the reaction may be determined by determining the amount of alkali present in the reaction mixture at any instant.

Reaction Mechanism

$$CH_3 - C \overset{O}{\underset{OC_2H_5}{\diagdown}} + OH^- \longrightarrow CH_3 - \overset{O^-}{\underset{OH}{\underset{|}{\overset{|}{C}}}} - OC_2H_5 \longrightarrow CH_3 - C \overset{O}{\underset{OH}{\diagdown}} + {}^-OC_2H_5$$

$$\downarrow$$

$$CH_3 - C \overset{O}{\underset{O^-}{\diagdown}} + HOC_2H_5$$

Procedure

(i) Take 100 ml of M/40 ethyl acetate and 200 ml of M/40 NaOH solution in a separate 250 ml conical flask. Cork them and keep in a thermostate maintained at room temperature. **Note:** Mol. wt. of ethyl acetate is 88.0 and density is 0.90. Prepare the molar solution by measuring it.

(ii) Accurately measure 100 ml of NaOH solution and pour it in ethyl acetate solution. Note the time (start the stop watch), when half of the volume of alkali has been poured into the ester. This is taken at zero time. Pipette out 10 ml of the reaction mixture and allow to run into a flask containing 25 ml of ice cold M/40 HCl solution.

(iii) Immediately titrate with M/40 alkali solution by using phenolphthalein as indicator.

(iv) Similarly, pipette out 10 ml the reaction mixture at successive interval of 5, 10, 15, 25, 40, 60 and 100 minutes and do the same as done in step (ii) and (iii).

(v) Record the titre value in Table 17.17.

Observation and Calculation

Table 17.17: Determination of rate constant		
t (min)	Volume of NaOH (ml)	$k = \dfrac{1}{t.a} \cdot \dfrac{x}{a-x}$
0	–	–
5	–	–
10	–	–
15	–	–
25	–	–
40	–	–
60	–	–
100	–	–

Calculation

(i) The experiment is based on back titration of the unreacted sodium hydroxide with the ester.

(ii) At zero time, t_o, no hydrolysis of ester occurs by M/40 NaOH, so it react with HCl. The remaining excess HCl reacts with the titrant (M/40 NaOH).

(iii) By time, M/40 NaOH reacts with the ester, therefore, the amount of reacting with HCl decreases. The amount of excess HCl that reacts with the titrant (M/40 NaOH) increases and therefore titre value increases.

(iv) According to the integrated rate law equation for second order reaction, when the concentrations are equal, is:

$$k = \frac{1}{t.a} \cdot \frac{x}{a-x}$$

where 'a' is the initial concentration of reactants $\frac{50}{100} \times \frac{M}{40}$ or $\frac{M}{80}$ in the present case

Volume of reaction mixture used = 10 ml
Volume of M/40 HCl used = 25 ml
25 ml of M/40 HCl = 25 ml of M/40 NaOH
Excess acid = v_t ml of M/40 NaOH
Acid used for residual NaOH in 10 ml of the reaction mixture

$$\equiv (25 - v_t) \text{ ml of M/40 NaOH}$$

Residual concentration of NaOH in the reaction mixture $= \frac{25 - v_t}{10} \cdot \frac{M}{40}$

Thus $a - x$ at time t

$$x = \frac{(25 - v_t)}{400} M$$

$$a = \frac{M}{80}$$

$$a - x = \frac{1}{80} - \frac{25 - v_t}{400} M$$

Note: For convenience, make the solution of acid and alkali in the same molarities.

(v) Calculate values of k by substituting a, x and $(a - x)$ in the integrated rate law equations.

(vi) Plot a graph of $\frac{1}{a - x}$ versus 't' and obtain the values of k from the stop of straight line.

REFRACTOMETRY

The speed of light in a vacuum is always the same, but when light moves through any other medium it travels more slowly since it is constantly being absorbed and reemitted by the atoms in the material. The ratio of the speed of light in a vacuum to the speed of light in another substance is defined as the **index of refraction (refractive index** or n) for the substance.

$$\frac{v_A}{v_B} = \frac{\sin \theta_A}{\sin \theta_B} = \frac{n_B}{n_A} \qquad \ldots(17.36)$$

Whenever light changes speed as it crosses a boundary from one medium into another its direction of travel also changes, i.e. it is refracted (Fig. 17.9). The relationship between light's speed in the two mediums (v_A and v_B), the angles of incidence (θ_A) and refraction (θ_B) and the refractive indexes of the two mediums (n_A and n_B) is shown below:

$$\frac{v_A}{v_B} = \frac{\sin \theta_A}{\sin \theta_B} = \frac{n_B}{n_A} \qquad \ldots(17.37)$$

Thus, it is not necessary to measure the speed of light in a sample in order to determine its index of refraction. Instead, by measuring the angle of refraction, and knowing the index of refraction of the layer that is in contact with the sample, it is possible to determine the refractive

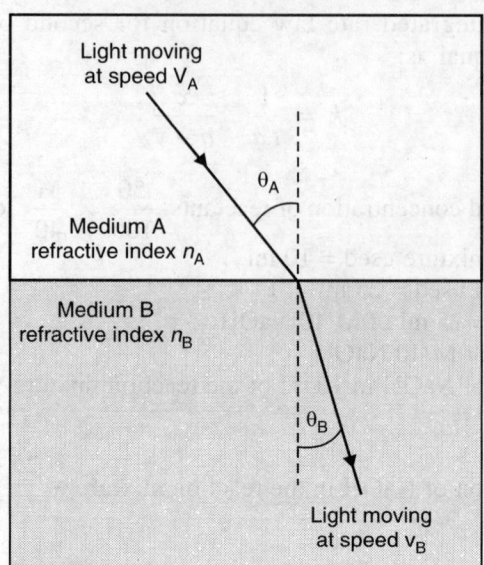

Fig. 17.9: Light crossing from any transparent medium into another in which it has a different speed, is refracted, i.e. bent from its original path. In the case shown, the speed of light in medium A is greater than the speed of light in medium B

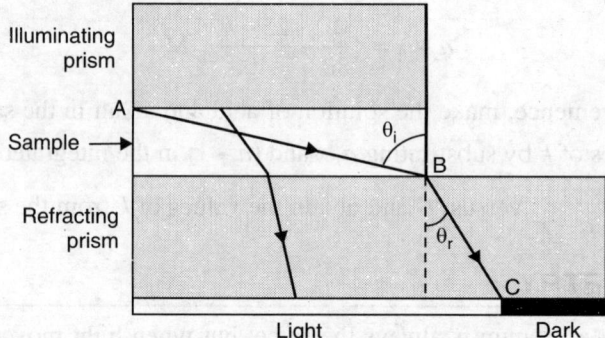

Fig. 17.10: Cross section of part of the optical path of Abbe refractometer

index of the sample quite accurately. Nearly all refractometers utilize the principle, but may differ in their optical design.

How to determine refractive index

Abbe refractometer is commonly used to measure refractive index.

In Abbe refractometer, the liquid sample is sandwiched into a thin layer between an illuminating prism and a refracting prism (Fig. 17.10). The refracting prism is made of a glass with a high refractive index (e.g. 1.75) and the refractometer is designed to be used with samples having a refractive index smaller than that of the refracting prism. A light source is projected through the illuminating prism, the bottom surface of which is ground (i.e. roughened like a ground-glass joint), so each point on this surface can be thought of as generating light rays travelling in all directions. Inspection of Fig. 17.10 shows that light travelling from point A to point B will have the largest angle of incidence (θ_i) and hence the largest possible angle of refraction (θ_r) for that sample. All other rays of light entering the refracting prism will have smaller θ_r and hence lie to the left of point C. Thus, a detector placed on the back side of the refracting prism would show a light region to the left and a dark region to the right. The scale at this point, shows a refractive index of the liquid.

Sample with different refractive indexes will produce different angles of refraction (see Eq. 17.36 above and recall that the angle of incidence and the refractive index of the prism are fixed) and this will be reflected in a change in the position of the borderline between the light and dark regions. By appropriately calibrating the scale, the position of the borderline can be used to determine the refractive index of any sample. In an actual Abbe refractometer, there is not a detector on the back of the refracting prism, and there are additional optics, but this is essential principle.

In most liquids and solids the speed of light, and hence the index of refraction, varies significantly with wavelength. (This variation is referred to as **dispersion**, and it is what cause white light moving through a prism to be refracted into a rainbow. Shorter wavelengths are normally refracted more than longer ones.) Thus, for the most accurate measurements it is necessary to use monochromatic light. The most widely used wavelength of light for refractometry is the sodium D line at 589 nm.

As mentioned earlier, the speed of light in a substance is slower than in a vacuum since the light is being absorbed and reemitted by the atoms in the sample. Since the density of a liquid usually decreases with temperature, it is not surprising that the speed of light in a liquid will normally increase as the temperature increases. Thus, **the index of refraction normally decreases as the temperature increases** for a liquid. For many organic liquids the index of refraction decreased by approximately 0.0005 for every 1°C increase in temperature. However, for water the variation is only about –0.0001/°C.

Many refractometers are equipped with a thermometer and a mean of circulating water through the refractometer to maintain a given temperature. Most of the refractive index measurements reported in the literature are determined at 20 or 25°C.

Specific Refraction, R

According to Lorenz and Lorenz, refractive index is related to specific refractive index, R, by an expression:

$$R = \frac{1}{d}\left[\frac{n^2 - 1}{n^2 + 2}\right] \qquad \ldots (17.38)$$

where R = specific refractivity of medium; d = density of medium; n = refractive index of medium

Molar refraction, R_m: Molar refraction is the product of specific refraction and molecular weight.

Significance

The refractive index is commonly determined as part of the characterization of liquid samples, in much the same way that melting points are routinely obtained to characterize solid compounds. It is also commonly used to:

- Help identify or confirm the identity of a sample by comparing its refractive index to known values.
- Assess the purity of a sample by comparing its refractive index to the value for the pure substance.
- Determine the concentration of a solute in a solution by comparing the solution's refractive index to a standard curve.

17.16. Determine the refractive index of a given liquid and find its specific and molar refraction

Procedure

(i) Remove both the prisms A and B (Fig. 17.10) from the refractometer, clean them gently with cotton moistened with alcohol.

(ii) Place 1–2 drops of the sample liquid on B and press both and clamp them back in the instrument.

(iii) Adjust the light lamp in such a way that light reflected by mirror of the instrument and travels toward prism.

(iv) Now view through the telescope to see the equal light and dark region.

(v) The reading on the scale shows the refractive index of the liquid.

Observation

Temperature: ...... °C

(i) Refractive index of liquid

(a) ....

(b) ....   Mean value (n) = ...

(c) ....

(ii) Density of sample liquid (d) $= \dfrac{W_3 - W_1}{W_2 - W_1} \times$ density of water

W_1 = weight of empty pyknometer
W_2 = weight of pyknometer and water
W_3 = weight of pyknometer and sample liquid

(iii) Molecular weight of sample liquid = M

(iv) Specific refraction, $R = \dfrac{1}{d}\left[\dfrac{n^2 - 1}{n^2 + 2}\right]$

(v) R_m = Mol. wt × R.

18
Chapter

Instrumental Spectroscopical Analysis

COLORIMETRIC ANALYSIS

Colorimetric analysis is a method of determining the concentration of a chemical element or chemical compound in a solution with the aid of a colour developing reagent. It is applicable to both organic compounds and inorganic compounds and may be used with or without an enzymatic stage. The method is widely used in medical laboratories for qualitative and quantitative purposes.

Experiment 18.1: Estimation of reducing sugar by dinitrosalicylic method (colorimetric analysis)

This method tests for the presence of free carbonyl group (C=O), the so-called reducing sugars, e.g. dextrose. This involves the oxidation of the aldehyde functional group present in, e.g. glucose and the ketone functional group in fructose. Simultaneously, 3,5-dinitrosalicylic acid (DNS) is reduced to 3-amino-5-nitrosalicylic acid under alkaline conditions. This strongly absorbs light at 540 nm.

$$\text{Aldehyde or keto group} \xrightarrow{\text{Oxidation}} \text{Carboxyl group}$$

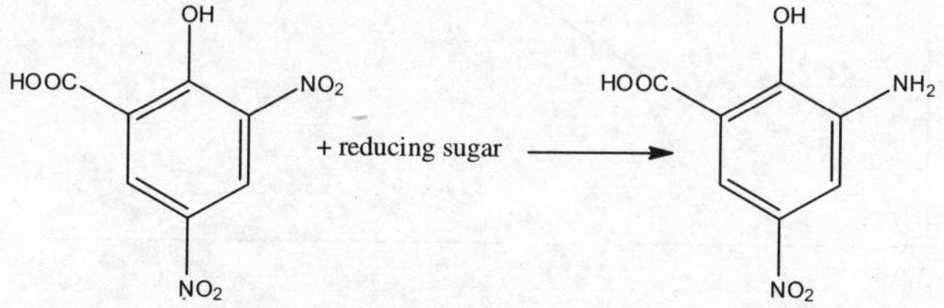

Because dissolved oxygen can interfere with glucose oxidation, sulphite, which itself is not necessary for the colour reaction, is added in the reagent to absorb the dissolved oxygen.

The above reaction shows that one mole of sugar will react with one mole of 3,5-dinitrosalicylic acid. However, it is suspected that there are many side reactions, and the actual reaction stoichiometry is more complicated than that previously described. The type of side reaction depends on the exact nature of the reducing sugars. Different reducing sugars generally yield different colour intensities; thus, it is necessary to calibrate for each sugar. In addition to the oxidation of the carbonyl groups in the sugar, other side reactions such as the decomposition of sugar also competes for the availability of 3,5-dinitrosalicylic acid.

Although this is a convenient and relatively inexpensive method, due to the relatively low specificity, one must run blanks diligently, if the colorimetric results are to be interpreted correctly and accurately.

Requirements

- Dinitrosalicylic acid reagent solution, 1%
- Potassium sodium tartrate solution, 40%

Procedure

1. Standard stock solution of glucose: Dissolve 100 mg of glucose in 100 ml of distilled water to prepare standard **stock solution**. Diluting 10 ml of stock solution to 100 ml with distilled water to prepare working **standard solution**.
2. Preparation of dinitrosalicylic acid (DNS) reagent: Dissolve one gram of dinitrosalicylic acid, 200 mg of crystalline phenol, and 50 mg of sodium sulphite simultaneously in 100 ml of 1% NaOH solution by stirring.
3. Preparation of standard curve: Standard curve was prepared by taking 0, 0.2, 0.4, 0.6, 0.8 and 1 ml of the working standard glucose solution and the volume was made up to 3 ml by adding distilled water. Add 3 ml of DNS reagent and heat the mixture for 5–10 minutes in a boiling water bath. After the development of the red-brown colour, add 1 ml of 40% Rochelle salt solution (in warm condition) to stabilize the colour and mix thoroughly. After cooling the tubes, the record the absorbance was recorded at a wavelength of 540 nm. Spectrophotometer. The standard curve so formed is shown in Fig. 18.1.
4. Plot the standard curve and calculate the amount in the sample from standard curve and calculate the contents.

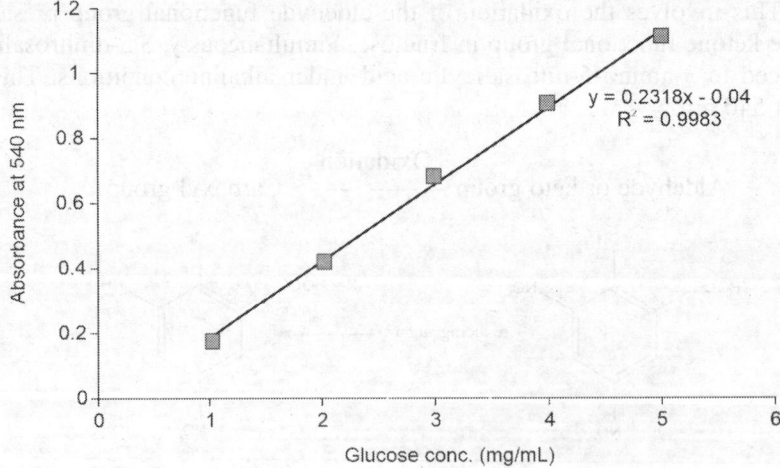

$$y = 0.2318x - 0.04$$
$$R^2 = 0.9983$$

Fig. 18.1: Standard curve of DNS colorimetric method

Experiment 18.2: Colorimetric method for estimation of sulphacetamide

Principle

This colorimetric method is based on diazotization of sulphacetamide by sodium nitrite in acidic medium followed by coupling with Bratton-Marshall reagent (N-(1-naphthyl) ethylene diamine dihydrochloride solution) to form the red colour. The absorbance is determined at its λ_{max}, 530 nm.*

---

* IJAPA, 3 (2), (2013), 30–36.

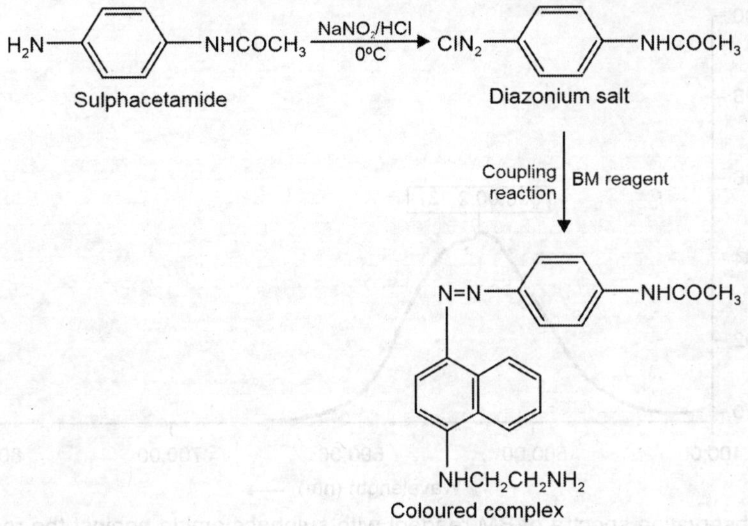

Sulphacetamide → Diazonium salt (NaNO₂/HCl, 0°C) → Coloured complex (Coupling reaction, BM reagent)

Preparation of reagents

1. Sodium nitrite solution (0.1%w/v): Dissolve 100 mg of sodium nitrite in distilled water and make up to 100 ml.
2. Hydrochloric acid (5N): Dilute 425 ml of concentrated HCl solution to 1000 ml with distilled water.
3. Ammonium sulphamate solution (0.1%w/v): Dissolve 500 mg of ammonium sulphamate in distilled water and make up to 100 ml with distilled water.
4. BM reagent (N-(1-naphthyl) ethylene diamine dihydrochloride solution) (0.1%w/v): Dissolve 100 mg of BM reagent in 100 ml of distilled water.
5. Sodium hydroxide solution (0.1N): Dissolve 400 mg sodium hydroxide in distilled water and make up to 100 ml with distilled water.

Preparation of standard solutions

Dissolve 100 mg of sulphacetamide in 100 ml of distilled water (stock solution I). Prepare 100 µg/ml working standard solution from the stock solution.

Procedure

1. Take 0, 0.1, 0.2, 0.4, 0.6, 0.8 and 1.0 ml working standard solution in 10 ml volumetric flask, cool down below 10°C temperature.
2. Add 1 ml of cold 5N concentrated HCl and 1 ml of 0.1% w/v sodium nitrite and shake for 5 minutes while maintaining the low temperature.
3. To this, add 1 ml of 0.5% w/v ammonium sulphamate followed by the addition of 1 ml of BM reagent (Scheme 1).
4. Make up the volume to 10 ml with distilled water.
5. Measure the absorbance of red colour at 530 nm against the reagent blank (Fig. 18.2).
6. Plot a calibration curve. The linearity range from 1 to 3 µg/ml (Fig. 18.3).
7. Similarly, adopt the same method to develop the colour and measure the absorbance of the unknown/sample solution.
8. Calculate the amount from the calibration graph.

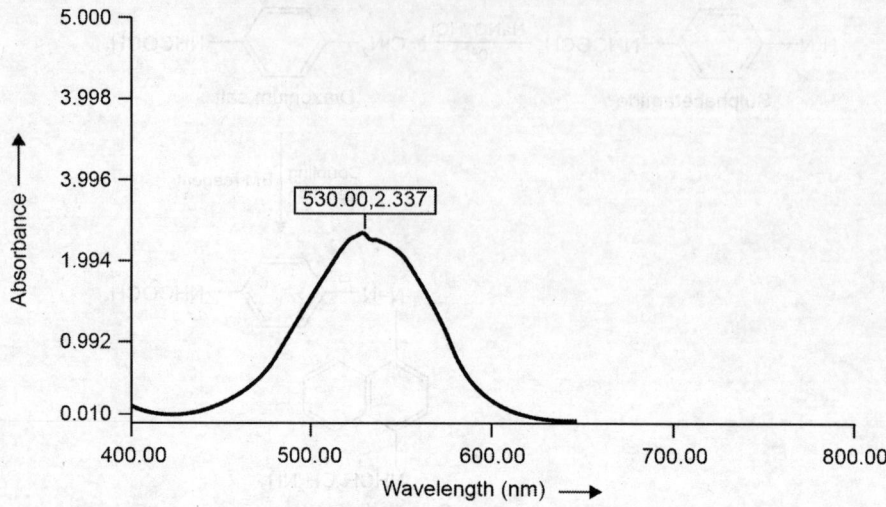

Fig. 18.2: Observation spectra of BM reagent with sulphacetamide against the reagent blank

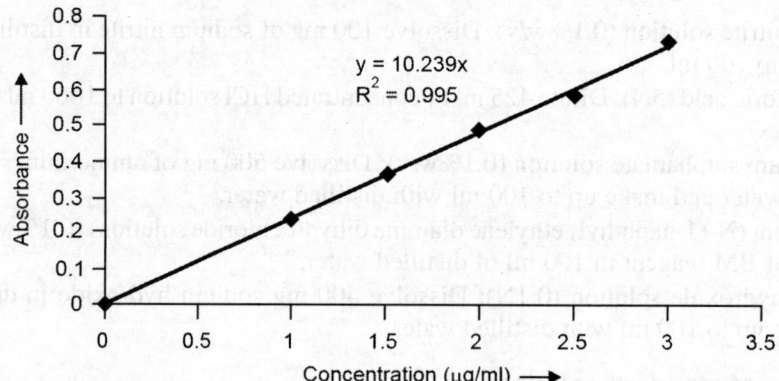

Fig. 18.3: Calibration graph of sulphacetamide by BM reagent

Experiment 18.3: Analysis of the effect of solvent on absorption maxima of drug

Introduction

Chromophores give rise to "characteristic" absorbance bands. Changes in their environment affect their energy levels which then affect the wavelength and the intensity of absorbance. There are many solvents but water, 95% ethanol and hexane are the most commonly used solvents in UV spectroscopy. Each is transparent in the region of UV-Vis spectrum. For preparing stock solutions, the sample is accurately weighed and made up to volume in volumetric flask. Aliquats are removed from this solution and appropriate dilutions are made to make solutions of desired concentration. For recording the spectrum 1 cm square quartz cell is commonly used. These require approx. 3 ml of solution. The quartz cell containing solution is placed in the path of light beam and spectrum is recorded by varying the wavelength of incident light.

Solvent effects

Highly pure, non-polar solvents such as saturated hydrocarbons do not interact with solute molecules either in the ground or excited state and the absorption spectrum of a compound in these solvents is similar to the one in a pure gaseous state. However, polar solvents, such as water, alcohols, etc. may stabilize or destabilize the molecular orbitals of a molecule either in the ground state or in excited state and the spectrum of a compound in these solvents may significantly vary from the one recorded in a hydrocarbon solvent.

1. $\pi\rightarrow\pi^*$ transitions: In case of $\pi\rightarrow\pi^*$ transitions, the excited states are more polar than the ground state and the dipole-dipole interactions with solvent molecules lower the energy of the excited state more than that of the ground state. Therefore, a polar solvent decreases the energy of $\pi\rightarrow\pi^*$ transition and absorption maximum appears ~10–20 nm red shifted in going from hexane to ethanol solvent.

2. $n\rightarrow\pi^*$ Transitions: In case of $n\rightarrow\pi^*$ transitions, the polar solvents form hydrogen bonds with the ground state of polar molecules more readily than with their excited states. Therefore, in polar solvents, the energies of electronic transitions are increased. For example, Fig. 18.4 shows that the absorption maximum of acetone in hexane appears at 279 nm which in water is shifted to 264 nm, with a blue shift of 15 nm.

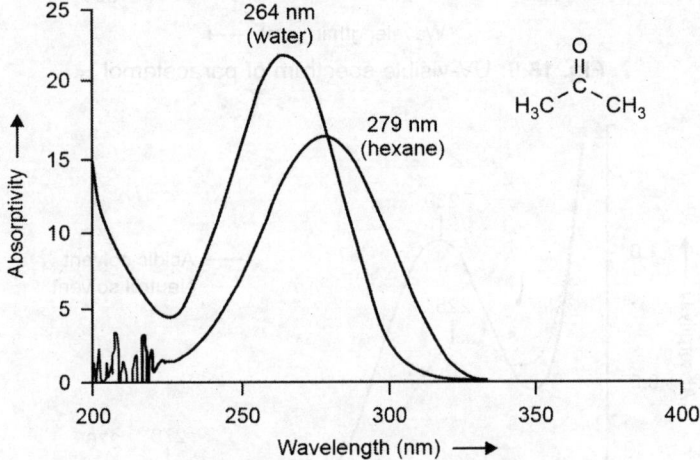

Fig. 18.4: UV spectra of acetone in hexane and in water

Procedure

1. Prepare five solutions of about 25 mg of paracetamol or aspirin or other available drugs in 25 ml of the given solvents.
   - n-Hexane
   - Chloroform
   - Ethanol
   - 1% HCl solution
   - 1% NaOH solution
2. Take the UV absorbance spectrum and observe the λ_{max}.

Note: The UV spectrum of paracetamol and aspirin are given for reference (Figs 18.5 and 18.6, respectively).

Experiment 18.4: Determination of paracetamol content in tablet

Paracetamol is a widely used over-the-counter analgesic (pain reliever) and antipyretic (fever reducer). It is commonly used for the relief of fever, headaches, and other minor aches and pains, and is a major ingredient in numerous cold and flu remedies.

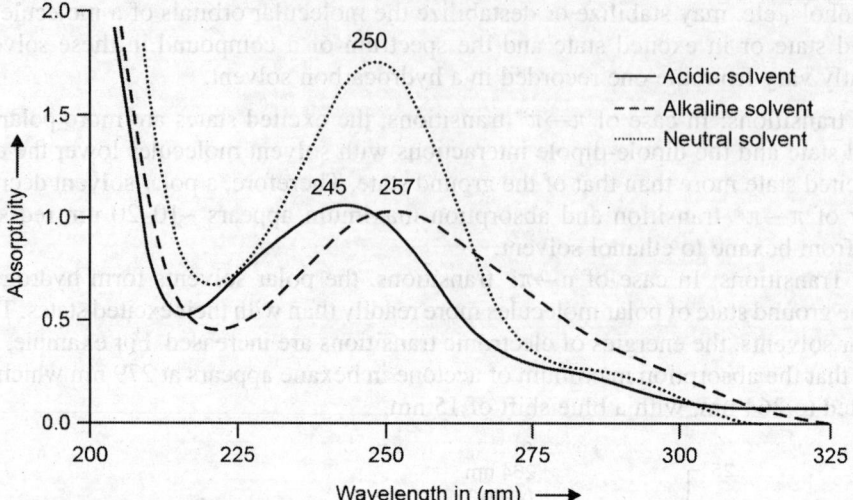

Fig. 18.5: UV-visible spectrum of paracetamol

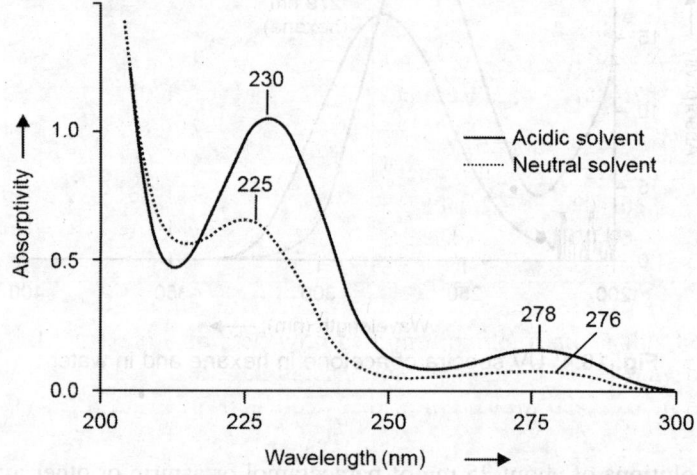

Fig. 18.6: UV-visible spectrum of aspirin

It shows three λ max at 242, 243 and 257 nm in neutral, acidic and alkaline media respectively. The present experiment is a estimation of paracetamol in alkaline media. Paracetamol shows maximum absorption at 257 nm due to presence of phenyl ring in alkaline media. The absorbance of different dilution of paracetamol is taken at this wavelength to make the calibration curve. The absorbance of unknown sample is taken and with the help of calibration curve, the concentration is read out.

NHCOCH₃ ... + NaOH ⟶ ... + H₂O

OH ... ONa

Paracetamol ... Sodium salt of paracetamol

Reagents required

1. Paracetamol reference substance.
2. NaOH.

Procedure

(i) Accurately weigh 100 mg of paracetamol reference substance into a 100 ml volumetric flask, dissolve with 50 ml of 0.1 M NaOH solution. Dilute to volume with water and mix well.

(ii) Separately transfer accurately 0.1, 0.2 .... to 1 ml of this solution into 10 different 10 ml volumetric flask and dilute with 0.1 M NaOH solution to the mark. The concentration range is 0.32~1.92 mg/ml.

(iii) Measure the absorbance of the each solution at 257 nm.

(iv) Weigh accurately and powder finely 10 tablets, weigh accurately a portion of the powder (equivalent to about 100 mg of paracetamol) into 100 ml volumetric flask, add 50 ml of 0.1 M NaOH solution, mix for 15 minutes.

(v) Filter if necessary. Make up the volume with 0.1 M NaOH solution.

(vi) Transfer 0.5 ml of this solution and dilute to 10 ml in volumetric flask.

Observation and calculation

Absorbance value of paracetamol		
	Concentration	**Absorbance**
1.	–	
2.	–	
3.	–	
4.	–	
5.	–	
6.	–	
Unknown	–	

Plot a calibration curve by plotting a graph between absorbance of different standard dilution and their concentration. Read out a concentration of unknown from calibration curve. Multiply the concentration with dilution factor to find out the initial concentration.

Note: Calculation can also be done by considering specific absorbance of paracetamol, 715 as specified in IP.

$$A = a.b.c$$

$$C = \frac{\text{Absorbance of unknown}}{715}$$

Experiment 18.5: UV spectrophotometric methods for simultaneous estimation of ibuprofen and paracetamol in tablet by simultaneous equation method

The ibuprofen [RS-2-(4-isobutyl-phenyl) propionic acid], is one of the most potent orally active antipyretic, analgesic and nonsteroidal anti-inflammatory drug (NSAID) used extensively in the treatment of acute and chronic pain, osteoarthritis, rheumatoid arthritis and related conditions. This compound is characterized by a better tolerability compared with other NSAIDs.

Ibuprofen   Paracetamol

Paracetamol is 4′-hydroxyacetanilide. It is antipyretic and analgesic.

Procedure

Procedure for calibration curve

1. Weigh accurately 10 mg of ibuprofen standard solutions and dissolve in water and make up the volume to 100 ml in volumetric flask (100 mg/ml). It will be a stock solution.
2. Prepare the different dilutions of ibuprofen in the concentration range of 4–14 µg/ml obtained by transferring (0.4, 0.6, 0.8, 1.0, 1.2, 1.4 ml) of ibuprofen stock solution (100 µg/ml) to the series of 10 ml volumetric flasks.
3. Similarly, prepare the stock solution of paracetamol and different dilution of standard solutions of paracetamol in the concentration range of 2–12 µg/ml by transferring (0.2, 0.4, 0.6, 0.8, 1.0, 1.2 ml) of paracetamol stock solution (100 µg/ml) to the series of 10 ml volumetric flasks.
4. Add methanol to each volumetric flask up to 10 ml.
5. Scan all dilutions in wavelength range of 200–400 nm. The absorbances were plotted against the respective concentrations to obtain the calibration curves (Figs 18.7 and 18.8).
6. A representative overlain spectrum of ibuprofen and paracetamol in methanol is shown in Fig. 18.9.

Formation of simultaneous equation

Set of two simultaneous equations were:

$Cx = (A_2 ay_1 - A_1 ay_2)/(ax_2 ay_1 - ax_1 ay_2)$ and

$Cy = (A_1 ax_2 - A_2 ax_1)/(ax_2 ay_1 - ax_1 ay_2)$,

where A_1 and A_2 are the absorbance of sample solutions at 224.0 nm and 248.0 nm, respectively.

C_x and C_y are concentrations of ibuprofen and paracetamol in mg/ml in sample solution.

By substituting the values of A_1 and A_2 the values of C_x and C_y can be calculated by solving the two equations simultaneously.

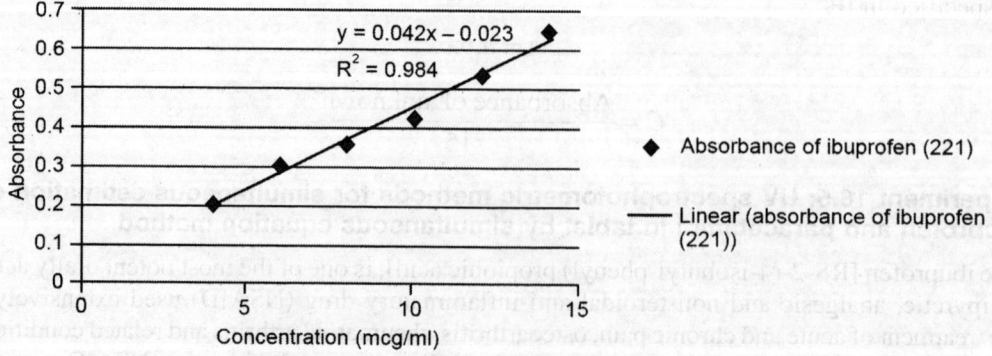

Fig. 18.7: Calibration curve of ibuprofen

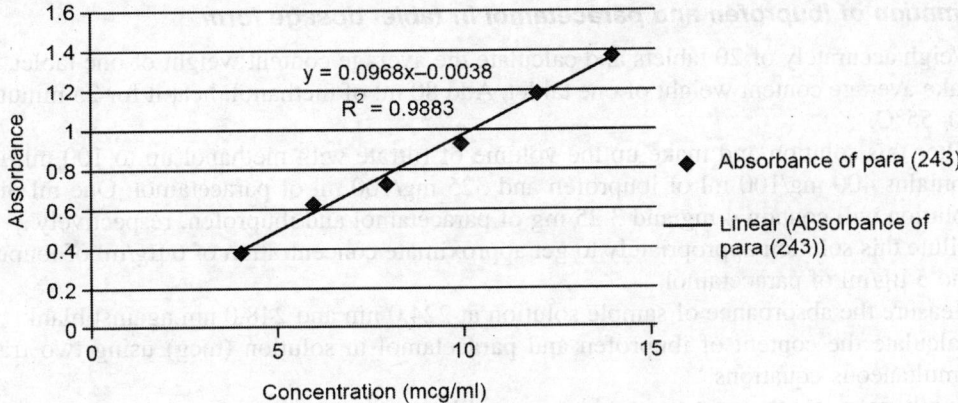

Fig. 18.8: Calibration curve of paracetamol

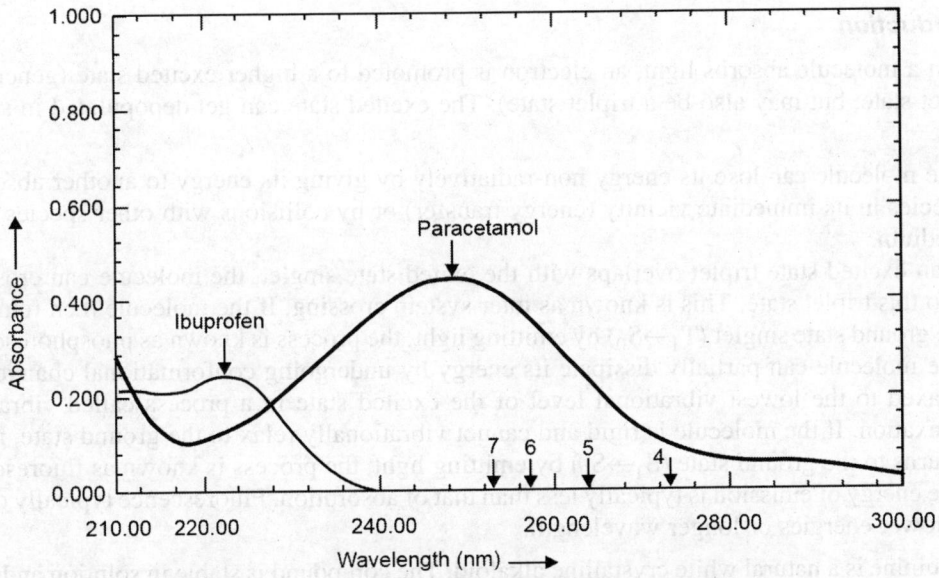

Fig. 18.9: Overlay spectra of ibuprofen and paracetamol

Here, ax_1 and ax_2 are the absorptivity coefficient of ibuprofen at 224.0 nm and 248.0 nm, respectively; ay_1 and ay_2 are the absorptivity coefficient of paracetamol at 224.0 nm and 248.0 nm, respectively.

To get absorptivity divide the absorbance by path length and concentration.

$$\varepsilon = A/lc$$

where A is the amount of light absorbed by the sample for a given wavelength, ε is the molar absorptivity, l is the distance that the light travels through the solution, and c is the concentration of the absorbing species per unit volume.

The standard units for molar absorptivity are liters per mole centimeter (L mol^{-1} cm^{-1}).

The linearity range for ibuprofen and paracetamol were 4–14 μg/ml and 2–12 μg/ml, respectively.

Estimation of ibuprofen and paracetamol in tablet dosage form

1. Weigh accurately of 20 tablets and calculate the average content weight of one tablet.
2. Take average content weight of one tablet. Add 80 ml of methanol; heat it for 25 minutes at 50–55°C.
3. Filter this solution and make up the volume of filtrate with methanol up to 100 ml, i.e. it contains 400 mg/100 ml of ibuprofen and 325 mg/100 ml of paracetamol. One ml of this solution will contain 4 mg and 3.25 mg of paracetamol and ibuprofen, respectively.
4. Dilute this solution appropriately to get approximate concentration of 6 µg/ml of ibuprofen and 5 µg/ml of paracetamol.
5. Measure the absorbance of sample solution at 224.0 nm and 248.0 nm against blank.
6. Calculate the content of ibuprofen and paracetamol in solution (mcg) using two framed simultaneous equations.
7. Finally calculate the content in tablet using dilution factor.

Experiment 18.6: Analysis of the quenching effect of iodide salt on fluorescence intensity of quinine sulphate

Introduction

When a molecule absorbs light, an electron is promoted to a higher excited state (generally a singlet state, but may also be a triplet state). The excited state can get depopulated in several ways.

- The molecule can lose its energy non-radiatively by giving its energy to another absorbing species in its immediate vicinity (energy transfer) or by collisions with other species in the medium.
- If an excited state triplet overlaps with the exited state singlet, the molecule can crossover into this triplet state. This is known as inter system crossing. If the molecule then returns to the ground state singlet ($T_1 \rightarrow S_0$) by emitting light, the process is known as phosphorescence.
- The molecule can partially dissipate its energy by undergoing conformational changes and relaxed to the lowest vibrational level of the excited state in a process called vibrational relaxation. If the molecule is rigid and cannot vibrationally relax to the ground state, it then returns to the ground state ($S_1 \rightarrow S_0$) by emitting light, the process is known as fluorescence.
- The energy of emission is typically less than that of absorption. Fluorescence typically occurs at lower energies or longer wavelength.

Quinine is a natural white crystalline alkaloid. The compound is stable in solution and emits blue light when it is excited in the near UV. It has antipyretic, antimalarial, analgesic properties and a bitter taste and has been used for over three centuries.

Quinine

It is a highly fluorescent and organic molecule that has been widely used as a fluorescence quantum yield standard. The fluorescence and absorption spectra of quinine are shown in Fig. 18.10. The observed fluorescence emission maximum is 437 nm. Addition of halide ions and other ions such as MnO_4^-, SO_4^{2-} and ClO_3^- can decrease the intensity of emission spectra due to quenching* without any effect on the position of emission maxima (Fig. 18.11). Also, the shape and full-width at half maximum (FWHM) of the absorption and emission bands remain unchanged. Hence, it may be considered that the process of quenching is dynamic in nature and a diffusion controlled bimolecular process is responsible for the observed quenching. This ruled out the possibility of a chemical reaction between anions and quinine. The study has revealed the order of two groups of quencher: NaI > NaBr > NaCl > NaF and $K_2Cr_2O_7$ > $KMnO_4$ > Na_2SO_4 > $NaClO_3$. Increasing anion size in the both groups leads to an increase in the quenching due to deactivation processes.

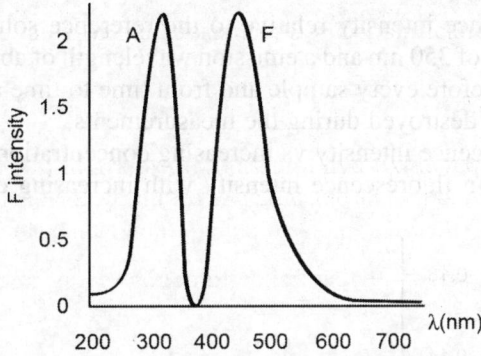

Fig. 18.10: The fluorescence (F) and absorbance (A) spectrum of quinine

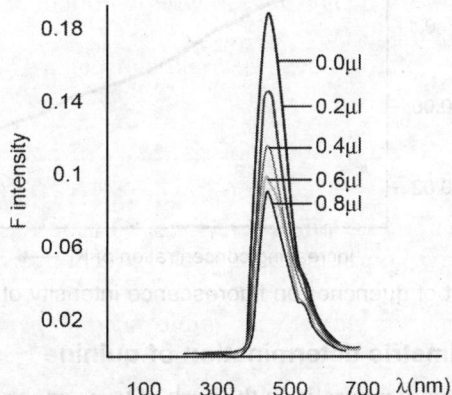

Fig. 18.11: The changing fluorescence emission spectra of quinine sulphate in aqueous solution with increasing addition of KI solution

Preparation of reagents

• Standard quinine sulphate solution: Dissolve 100 mg of quinine sulphate in 100 ml of 0.1N or 0.05M H_2SO_4 solution. Now take 10 ml of this solution and dilute to 1000 ml with 0.1N H_2SO_4 solution. This will be the working standard.

• KI solution: Dissolve 200 mg of KI in 100 ml of distilled water. This will give the concentration of 2 mg or 2,000 microgram/ml. Dilute 1 ml of this solution to 100 ml with distilled water to get concentration of 20 microgram/ml. Now finally dilute this concentration to 100 ml to get the working standard (0.2 microgram/ml).

---

* Quenching refers to any process which decreases the fluorescence intensity of a given substance. A variety of processes can result in quenching, such as excited state reactions, energy transfer, complex-formation and collisional quenching.

Procedure

1. Prepare the following dilution in 10 ml volumetric flask as shown in the table given below.

Flask No.	1	2	3	4	5	6
Working standard of quinine sulphate (ml)	5	5	5	5	5	5
KI solution (ml)	0	1	2	3	4	5
0.1N or 0.05M H_2SO_4 solution (ml)	5	4	3	2	1	0

2. Measure the fluorescence intensity relative to the reference solution (no quencher) at an irradiation wavelength of 350 nm and a emission wavelength of about 450 nm. The reference solution is measured before every sample and from time to time a new reference sample is made, since quinine is destroyed during the measurements.
3. Plot a graph of fluorescence intensity vs increasing concentration of KI.
4. Observe the decrease in fluorescence intensity with increasing concentration of quencher (Fig. 18.12).

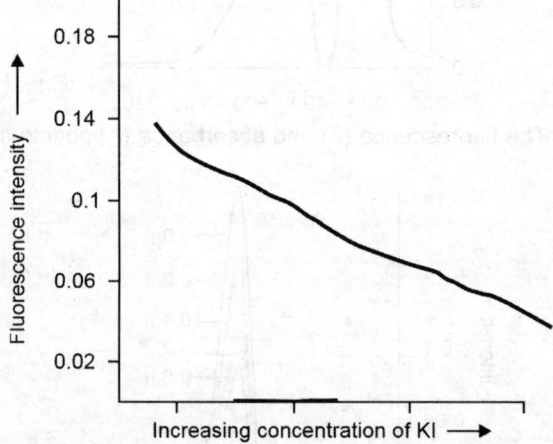

Fig. 18.12: Effect of quencher on fluorescence intensity of quinine sulphate

Experiment 18.7: Fluorimetric determination of quinine

Quinine is an alkaloid occurring naturally in the bark of trees or shrubs of the various species of two Rubiaceous genera. It is used as antimalarial drug.

Experimental overview

Quinine shows the fluorescence which is the basis of its estimation. Molecular fluorescence occurs when a compound absorbs radiation, causing electrons to be promoted to excited states. As these excited states relax back to the ground state, light is emitted at wavelengths characteristic of the energy differences between the ground and excited states. At low concentrations the intensity of the fluorescence is proportional to concentration.

However, a variety of conditions adversely affect the linear relationship:
- Self quenching.
- External quenching.
- Decreased quantum efficiency.

At high concentrations, however, the compound will absorb some of the fluoresced light, resulting in a non-linear dependence of the fluorescence intensity on the concentration.

Quinine

Reagents required

1. Quinine sulphate.
2. Sulphuric acid.

Procedure

1. **Preparation of standard quinine sulphate solution:** Weigh accurately 10 mg of quinine sulphate, dissolve in sufficient quantity of 0.5 M H_2SO_4 solution and make up the volume to litre in volumetric flask.
2. Pipet out 0.1, 0.2, 0.3, 0.4, 0.5 to 1.0 ml from the above stock solution in 10 ml volumetric flask and make up the volume with 0 M H_2SO_4 solution.
3. **Preparation of test sample:** Dissolve about 10 mg of the sample and dissolve in sufficient quantity of 0.5M H_2SO_4 solution and make up the volume to litre in volumetric flask. Pipet out 0.4 ml from this solution in 10 ml volumetric flask and make up the volume with 0 M H_2SO_4 solution.
4. Follow the general direction by the teacher for the use of spectrofluorometer.
   Set the excitation wavelength to 350 nm and emission wavelength to 450 nm in the spectrofluorometer. Record the fluorescence intensity of all the ten standard solution by using sulphuric acid as blank solution.
5. Similarly, record the fluorescence intensity of sample solution (Table 18.1).
6. Plot a calibration curve by plotting a graph between the concentration and emission intensity. Read out the concentration of unknown solution from the calibration curve. Multiply with dilution factor to get the concentration in the sample.

Table 18.1: Fluorescence intensity of quinine sulfate solution

	Concentration (mg)	Fluorescence intensity
1.	0.1	–
2.	0.2	–
3.	0.3	–
4.	0.4	–
5.	0.5	–
6.	0.6	–
7.	0.7	–
8.	0.8	–
9.	0.9	–
10.	1.0	–
11.	Unknown	–

Experiment 18.8: Determination of sodium and potassium ion concentrations in solution

Experimental overview

Flame photometry is a relatively old instrumental analysis method. Its origins date back to Bunsen's flame-color tests for the qualitative identification of select metallic elements. As an analytical method, atomic emission is a fast, simple, and sensitive method for the determination of trace metal ions in solution. Because of the very narrow (0.01 nm) and characteristic emission lines from the gas-phase atoms in the flame plasma, the method is relatively free of interferences from other elements.

The method is suitable for many metallic elements, especially for those metals that are easily excited to higher energy levels at the relatively cool temperatures of some flames—Li, Na, K, Rb, Cs, Ca, Cu, Sr, and Ba. Metalloids and nonmetals generally do not produce isolated neutral atoms in a flame, but mostly as polyatomic radicals and ions. Therefore, nonmetallic elements are not suitable for determination by flame emission spectroscopy, except for a very few and under very specialized conditions.

Reagents required

Standard sodium stock solution, 100.0 ppm

1. Accurately weigh out by difference 0.1271 g of reagent grade NaCl into a small weighing bottle. It is very difficult and time consuming to weigh out exactly this amount. Get it as close as you reasonably can, record the exact mass, and correct your concentrations accordingly.

   Note: Mol. weight of NaCl = 58.5

         58.5 g NaCl/litre = 1000 ppm of NaCl

         58.5/23 g NaCl/litre = 1000 ppm for Na

         0.1271 g of NaCl/500 ml = 100 ppm of Na

2. Carefully transfer the salt quantitatively into a 500 ml volumetric flask. Use a few squirts of deionized water from your wash bottle on the weighing bottle and the sides of the flask to wash all of it down into the flask.

3. Add about 100 ml of deionized water to the flask, swirl several times, and dissolve all of the salt before diluting to volume with deionized water. This is critical.

Standard potassium stock solution, 100.0 ppm

Similarly make the stock solution for potassium (atomic weight of K = 39 and Cl = 33.5).

Unknown solution

Obtain the unknown sample and carefully dilute to 100 ml mark with deionized water.

Procedure

Preparation of standard calibration solution: Pipet 10.00, 20.00, 30.00, 40.00, 50.00, 60.0, 70.0, 80.0, 90.0 ml of the standard 100 ppm sodium solution into different volumetric flasks. This will give the concentration range of 10 to 90 ppm respectively. Dilute carefully to the mark with deionized water and mix thoroughly.

Instructions for use of the flame photometer

1. Ensure that the photometer drain is leading into a sink and that the instrument is connected to gas, air and electricity supplies. Ensure the mains supply gas tap is off.

2. Turn the "sensitivity" and instrument "gas" controls fully counterclockwise.
3. Insert the sodium optical filter (589 nm).
4. Switch on the instrument and unclamp the galvanometer by turning counterclockwise.
5. Open the mica window, turn on the mains gas supply, light the gas and close the window.
6. Turn on the air supply control and adjust the air pressure to 10 lb/in^2. Leave for 1–2 minutes to stabilize.
7. Place a beaker of distilled water into position at the left hand side of the instrument and insert the narrow draw tube into it to allow water to pass through the photometer.
   Note: Once set up, the photometer must have water running through it at all times when a salt solution is not being measured. The rate of uptake is fast, so make sure there is always enough water in the beaker.
8. Adjust the gas control to give a flame with a large central blue cone then, with water passing through the instrument, slowly close the gas control until ten separate blue cones just form.
9. Set the galvanometer to zero using the "set zero" control.
10. Replace the distilled water with the NaCl solution (100 ppm standard) and adjust the "sensitivity" control till the galvanometer reads 100.
11. Quickly but carefully, replace the NaCl standard with standards of decreasing concentration and note the readings in the Table below.
12. Run water through the instrument again for 1–2 minutes, then place the draw tube into a beaker containing the unknown sachet solution and note the galvanometer reading.
13. Run water through the instrument again and replace the sodium with the potassium filter (766 nm).
14. Repeat the above procedure with the KCl standards, setting to 100 with most concentrated KCl standard, then reading the others in reverse order. Then, read the unknown solution.
15. Finally, run water through the instrument until the flame appears free of color again.
16. When the instrument is no longer required, switch off in the following sequence:
   (i) Turn off the gas control and the mains gas supply
   (ii) Wait for the flame to die out.
   (iii) Turn off the air supply.
   (iv) Switch off the electricity
   (v) Clamp the galvanometer.

Observation and calculation

Galvano reading			
Conc. of sodium (ppm)	Emission intensity	Conc. of potassium (ppm)	Emission intensity
1. 10	–	10	–
2. 20	–	20	–
3. 30	–	30	–
4. 40	–	40	–
5. 50	–	50	–
6. 60	–	60	–
7. 70	–	70	–
8. 80	–	80	–
9. 90	–	90	–
10. 100	–	100	–
11. Unknown	–	Unknown	–

Plot a calibration curve by plotting the emission intensities as a function of Na concentration and potassium concentration separately. Determine the concentration of sodium and potassium unknown sample from the calibration curve.

Multiply with the dilution factor to get the concentration in original solution.

Result

The given solution contains sodium .... ppm and potassium .... ppm.

Experiment 18.9: Determination of sulphate by nephelometric titration

When electromagnetic radiation (light) strikes a particle in solution, some of the light will be
- Absorbed by the particle
- Transmitted through the solution
- Scattered or reflected

The amount of light scattered is proportional to the concentration of the insoluble particle. In turbidimetry, the intensity of the light transmitted though the medium, the unscattered light is measured. Turbidimetric measurements are made at 180° from the incident light beam. In nephelometry, the intensity of scattered light is measured, at the right angles to the light beam. The turbidimetry standard unit is called nephelometric turbidimetric unit (NTU).

Principle

In this experiment, unknown sample of sulphate ion is analyzed with turbidimetry. An excess of barium chloride is added to an acidified sample. The barium chloride combines with sulphate in the sample to yield suspension of barium sulphate. This method is much faster and sensitive as compared to the gravimetric method.

$$SO_4^{2-} + BaCl_2 \rightarrow BaSO_4\downarrow + 2Cl^-$$

In highly acidic medium, only common ion which form precipitate with sulphate is only barium. Glycerol-alcohol solution is added to stabilize the precipitate. Sodium chloride–HCl is added before the addition of barium chloride. This is to inhibit the growth of microcrystals of barium sulphate.

Preparation of reagents

1. **Standard sulphate solution:** Dry the potassium sulphate in a 110°C oven for at least 1 hour. Allow the salt to cool to room temperature. Weigh 0.18 g of the cooled salt to the nearest 0.1 mg, and transfer it to a 1 litre volumetric flask. Dissolve the salt in deionized water and dilute the solution to the mark. The stock solution prepared in this step contains 100 mg/L sulphate or 100 ppm of sulphate ion.
2. **NaCl–HCl reagent:** Dissolve 12 g of NaCl in 40 ml distilled water, add 1 ml of concentrated HCl solution and the then dilute to 50 ml with distilled water.
3. **Glycerol–alcohol solution:** Prepare a mixture of 25 ml glycerol and 50 ml of ethanol.
4. **Barium chloride.**

Procedure

1. Prepare a solution in 25 ml volumetric flask as given in the following Table.
2. Add 0.2 g BaCl₂ solution to each flask, shake for 1 minute to dissolve barium chloride completely.
3. Allow the each flask to stand 2–3 minute and measure the turbidity against the reagent blank.
4. Plot a calibration curve.
5. Determine the sulphate of sample solution from the calibration curve.

	Conc. (ppm)	Volume (ml) taken from stock solution (100 ppm)	$V_{NaCl, HCl}$	$V_{Glycerol, alc}$	Volume of water to make 25 ml $V_{vol\ flask\ (ml)}$
Blank	0	0	2.5	5	17.5
1.	10	2.5	2.5	5	15
2.	15	3.75	2.5	5	13.75
3.	20	5.00	2.5	5	12.5
4.	25	6.25	2.5	5	11.25
5.	30	7.25	2.5	5	11
Sample	x	y	2.5	5	z

Experiment 18.10: Determination of small amount of chloride by nephelometric titration

Principle of nephelometer

Nephelometry and turbidimetry are used for continuous monitoring of air and water pollution. In water, turbidity is monitored whereas in air, smoke and dust are monitored. The techniques are also used in food, beverages and in the determination of molecular weight of high polymers which are settled down on earth from factories. The CO_2 can also be determined by this technique.

Nephelometric analysis is based on measuring the intensity of a luminous flux scattered by solid particles suspended in solution. Nephelometric analysis is based on measuring the weakening of intensity of a luminous flux when it passes through a solution containing particles in suspension. The intensity decreases owing to absorption and scattering of light.

Reagents

- Stock chloride solution: Dissolve 4.12 g of sodium chloride in 1 litre distilled water.
- Diluted chloride solutions: Dilute 10 ml of the stock solution diluted to 1 litre with distilled water. This solution contains 25 mg of chloride per litre. Dilute 1 ml of this to 50 ml. It will give a solution corresponding to 0.5 ppm of chloride ion.
- Nitric acid–silver nitrate reagent: Dissolve 1.70 g of silver nitrate in 0.2N nitric acid solution and make up the volume to 1 litre with distilled water.
- Absolute ethanol.

Calculation

4.12 g of sodium chloride contains 2.5 'g' of chloride, when it is dissoved in 1 litre of water, produces 2.5 g/litre or 2.5 mg/ml chloride solution. Further, its 10 ml of solution is diluted to 1 litre to get 25 mg/litre or 25 μg/ml chloride solution which is equivalent to 25 ppm chloride solution. 1 ml of the solution diluted to 50 ml with water corresponds to 0.5 ppm of chloride ion.

Procedure

1. Take the diluted chloride solution corresponding to 0 to 5 ppm chloride as shown in the below given table in the 50 ml volumetric flask. Adjust the neutral pH with either 1N nitric acid or 1N NaOH solution. Add distilled water until the volume approximates 20 ml. Add 20 ml of absolute ethanol and then add drop-wise 5 ml of the nitric acid–silver nitrate reagent while swirling the contents of the flask. Make up the volume with absolute ethanol. Place the volumetric flask in a water-bath at 40°C for 30 minutes and then cool rapidly to room temperature. Read out the turbidity of each dilution by nephelometer.

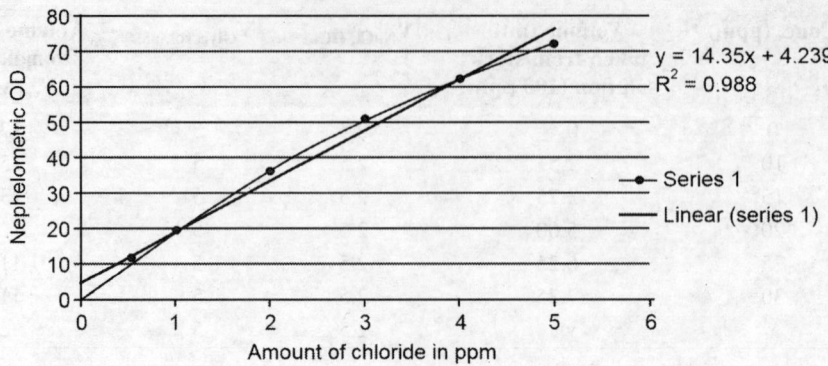

Fig. 18.13: Standard curve for chloride in nephelometric determination

Note: A blank determination must be made in order to eliminate the possibility of chloride contamination from the reagents.

2. Make a calibration curve as shown in Fig. 18.13.
3. Transfer the sample (0.5 g) sufficient distilled water to a 50 ml volumetric flask, adjust the pH with either 1N nitric acid or 1N sodium hydroxide until the solution is just neutral to phenolphthalein.
4. Add distilled water until the volume approximates 20 ml.
5. Add 20 ml of absolute ethanol and then, drop-wise from a pipette, 5 ml of the nitric acid–silver nitrate reagent while swirling the contents of the flask.
6. Make up to the mark with absolute ethanol and shake. If any initial turbidity is found before the addition of the nitric acid-silver nitrate reagent, the sample must be rejected, because turbidity at this point indicates contamination.
7. Place the volumetric flask in a water bath at 40°C for 30 minutes, and then cool the sample rapidly to room temperature. Find out the intensity of turbidity from nephelometer.
   Note: The sample should be read within 30 minutes after it has been cooled to room temperature.
8. Compare the reading and find out the chloride content from the standard curve (Fig. 18.13), and calculate the amount of chloride.

$$\% \text{ of chloride} = \frac{\text{ppm of chloride (from the curve)} \times 0.005}{\text{Weight of sample, in grams}}$$

Observation table

Chloride (ppm)	Standard solution (25 ppm) in ml	Readings
5	10	
4	8	
3	6	
2	4	
1	2	
0.75	1.5	
0.5	1.0	
0.25	0.5	
0	—	
Unknown	x	

Result

The amount of chloride is found to be = ... % w/w.

Precautions

1. The greatest source of error in nephelometry is practically an instrumental, so instrument must be calibrated before measurement precisely to get the reproducible results.
2. Since adsorption phenomena are of great influence upon the crystallization velocity, it may be expected that the homogeneity of the medium during the formation of the slightly soluble substance will be of great importance in obtaining good results.
3. The time elapsed between the moment of mixing the solutions and their nephelometric measurement, which can affect the reading of nephelometer therefore the prepared sample should not be kept for more than 1 hour before measurement.
4. Nephelometry is used for determination of small amount of chloride present in sample. For samples of higher amount assay should be shifted on turbidimetry.

Quantitative Organic Analysis

ACID VALUE

Definition

Acid value is defined as the number of milligrams of potassium hydroxide required to neutralize the free fatty acids in 1 gram of an oil or fat.

Significance

Acid value indicates the amount of non-esterified fatty acids (or free fatty acids) present in oil or fat. Acid value is a valuable test for freshness. Stale/rancid fats or oils have abnormally high acid value. Fats/oil contain glycerides of fatty acid. Owing to liberation of free acid, a high acid value would be expected in a rancid fat/oil.

Procedure for Determination of Acid Value

1. Unless otherwise specified in the individual monograph, dissolve an accurately weighed quantity of the substance (10 g) (Table 19.1) being examined in a mixture of equal volumes of mixture (50 ml) of 95% ethanol and ether, previously neutralized with 0.1M potassium hydroxide solution to phenolphthalein solution.

Table 19.1	
Acid value	**Weight (g) of the sample**
Less than 5	10
5 to less than 15	5
15 to less than 50	3
50 to less than 120	1
More than 120	0.5

2. If the sample does not dissolve in the cold solvent, connect the flask with a reflux condenser and warm slowly, with frequent shaking, until the sample dissolve.
3. Add phenolphthalein indicator solution (1 ml) and titrate with 0.1M potassium hydroxide solution until the solution remains faintly pink after shaking for 30 seconds.

Note: If the oil has been saturated with carbon dioxide for the purpose of preservation gently reflux the solution of the oil in ethanol (95%) and ether for 10 minutes before titration.

The oil may be freed from the carbon dioxide by exposing it in a shallow dish in a vacuum desicator for 24 hours before weighing the sample.

Formula

$$\text{Acid value} = \frac{A \times M \times 5.61}{W}$$

where A = Volume (ml) of potassium hydroxide solution consumed; W = Weight (g) of substance or the oil taken; M = Molarity of KOH.

Standard Values

Fat/oil	Acid value	Fat/oil	Acid value
Lard oil	0.5–0.8	Soybean oil	1.1
Mustard oil	1.5 max	Wool fat	59.8
Seasame oil	9.8	Butter fat	0.4–35.4
Corn oil	1.37–2.02	Olive oil	0.3–1.0
Castor oil	0.12–0.80	Linseed oil	1–3.5
Cotton seed oil	0.6–0.9	**Wax**	
Palm oil	10	Spermaceti	Below 1
Cod liver oil	5.6	Carnauba	4–7
Coconut oil	0.37	Beeswax	18–24
Sunflower oil	0.263		

SAPONIFICATION VALUE

Definition

Saponification value is defined as the number of milligrams of potassium hydroxide required to completely saponify 1 g of the oil or fat.

Significance

1. Saponification value is a measure of the size of the fat molecule or the size/molecular weight of fatty acids in the fat. (**Note:** Each molecule of fat regardless of its size requires three molecules of potassium hydroxide for saponification).
2. The saponification value indicates the quantity of alkali which must be used to convert a blend of fats to form soap. Handmade soap makers who aim for bar soap use NaOH sap values which are derived from the saponification values calculated in lab (KOH sap values). To convert KOH values to NaOH values, divide the KOH values by the ratio of the mol. wt. of KOH and NaOH (1.403).
3. Saponification value is also useful for detecting adulteration of a given fat by one of the higher or lower saponification value.

Procedure for Determination of Saponification Value

1. Introduce an accurately weighed quantity of the substance (about 2 g) being examined into a 250 ml flask of borosilicate glass, fitted with a reflux condenser.
2. Add alcohol 0.5M KOH solution (25 ml), little pumice powder and boil under reflux on a water bath for 30 minutes.
3. Add phenolphthalein solution (1 ml) and titrate immediately with 0.5M hydrochloric acid ('a' ml).
4. Repeat the operation omitting the substance being examined ('b' ml).

The sample is first saponified by adding standard KOH and then excess of KOH is titrated with standard HCl.

$$RCOOH + KOH \longrightarrow RCOOK + H_2O$$

$$KOH + HCl \longrightarrow KCl + H_2O$$

Formula

$$Saponification\ value = \frac{b - a}{Weight\ (g)\ of\ sample} \times 28.05$$

where b = Volume (ml) of 0.5M potassium hydroxide for blank (without sample of oil or fat); a = Volume (ml) of 0.5M potassium hydroxide consumed with the sample (oil or fat).

0.5M Alcoholic KOH solution: Dissolve 28.06 g of KOH in sufficient quantity of 60% alcohol. Dilute to 1000 ml with 60% alcohol in a volumetric flask.

Standard Values

Fat/oil	Saponification value	Fat/oil	Saponification value
Almond oil	183–208	Palm oil	248
Olive oil	185–196	Lard	192–198
Coconut oil	190–198	Linseed oil	188–195
Theobroma	193–195	**Wax**	
Cod liver oil	180–190	Spermaceti	120–136
Mustard oil	168–177	Wool fat	90–106
Castor oil	175–183	Carnauba	70–95
Arachis oil	188–196		

Note: If the oil has been saturated with carbon dioxide, remove this before making the solution of the oil in 95% ethanol and ether before titration. The oil may be freed from the carbon dioxide by exposing it in a shallow dish in a vacuum desicator for 24 hours before weighing the sample.

IODINE VALUE

Definition

Iodine value is defined as the number of grams of iodine that combine with 100 g of an oil or fat. The iodine value is a measure of the degree of unsaturation of an oil or fat. The unsaturation is due to presence of glycerides of unsaturated fatty acids like linolenic, linoleic, oleic, recinoleic acids. Oils are classified on the basis of iodine value (Table 19.2) in drying, semidrying and non-drying oils.

Table 19.2: Classification of oils on the basis of iodine value

Oil class	Iodine value
Drying oil	> 140
Semidrying oil	125–140
Non-drying oil	< 125

Significance

1. Iodine value is regarded as a measure of its degree of unsaturation and gives an idea of its drying characters. Drying and semidrying oils finds uses in surface coating properties where drying oils are essential in paints, resins, printing inks.
2. Iodine value is also helpful in finding adulteration in fats and oils and judging its suitability in paint industry.

Standard Values

The standard iodine value for some of the fats or oils are given below.

Fat/oil	Iodine value	Fat/oil	Iodine value
Almond oil	99–103	Lard	50–66
Castor oil	84	Cod liver oil	155–180
Olive oil	79–88	Linseed oil	175–202
Arachis oil	86–106	**Wax**	
Coconut oil	7–11	Wool fat	18–32
Mustard oil	168–177	Beeswax	8–11
Cottonseed oil	109–116	Spermaceti	below 5
Theobroma	33–42	Carnauba	10–14

Determination of Iodine Value

Iodine value is determined by the following methods.

A. Iodine Monochloride Method or Wij's Method

This method was devised by Wij. It uses the solution of iodine monochloride in a mixture of carbon tetrachloride and glacial acetic acid. Fats or oils due to presence of double bonds combine with iodine and the result is calculated as equivalent to iodine.

Procedure

1. Dissolve an accurately weighed quantity of the substance being examined in a dry 500 ml iodine flask in carbon tetrachloride (10 ml).
2. Add iodine monochloride solution (20 ml), and allow to stand in the dark at a temperature between 15°C and 25°C for 30 minutes.
3. Introduce potassium iodide solution (15 ml). Carefully remove the stopper, rinse the stopper and the sides of the flask with water (100 ml).
4. Shake and titrate with 0.1M sodium thiosulphate solution using starch solution as indicator added toward the end of the titration.
5. Similarly carry out the blank titration.

Formula

$$\text{Iodine value} = \frac{(b - a) \times 1.269}{\text{Weight (g) of sample}}$$

where b = Volume (ml) of 0.1M sodium thiosulphate solution consumed in blank titration; a = Volume of 0.1M sodium thiosulphate solution consumed in sample titration.

Note: The approximate weight in 'g' of a substance to be taken may be calculated by dividing 20 by the highest expected iodine value. If more than half the available halogen is absorbed, the test must be repeated with smaller amount of the substance (oil/fat).

There are two ways for preparing Wij's solution:

(a) Chlorine is passed through a solution of iodine in a mixture of carbon tetrachloride and glacial acetic acid. The completion of reaction is completed as shown by the titre value of solution with sodium thiosulphate, after the addition of potassium iodide.

$$Cl_2 + I_2 \longrightarrow 2ICl$$

$$ICl + KI \rightleftharpoons KCl + I_2$$

(b) Interaction of iodine trichloride in glacial acetic acid with iodine in carbon tetrachloride yield iodine monochloride. The mixture is then diluted with glacial acetic acid.

$$I_2 + ICl_3 \rightleftharpoons 3ICl$$

B. Pyridine Bromide Method

This method makes use of additive compound of pyridine bromide and sulphuric acid. This reagent forms additive compound with unsaturated glyceride without any substitution or oxidation and the excess of pyridine bromide can subsequently be determined by the addition of potassium iodide followed by titration with standard sodium thiosulphate solution. This method is said to give more consistent results then iodine monochloride method with oils.

Procedure

1. Dissolve an accurately weighed quantity of the substance being examined in a dry iodine flask in carbon tetrachloride (10 ml).
2. Add pyridine bromide solution (25 ml), allow to stand for 10 minutes in the dark and transfer potassium iodide solution (15 ml) in the cuptop.
3. Carefully remove the stopper, rinse the stopper and sides of the flask with water (100 ml).
4. Shake and titrate with 0.1M sodium thiosulphate solution using starch mucilage as indicator, added towards the end of the titration.
5. Similarly carry out the blank titration.

Formula

$$\text{Iodine value} = \frac{(b - a) \times 1.269}{\text{Weight (gm) of sample}}$$

where b = Volume (ml) of 0.1M sodium thiosulphate solution consumed in blank titration; a = Volume (ml) of 0.1M Sodium thiosulphate solution consumed in sample titration.

Note: The approximate weight in g, of the substance to be taken may be calculated by dividing 12.5 by the highest expected value. If more than half the available halogen is absorbed, the test must be repeated with smaller quantity of substance.

Preparation of pyridine bromide solution

Dissolve pyridine (8 g) and sulphuric acid (5.4 ml) in glacial acetic acid (20 ml). Keeping the mixture cool, add bromine solution (2.6 ml) dissolved in glacial acetic acid (20 ml) and then dilute the solution to 1000 ml with acetic acid.

C. *Iodine Monobromide Method*

1. Place an accurately weighed quantity of substance in a 250 ml iodine flask.
2. Dissolve in chloroform and add slowly from a burette iodine monobromide solution (25 ml).
3. Insert the stopper and allow to stand in the dark for 30 minutes with occasional shaking.
4. Add potassium iodide solution (10 ml) and water (100 ml) and titrate with 0.1M sodium thiosulphate solution using starch solution (indicator), added towards the end of titration.
5. Calculate the iodine value from the formula as given in previous method.
6. Similarly, carry out the blank titration.

Note: The approximate weight of the substance to be taken unless otherwise directed in the monograph is calculated as follows: Presumed iodine value less than 20, 1.0 g; presumed iodine value 60–100, 0.15–0.25 g; presumed iodine value more than 100, 0.10–0.15 g.

HYDROXYL VALUE

Definition

Hydroxyl value is defined as the number of milligrams of potassium hydroxide equivalent to hydroxyl group present in 1 'g' of alcoholic substance.

Procedure for Determination of Hydroxyl Value

Method A

1. Weight accurately the quantity of the substance as specified in Indian Pharmacopoeia being examined in a 250 ml flask fitted with a condenser.
2. Add the appropriate quantity of pyridine acetic anhydride reagent.
3. Boil for 1 hour on a water bath, adjusting the level of the water to maintain it 2 to 3 cm above the level of the liquid in the flask.
4. Cool, add water (5 ml) through the top of condenser. If this causes cloudiness, add pyridine to produce a clear liquid, shake, replace in the water bath for 10 minutes, remove and cool.
5. Rinse the condenser and walls of the flask with 95% ethanol (5 ml) previously neutralized to dilute phenolphthalein solution.
6. Titrate with 0.5M alc. potassium hydroxide using dilute phenolphthalein solution as indicator.
7. Similarly perform a blank determination.

Formula

Hydroxyl value may be calculated from the following formula:

$$\text{Hydroxyl value} = \frac{V \times 28.05}{W} + \text{Acid value}$$

where V = Difference in ml between the two titrations; W = Weight in 'g', of the substance.

Preparation of pyridine–acetic anhydride reagent

Add cautiously with cooling freshly distilled acetic anhydride (25 ml) to freshly distilled anhydrous pyridine (50 ml). Cool down and dilute with freshly dry pyridine to 100 ml.

Method B

1. Weigh accurately the specified quantity of the substance being examined into a flask fitted with a reflux condenser.
2. Add stearic anhydride (12 g) and xylene (10 ml) and heat under reflux for 30 minutes.

3. Cool, add the mixture of pyridine (40 ml) and water (4 ml), heat under reflux for further 30 minutes and titrate the hot solution with 1M potassium hydroxide solution using phenolphthalein as indicator.
4. Similarly carry out the blank titration.

Note: Acid value is determined by usual procedure mentioned earlier.

PEROXIDE VALUE

Definition

It is the number which expresses in milliequivalents of active oxygen, the amount of peroxide contained in 1000 g of the substance.

Procedure for Determination of Peroxide Value

1. Weigh 5.0 ± 0.05 g of substance into a 250 ml glass stoppered conical flask.
2. Add mixture of 3 volumes of glacial acetic acid and 2 volumes of chloroform (30 ml) and swirl until dissolved.
3. Add saturated potassium iodide solution (0.5 ml).
4. Allow to stand exactly for 1 minute, with occasional shaking, add water (30 ml) and titrate gradually with continuous and vigorous shaking with 0.1N sodium thiosulphate solution until the yellow colour appears.
5. Add starch solution (0.5 ml) and continue the titration, shaking vigorously until the blue colour just disappears ('a' ml).
6. Carry out the blank determination ('b' ml).
7. Calculate the peroxide value from the expression.

Formula

$$\text{Peroxide value} = \frac{(a - b) \times 10}{W}$$

where W = Weight of the substance (in g).

ACETYL VALUE

Definition

It is the number which expresses in milligrams the amount of potassium hydroxide required to neutralize the acetic acid liberated by the hydrolysis of 1.0 g of the acetylated substance.

Procedure for Determination of Acetyl Value

1. Determine the saponification value (a) of the substance as mentioned earlier.
2. Acetylate the substance being examined by the following method.
3. Place the substance (10 g) with acetic anhydride (20 ml) in long neck round bottom flask attached to a reflux air condenser.
4. Support the flask on a sheet of heat resistant material in which a hole of about 4 cm in diameter has been cut and heat it with a small, nacked, not more than 25 mm in height and which does not impinge on the bottom of the flask.
5. Boil gently for 2 hours, allow to cool, pour into water (600 ml) contained in larger beaker, add pumice powder (0.2 g) and boil for 30 minutes.
6. Cool, transfer to a separator and discard the lower layer. Wash the acetylated product with 3 or more quantities each of 50 ml, of a warmed saturated sodium chloride solution (each of 50 ml) until the washings are no longer acidic to litmus paper.

7. Finally shake with warm water (20 ml) and remove the aqueous layer as completely as possible.
8. Pour the acetylated substance into a small dish, add anhydrous sodium sulphate (1 g), stir thoroughly and filter.
9. Determine the saponification value (b) of the acetylated substance.
10. Calculate the acetyl value as per formula given below.

Formula

$$\text{Acetyl value: } 1335\,(b-a)\,(1335-a)$$

where a = Saponification value of the substance; b = Saponification value of the acetylated substance.

ESTER VALUE

Ester value is the number of milligrams of potassium hydroxide required to saponify the ester present in 1.0 g of the substance. Determine the acid value and saponification value as mentioned earlier and calculate the ester value from the expression.

$$\text{Ester value} = \text{Saponification value} - \text{Acid value}$$

REICHERT MEISSEL VALUE

Reichert Meissel value is the number of ml of 0.1N KOH solution required to neutralize soluble volatile acids obtained by distillation of 50 g of oil or fat. The RM value indicates the amount of steam volatile fatty acids present in oil or fat. It is of special importance to test the purity of butter or ghee since the RM value of adulterated ghee or butter is usually lower than that of pure butter and ghee.

Procedure for Determination of Reichert Meissel Value

1. Weigh 5.00 ± 0.01 g of the fat into the flask.
2. Add 20 g (16 ml) of glycerol and 2 ml of the sodium hydroxide solution (44%).
   Note: *For supplying the sodium hydroxide solution, use a burette protected from the entry of carbon dioxide.*
3. Heat the flask over a naked flame, avoiding overheating and shaking continuously until the liquid no longer foams and becomes clear.
4. Allow the flask to cool to about 90°C, add 90 ml of recently boiled distilled water of about the same temperature and mix. The liquid should remain clear.
5. Add 0.6 to 0.7 g of the pumice and then 50 ml 1N sulphuric acid solution.
6. Connect the flask immediately to the distillation apparatus and warm it gently until the free fatty acids form a clear surface layer.
7. Start heating and regulate the flame so as to collect in the measuring flask 110 ml of distillate in 19–21 minutes, taking the moment when the first drop forms in the condenser as the beginning of the distillation period.
8. Regulate the water flowing in the condenser so as to maintain the temperature of the water leaving the condenser at 20 ± 1°C.
9. When exactly 110 ml of distillate have been collected, remove the burner immediately and substitute a small beaker for the measuring flask.
10. Mix the contents of the measuring flask by gentle shaking and immerse the flask in a water bath at 20 ± 1°C for 10 to 15 minutes, the 110 ml mark on the flask being 1 cm below the level of the water in the water bath and the flask being turned from time to time.

11. Stopper the flask and mix by inverting it 4 to 5 times without shaking.
12. Filter the 110 ml of distillate through a dry medium speed filter paper (diameter 80–90 mm) which fits snugly into the funnel. The filtrate should be clear.
13. Pipette 100 ml of the filtrate into 250 ml conical flask, add 0.5 ml of phenolphthalein indicator solution and titrate with the standardized aqueous alkali solution (0.1N) to a pink colour persistent for 1/2 to 1 minute.
14. Conduct a blank test without fat and instead of saponifying over a naked flame, heat over a boiling water bath for 15 minutes.

Note: *Not more than 0.5 ml of the standardized alkali solution should be required for the titration. Otherwise, new reagent solutions should be prepared.*

Formula

$$\text{Reichert value} = 11.t\,(v_1 - b)$$

where v_1 = number of millilitres standardized alkali solution (0.1N) required for the sample; b = number of millilitres standardized alkali solution (0.1N) required for the blank test; t = exact normality of the standardized alkali solution (0.1N).

DETERMINATION OF THE NUMBER OF HYDROXYL GROUPS IN PHENOL

Procedure

1. Dissolve an accurately weighed quantity (about 1.0 g) of phenol in a mixture of definite volume of acetic anhydride and pyridine (1: 4) (10 ml) and heat under refluxing condition for 40 minutes for acetylation.
2. Cool down, add water (100 ml) to convert the unreacted acetic anhydride to acetic acid.

$$R(OH)_n + nCH_3CO.O.COCH_3 \longrightarrow R(OCOCH_3)_n + nCH_3COOH$$

3. Titrate the total free acetic acid with 1N sodium hydroxide solution by using phenolphthalein as indicator.
4. Similarly, perform the blank titration.
5. The difference in the volumes of sodium hydroxide solution required in the two experiments is equivalent to the difference in the amount of acetic acid formed, i.e. the acetic acid used in the acetylation. If the molecular weight of phenol is known, the number of hydroxyl groups can then be calculated.

Formula

$$\text{No. of hydroxyl group} = \frac{(b - a) \times \text{Mol. wt. of compound}}{\text{Weight of compound}}$$

where b = Volume (ml) of 1N NaOH consumed in blank titration; a = Volume (ml) of 1N NaOH consumed in test titration.

DETERMINATION OF THE NUMBER OF HYDROXYL GROUPS IN POLYHYDRIC ALCOHOL

Glycol C_2H_4 (OH)$_2$ (mol. wt. 62): The procedure for glycol is same as for phenol but add about 0.5 ml of glycol to acetylating mixture and weigh as before.

Glycerol C_3H_5 (OH)$_3$ (mol. wt. 92): Use approximately 0.5 ml of glycerol, and cork the flask when weighing the glycerol. Heat on water bath for 60 minutes instead of 30 minutes. Anhydrous glycerol will give excellent results.

Mannitol C_6H_8 (OH)$_6$ (mol. wt. 182): Take approximately 0.5 g of finely powdered mannitol in the flask. Heat on water bath for 60 minutes, During the titration with sodium hydroxide solution, a fine precipitation of hexacetyl mannitol may occur, but will not affect the titration.

Glucose C_6H_7O (OH)$_5$ (mol. wt. 180): Use approximately 0.5 g of finely powdered anhydrous glucose, heating for 60 minutes. Slightly low results are obtained.

DETERMINATION OF THE % OF ACETYL GROUPS IN AN ACETYL ESTER

Procedure

1. Hydrolyse an accurately weighed (about 1.0 g) of acetyl ester by heating under refluxing condition with 1M sodium hydroxide solution (25 ml) for 30 to 45 minutes. This volume being in excess of that required for complete hydrolysis.
2. Titrate the excess of sodium hydroxide with 1M hydrochloric acid or M/2 sulphuric acid solution ('a' ml) by using phenolphthalein as indicator.

$$R(O.COCH_3)_n + nNaOH \rightarrow R(OH)_n + nCH_3COONa$$

3. Similarly carry out the blank titration (b ml). The difference in both the volume indicates the actual amount of sodium hydroxide used to hydrolyze the acetylated compound.

Formula

$$\% \text{ of acetyl group} = \frac{(b - a) \times \text{Molarity of NaOH} \times 43.04 \times 100}{\text{Weight of sample} \times 1000}$$

Determination of the % of Acetyl Groups in Triacetyl Glycerol C_3H_5 (OCOCH$_3$)$_3$ (Mol. wt. 218)

1. Fix two 250 ml conical flasks, A and B, with reflux water condenser.
2. Weigh the flask A, add triacetylglycerol (about 1 ml) and weigh again.
3. Add 1M sodium hydroxide solution (25 ml) to each flask (flask B acting as blank) and add a few fragments of unglazed porcelain to each flask.
4. Boil each flask gently for 30 minutes, stop the heating, add distilled water (about 10 ml) and then cool in cold water.
5. Titrate the contents of each flask with 1M hydrochloric acid solution, using phenolphthalein as an indicator.

Determination of the % of acetyl groups in

1. **Hexaacetylmannitol C_6H_8 (OCOCH$_3$)$_6$ (mol. wt. 434):** The procedure for hexacetyl-mannitol is same, but since hexaacetylmannitol is a crystalline compound, weigh out 1.0 to 1.2 g of powdered substance in the flask A.
2. **Pentaacetylglucose C_6H_7O (OCOCH$_3$)$_5$ (mol. wt. 390):** A modification of the above method is required for acetylated sugars because on alkaline hydrolysis the liberated sugar, e.g. glucose undergoes slight resinification, giving a brown solution, in which endpoint of the titration is difficult to detect accurately. If, however, M/2 sulphuric acid solution is used instead of 1M sodium hydroxide solution, hydrolysis occurs rapidly and acidic solution remains colourless giving an excellent endpoint when the mixture of acetic acid and unchanged sulphuric acid is back titrated with 1M sodium hydroxide solution using phenol-phthalein as an indicator.

Procedure

1. Weigh the powdered pentaacetylglucose (1.5 g) in the flask A, and then add M/2 sulphuric acid solution (25 ml) to each of the flasks A and B, together with small amounts of porcelain.

2. Boil under reflux gently for 30 minutes, add distilled water (10 ml) and then cool down the solutions.
3. Titrate with 1M sodium hydroxide solution.

DETERMINATION OF NUMBER OF AMINO GROUP

Number of amino group is determined in the same way as number of hydroxyl group as mentioned earlier. Trace amounts of amines are generally determined by calorimetric methods. For primary amines, formation of Schiff bases with salicyldehyde and subsequent determination of absorbance at 410 nm is a good calorimetric method.

DETERMINATION OF % OF ESTER GROUP

Procedure

1. Boil a convenient quantity of ethanol (95%) thoroughly to expel carbon dioxide and neutralize it to phenolphthalein solution.
2. Dissolve an accurately weighed quantity (about 2.0 g) of the substance being examined in ethanol (5 ml).
3. Neutralize the free acid by titrating with 0.1M alcoholic potassium hydroxide solution until just pink to phenolphathalein.
4. Add 0.5M alc. potassium hydroxide solution (25 ml) and boil under reflux condenser on a water bath for 1 hour.
5. Cool down, add water (20 ml) and titrate the excess of alkali with 0.5M hydrochloric acid using a further 0.2 ml of phenolphthalein solution as indicator.
6. Repeat the operation without the substance being examined (blank titration). The difference between the titrations represent the alkali required to saponify the esters.

$$R\text{–}COOR^1 + KOH = R\text{–}COOK + R^1\,OH$$

$$R\text{–}COOR^1 = KOH = 2000 \text{ ml of } 0.5M \text{ KOH}$$

The number of ester group can be calculated in the same way as in acetyl group.

Note: The number of ester group can be determined in benzyl benzoate, methyl salicylate, ethyl oleate, etc., in this way.

DETERMINATION OF NUMBER OF CARBOXYLIC GROUPS

The number of carboxylic groups which is equivalent to basicity of acid is determined by the following:

$$\text{Basicity} = \frac{\text{Mol. weight}}{\text{Eq. weight}}$$

Thus, if molecular weight is known, number of carboxylic acid can be determined with the determination of equivalent weight. The equivalent weight of water soluble acid can be determined by titration method.

This method is based on the fact that 1 equivalent alkali neutralizes 1 equivalent of the acid.

$$1N \text{ NaoH} = 1 \text{ eq. wt. of acid}$$

Determination of Equivalent Weight

A. Procedure for Soluble Acid

1. Dissolve an accurately weighed quantity of soluble acid (about 3.0 g) in water and volume is made up to 100 ml.

2. Pipette out 20 ml of this solution and titrate with 0.5N NaOH solution using phenolphthalein as indicator.
3. Take at least three concordant reading.
4. Calculate the number of carboxylic groups as per the formula given below.

Observation and calculation

$$\text{Equivalent weight of acid} = \frac{x \times 2}{5 \times V} \times 1000$$

where x = weight of acid; V = volume of 0.5N NaOH consumed.

B. Procedure for Insoluble Acid

Insoluble acid can be titrated as such after dissolving in water.

1. Suspend an accurately weighed quantity of acid (3.0 g) in water.
2. Titrate with 1.0N NaOH solution by using phenolphthalein indicator.
3. Calculate the number of carboxylic group as per the given formula.

Formula

$$\text{Equivalent weight of acid} = \frac{x}{V} \times 1000$$

where x = Weight of acid; V = Volume of 1.0N NaOH solution.

ESTIMATION OF % OF GLUCOSE IN THE GIVEN SAMPLE

Estimation of glucose is based upon the presence of aldehydic group in glucose owing to which it reduces the Fehling's solution (blue colour) into cuprous oxide (red colour). Fehling's solution is obtained by mixing an aqueous copper sulphate solution (Fehling's solution A) and alkaline solution of sodium potassium tartarate (Fehling's solution B).

$$Cu(OH)_2 + C_6H_{12}O_6 \longrightarrow \underset{\text{Gluconic acid}}{\begin{array}{c} COOH \\ | \\ (CHOH)_4 \\ | \\ CH_2OH \end{array}} + \underset{\substack{\text{Cuprous oxide} \\ \text{(Red precipitate)}}}{Cu_2O}$$

$$\underset{\text{Glucose}}{}$$

Procedure

1. Weigh accurately the sample (about 1.25 g), dissolve in water and make up 250 ml in volumetric flask.
2. Pipette out 25 ml of Fehling's solution (Equal volume of Fehling's A and B solution), dilute with water and boil gently over a gauze.
3. Now titrate this solution with glucose solution untill blue colour entirely disappeared.
4. Repeat the titrations until consistent values are obtained.

According to theoretical concept, 1 ml of Fehling's solution contain = 0.005 g of pure glucose.

V (titration reading) vol. of glucose solution contain = 25 × 0.005 g of pure glucose.

$$\text{Percentage of glucose} = \frac{25 \times 0.005 \times 250}{V \times \text{wt. of sample}} \times 100$$

Fehling's solution A

Dissolve crystalline copper sulphate (17.32 g) in water and make up the volume to 250 ml in volumetric flask.

Fehling's solution B

Dissolve crystalline sodium potassium tartarate (86.5 g) in warm water. Dissolve pure sodium hydroxide (30 g) in water. Mix the tartarate and sodium hydroxide solution, cool and make up to 250 ml in volumetric flask.

When the Fehling's solution is required, transfer equal volumes of solution A and B to a dry flask and mix thoroughly by shaking.

ESTIMATION OF GLYCINE

Procedure

1. Weigh accurately glycine (about 2 g), dissolve in water and make up the volume to 250 ml in volumetric flask with water.
2. Pipette out 25 ml of the solution, add 2 drops of phenolphthalein and then add dilute sodium hydroxide solution very carefully until the solution is just faintly pink.
3. **Neutralization of formalin solution:** Place about 50 ml of formalin solution, add 2 drops of phenolphthalein indicator. Now add carefully NaOH solution until the solution is just pink.
4. Now add about 10 ml of neutralized formaldehyde solution.
5. Titrate with 0.1M NaOH solution until pink colour just restored.
6. Repeat the procedure till consistent readings are obtained.

$$\% \text{ of glycine} = \frac{\text{Vol. of Sod. Hydroxide consumed} \times \text{Mol. wt. of Glycine} \times 100}{1000 \times \text{wt. of sample}}$$

Amino acid as glycine cannot be estimated by direct titration with standard alkali solution due to presence of acidic and basic groups together. If, however, the amino acid is first treated with neutral formaldehyde solution to protect the amino group, it can be directly titrated with standard sodium hydroxide solution.

$$HCHO + H_2NCH_2COOH \longrightarrow CH_2 = NCH_2COOH + H_2O$$

Glycine is present in aqueous solution as the "zwitterion" $H_3\overset{+}{N}CH_2COO^-$ which is incapable of reacting with formaldehyde. When hydroxide solution is added, the glycine is converted into $H_2NCH_2COO^-$ ion which react with formaldehyde to give stable cation.

$$H_3N^+CH_2COO^- + OH^- \longrightarrow H_2NCH_2COO^- + H_2O$$

$$H_2NCH_2COO^- + CH_2O \longrightarrow CH_2 = NCH_2COO^- + H_2O$$

Since formaldehyde solution invariably contain formic acid and amino acid themselves exactly neutral. It is important that both the formaldehyde solution and glycine solution should be brought to the same pH and for this purpose each solution is first made alkaline to phenolphthalein by means of dilute sodium hydroxide solution.

DETERMINATION OF NUMBER OF KETO GROUPS

Ketones can be determined quantitatively by conversion to the 2,4-dinitrophenylhydrazone which is collected and weighed. The weight of the precipitate is correlated with number of keto groups.

Ketone — 2,4-Dinitrophenyl hydrazine → 2,4-Dinitrophenyl hydrazone

Reagents Required

Methanol

This must be free from ketones, if necessary reflux 1 litre of purest material available for 2 hours with 2,4-dinitrophenylhydrazine (5 g) and 5 drops of concentrated hydrochloric acid. Then, distil methanol through fractionating column and collect the fraction boiling at 64.5–65.5°C.

2,4-Dinitrophenylhydrazine solution

Prepare a saturated solution of 2,4-dinitrophenylhydrazine in 20 ml of purified methanol. This solution should be discarded after 1 week.

Potassium hydroxide

Dissolve 10 g of solid in distilled water (20 ml) and then make up to 100 ml with purified methanol.

Procedure

1. Dissolve the sample (about 0.1 g) in purified methanol (10 ml) and transfer 1 ml of this solution to a stoppered test tube.
2. Add 2,4-dinitrophenylhydrazine solution (1 ml) and 1 drop of concentrated hydrochloric acid, then place the stoppered tube in a beaker of boiling water for 5 minutes.
3. Cool down, collect the precipitate and dry them to constant weight.
4. The weight of the precipitate is correlated with number of keto groups. (Alternatively, the estimation may be made spectrophotometric method. For this, add potassium hydroxide solution (5 ml) and measure absorbance of the solution at 480 nm against a blank obtained by subjecting 1 ml of purified methanol to the above procedure).

Formula

$$\text{Percentage of keto compound} = \frac{W}{X} \times \text{gravimetric factor} \times 100$$

where X = Weight of keto compound; W = Weight of precipitates.

Note: The colour of precipitate is yellow but on adding alkali solution to the precipitate, an intense yellow colour is developed. It may be due to resonance delocalization of negative charge resulting from removal of a proton.

Intense yellow colour

Chromatography

Chromatography is the separation and purification techniques employed for organic as well as for inorganic compounds. Two or more compounds or ions are separated by the distribution between two phases, one, which is moving, and the other, which is stationary. These two phases can be solid-liquid, liquid-liquid or gas-liquid. Although, there are many different variations of chromatography, the principles is essentially the same.

Types of chromatography

These are classified as follows:

1. *Gas Chromatography*:
   (a) Gas liquid chromatography
   (b) Gas solid chromatography
2. *Liquid Chromatography*:
   (a) Liquid-liquid chromatography
   (b) Liquid solid chromatography
   (c) Ion exchange chromatography
   (d) Exclusion chromatography

Physical surface forces are mainly involved in the retentive ability of the stationary phase in most of the chromatographic procedures. When the stationary phase is liquid and mobile phase is either liquid or gas, the process is called partition chromatography. In contrast, when the stationary phase is solid and mobile phase is either liquid or gas, it is categorized under adsorption type of chromatography.

Two other liquid chromatographic methods differ somewhat in their mode of action. For example, in Ion-exchange chromatography (IEC), ionic components of the sample are separated by selective exchange with ions of the stationary phase. Exclusion chromatography (EC) is also referred to gel permeation chromatography by polymer chemists and as gel filtration by biochemists. In this, components are separated on the basis of their particle size.

In this chapter, only experiments related with two techniques, thin layer chromatography and paper chromatography are illustrated.

THIN LAYER CHROMATOGRAPHY (TLC)

Thin layer chromatography or TLC is a solid-liquid form of chromatography where the stationary phase is normally a polar absorbent, usually finely ground alumina or silica particles. This absorbent is coated on a glass slide or plastic sheet creating a thin layer of the particular stationary phase. By manipulating the mobile phase, organic compounds can be separated. The mobile phase can be a single solvent or combination of solvents. TLC is a quick, inexpensive microscale technique that can be used to:

- Determine the number of components in a mixture
- Verify a substance's identity
- Monitor the progress of a reaction
- Determine appropriate conditions for column chromatography
- Analyze the fractions obtained from column chromatography

Experimental procedure

Stationary Phase

As stationary phase, a special finely ground matrix (silica gel, alumina, or similar material) is coated on a glass plate, a metal or a plastic film as a thin layer (~0.25 mm in thickness). In addition, a binder like gypsum as in Silica gel G is mixed into the stationary phase to make it stick better to the slide. In many cases, a fluorescent powder is mixed into the stationary phase to simplify the visualization later on (e.g. bright green when you expose it to 254 nm UV light). Uniform thin layer of adsorbent is placed on the support by various techniques. These are mainly:

(a) Spreading
(b) Dipping
(c) Spraying

After placement of layer of adsorbent, the plate is dried in air for 5–10 minutes and then in oven for half an hour at 110°C temperature.

Preparation of TLC plate

Do not touch the TLC plate on the side with the white surface. In order to obtain an imaginary start line with pencil, make two notches on each side of the TLC plate (Fig. 20.1). Do not use pen.

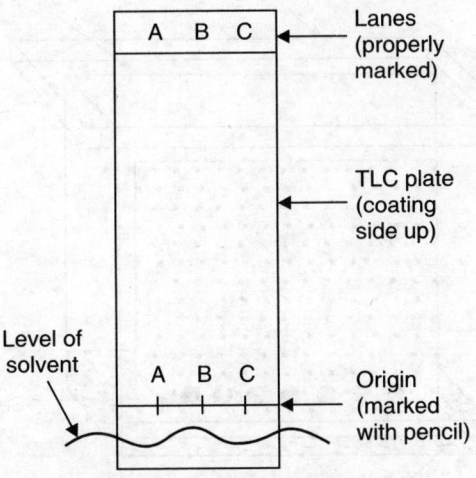

Fig. 20.1: Preparation of TLC plate

Capillary spotters

Place a fine capillary tube in the dark blue part of the Bunsen burner flame. Hold it there until it softens and starts to sag. Quickly remove the capillary from the flame and pull on both ends to about 2–3 times its original length. If you pull the capillary inside the flame, you will have a "piece of art", but not a good spotter. Allow the capillary to cool down, and then break it in the middle. Make sure that you break off the closed end on one of them.

Spotting of the TLC plate

The main advantage of TLC over other separation methods is that it is truly a microscale technique. Only a few micrograms of material in solution is necessary to observe the solute on a TLC plate. Dissolve a few milligrams of material in a solvent (preferably volatile) creating a dilute solution. Once the sample is prepared, a spotting capillary must be used to add the sample to the plate. The solution can be drawn up the tube by capillary action and spotted on the plate at the place marked by pencil. This is known as the origin.

Notice that pencil is always used to mark a TLC plate since the graphite carbon is inert. If organic ink is used to mark the plate, it will chromatograph just as any other organic compound and give incorrect results. To spot the plate, simply touch the end of the capillary tube to the coated side of the plate. The solvent should evaporate quickly leaving the mixture behind on the plate. You may have to spot the plate a couple of times to ensure the sufficient quantity of sample, but do not spot too much sample. If too much solute is added to the plate, a poor separation will result. Smearing, smudging and spots that overlap will result making identification of separated components difficult.

Development

Once the dilute solution of the mixture has been spotted on the plate, the next step is the development of the plate. The bottle (chamber) is filled with a small amount of the mobile phase and cover it (Fig. 20.2). In addition, a piece of filter paper is put in the chamber to help create an atmosphere saturated with solvent. Also make sure the origin spots are not below the solvent level in the chamber. If the spots are submerged in the solvent, they are washed off the plate and lost.

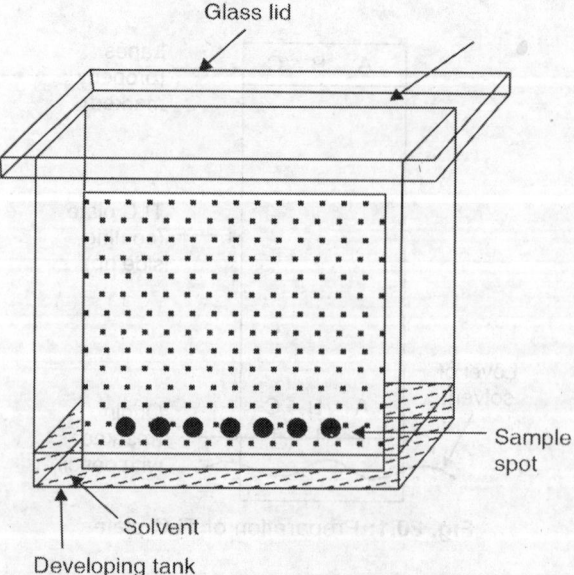

Fig. 20.2: TLC development chamber

Visualization

If organic compounds are coloured such as dyes, inks or indicators, then visualization of the separated spots is easy. However, since most organic compounds are colourless, this method does not work.

In most cases observing the separated spots by UV light works well. TLC plates normally contain a fluorescent indicator which makes the TLC plate glow green under UV light of wavelength 254 nm. Compounds that absorb UV light will quench the green fluorescence yielding dark purple or bluish spots on the plate. Simply put the plate under a UV lamp, and the compounds become visible to the naked eye. Lightly circle the spots to have a permanent record of their location for later calculations.

Another useful visualizing technique is an iodine (I_2) chamber. Iodine sublimes and will absorb to organic molecules in the vapor phase. The organic spots on the plate will turn brown and can be easily identified. Also circle these observed spots, since the iodine adsorbed spots eventually fade away from the plate. Sometimes, a combination of both a UV lamp and iodine is needed to observe all the spots. Some compounds are not "UV active", that is, they do not absorb light at the wavelength of 254 nm. Using both methods will ensure correct identification of all the spots on the TLC plate.

R_f Value

In addition to qualitative results, TLC can also provide a chromatographic measurement known as an R_f value. The R_f value is the "retardation factor" or the "ratio-to-front" value expressed as a decimal fraction.

The R_f value can be calculated as:

$$R_f \text{ value} = \frac{\text{Distance from the origin to ensure of spot}}{\text{Distance from the origin is solvent front}}$$

This number can be calculated for each spot observed on a TLC plate. Essentially, it describes the distance travelled by the individual components. If two spots travel the same distance or have the same R_f value then it might be concluded that the two components are the same molecule. For R_f value comparisons to be valid; however, TLC plates must be run under the same exact conditions. These conditions include the stationary phase, mobile phase, and temperature. Just as many organic molecules have the same melting point and colour, many can have the same R_f value, so identical R_f values do not necessarily mean identical compounds. Additional information must be obtained before this conclusion can be made. It is important to restate that R_f value is only significant when the same chromatographic conditions are used.

Experiment 20.1: Identify the amino acid with the help of thin layer chromatography. Calculate its R_f value of individual amino acid

Reagents Required

(i) Preparation of amino acids solution

Prepare a 0.5 or 1% solution of standard amino acid like glycine, aspartic acid, glutamic acid, etc. in water or ethanol. Similarly prepare a solution of unknown amino acid which is to be identified.

(ii) Developer (mobile phase)

Prepare a mixture of glacial acetic acid, water and butan-1-ol in a proportion of 20, 20 and 60 by volume.

(iii) Spraying agent

Prepare a 0.2% ninhydrin solution in 95 volume of butan-1-ol and 5 volume of acetic acid.

Procedure

1. Clean the glass plate (support for adsorbent).
2. Make a suspension or slurry of silica gel G in distilled water and spread on given glass plate that is rested on an absolutely labelled surface. Spread the slurry or suspension on the surface of plate by the backward and forward movement.
3. Dry the plate at room temperature for 5–10 minutes and then in oven at 110°C for half an hour.
4. Meanwhile prepare a mobile phase (developer) and pour into jar. Place a filter paper around the wall of jar. Cover the jar properly (Fig. 20.2) and allow to saturate the jar with the vapours of mobile phase for better development.
5. Draw an imaginary start line with pencil, make two notches on each side of the TLC plate (Fig. 20.1).
6. Draw a solution of amino acid with the help of capillary and simply touch the end of the capillary tube to the coated side of the plate for spotting. Allow the solvent to evaporate quickly leaving amino acid behind on the plate. Spot the plate a couple of times to ensure the material is present, but do not spot too much sample. Like this, spot the other amino acids and unknown amino acid on the same imaginary line on the plate with 1 cm apart.
7. Insert the plate in the developing chamber containing mobile phase but make sure the origin spots are not below the solvent level in the chamber. **If the spots are submerged in the solvent, they will be washed off the plate and lost.**
8. Take out the plate gently when the mobile phase is about to touch the upper side of the plate. Mark the solvent front with pencil and dry the plate in well-ventilated area or in oven.
9. Spray the plate with spraying agent, dry the plate in oven and mark the spot.
10. Calculate the R_f value and compare the R_f value of unknown amino acid with standard amino acid.

Observations

Amino acid	Distance travelled by amino acid	Distance travelled by solvent front	R_f value
1. Glycine			
2. Aspartic acid			
3. Glutamic acid			
4. Unknown			

Result

On the basis of same R_f value, the unknown amino acid is found to be ———

Experiment 20.2: Identify the drug among the aspirin, acetaminophen, ibuprofen and caffeine with the help of thin layer chromatography. Calculate its R_f value.

Reagents required

(i) Solution

Prepare a 0.5 or 1% solution of aspirin, acetaminophen, ibuprofen and caffeine, in water or ethanol. Similarly prepare a solution of unknown drug to be identified.

(ii) Developer

Prepare a mixture of hexane and ethyl acetate in equal proportion by volume.

(iii) Visualizing agent

Iodine vapours.

Procedure

It is similar to exercise No. 20.1 but in this, keep the developed plate after drying in iodine chamber. Mark the brown coloured spot and calculate the R_f value and compare the R_f value of unknown drug with aspirin, acetaminophen, ibuprofen and caffeine.

Experiment 20.3: Identify the sulpha drug among the sulphadiazine, sulphacetamide, sulphathiazole with the help of thin layer chromatography. Calculate its R_f value.

Reagents Required

(i) Solution of sulpha drugs

Prepare a 0.5 or 1% solution of sulphadiazine, sulphacetamide, sulphathiazole and unknown sulpha drug, in water or ethanol.

(ii) Developer

Prepare a mixture of acetone, diethyl amine and methanol in 20, 4 and 3 proportion by volume or chloroform, methanol and water in 32, 8 and 5 proportion by volume.

(iii) Visualizing agent

0.05% $NaNO_2$ solution.

Procedure

It is similar to exercise No. 1 but in this, keep the developed plate after drying in UV chamber or spray with 0.05% $NaNO_2$ solution followed by N-(1-napthyl) ethylenediamine dihydrochloride (0.1 g) in H_2O (300 ml) and HCl (30 ml). Mark the brown coloured spot and calculate the R_f value and the compare the R_f value of unknown drug with sulphadiazine, sulphacetamide and sulphathiazole.

PAPER CHROMATOGRAPHY

It is a technique in which the analysis of unknown substances is carried out mainly by the flow of solvents on specially designed filter paper. There are two types of paper chromatography.

1. *Paper adsorption chromatograph* in which paper impregnated with silica or alumina act as adsorbent (stationary phases) and solvent as mobile phases.
2. *Paper partition chromatograph* in which moisture/water present in the pores of cellulose fibers present in filter paper act as stationary phases and another mobile phase is used as solvent.

In general, paper chromatograph refers to paper partition chromatograph only since most separations are based on partition type only.

Principles of separation

Paper chromatography is, in the general principle, quite similar to thin-layer chromatography. As in TLC, R_f values are often used to characterize compounds separated by a given solvent and sorbent combination, and are, in fact, even more reproducible and widely used. The main differences between the two techniques are:

1. The use of paper (i.e. cellulose fibers) as sorbent;
2. Lack of backing as support; and
3. The use of more polar solvents for separation of more polar constituents.

The principle of separation is mainly partition rather then adsorption. A cellulose layer in filter paper contains moisture that act as stationary phase. Organic solvents or buffers are used as mobile phases. Instead of water as stationary phase, other organic solvents can be used by suitable modification.

Chromatographic paper is available most commonly in 20 × 20 cm sheets. The underlying principle behind the use of paper as a sorbent is that water molecules that associate with cellulose fibers interact with molecules in the mobile phase via hydrogen bonding. As a result, more polar molecules are resolved by PC, and more polar solvents are employed. (discussed below). In addition to solvent, the use of an electric field has been employed in so-called paper electrophoresis.

In addition, descent paper-chromatography in which solvent is provided to the top of the chromatogram has been widely employed. Other variations include circular or horizontal paper-chromatography for which apparatuses are available.

Experimental procedure

Stationary Phase

Cut a piece of chromatographic paper to fit into your development chamber of particular size. Mark a line on the bottom edge of the paper with the help of pencil. On this line, spotting of the sample can be done. Any notes or marks you make on the chromatography paper other than your sample spots must be made with pencil.

For very crude separations, separations can be done using high-grade filter paper as the stationary phase. Paper of chromatographic grade consists of α-cellulose—98.99%, β-cellulose 0.3%, pentosans—0.4–0.8%, ether soluble matter—0.015–0.02%, ash—0.01–0.07%. Whatmann filter papers of different grade like No. 1, No. 2, No. 3, No. 4, No. 17, No. 20, etc. are used. These papers differs in sizes, shapes porosities and thickness. Choice of filter paper depends upon thickness, flow rate, purity, technique, etc.

Development

Choose a developing chamber that can be sealed well. The chamber should be large enough to hold the paper that is to be developed. Add the mobile phase to the chamber so that it is about 2 cm deep. Seal the chamber tightly and let the chamber stand until the atmosphere becomes saturated. A saturated atmosphere allows for more effective development of the chromatograms.

Mobile Phase

Pure solvents, buffer solutions, or mixtures of solvents are used. Some of the examples of hydrophilic mobile phase:

- Isopropanol : liquid ammonia : water (9 : 1 : 2)
- N-butanol : glacial acetic acid : water (4 : 1 : 5)
- Methanol : water (3 : 1 or 4 : 1)
- t-butonal : water : formic acid (40 : 20 : 5)

Loading of the Sample on the Paper

Each sample should be dissolved in an appropriate solvent to make about 1% solution. Less than 1 millilitre of solution is required for the experiment. Touch the tip of a clean drawn-out capillary tube to the sample and let about 3 mm of the sample rise into the tube. If too much solution is drawn into the capillary, touch the tip to a piece of clean filter paper. To spot the sample, touch the capillary to the line (as marked with pencil) on the chromatogram. Make sure the spot does not exceed 1 cm in diameter. Allow the solvent to evaporate. More than one sample can be loaded onto a single piece of chromatography paper. However, all spots on the chromatogram should be 2 to 2.5 cm away from the edges of the paper and from each other.

If a larger quantity of sample is needed for the experiment than is provided by one application, the solution may be re-spotted. When the original spot has dried, draw solution into the capillary as before. Apply this solution over the top of the first spot, but do not allow the diameter of the circle to grow larger than that of the original spot. Repeat if necessary, allowing each spot to dry before the next application.

Development of the Chromatogram

After preparing the chamber and spotting the samples, the paper is ready to be developed. Be careful to handle the paper only by its edges to prevent contamination. Initially, the chromatogram should be suspended in the chamber without touching the solvent. To suspend the chromatogram, thread a piece of string through a paper clip at the top of it. Then tape the string to the outside of the chamber to hold the chromatogram in place. After the chromatogram has hung in the chamber for 10 minutes, immerse the paper's bottom edge into the developing solvent.

Ascending development

Like conventional type, the solvent flows against gravity. The spots are kept at the bottom portion of paper and kept in a chamber with mobile phase solvent at the bottom.

In a chromatographic chamber, the solvent rises up the paper by capillary action and allows a separation of the components as it ascends. Very simple equipment are required. However, the solvent will rise only 20–25 cm and separations of the analytes are limited.

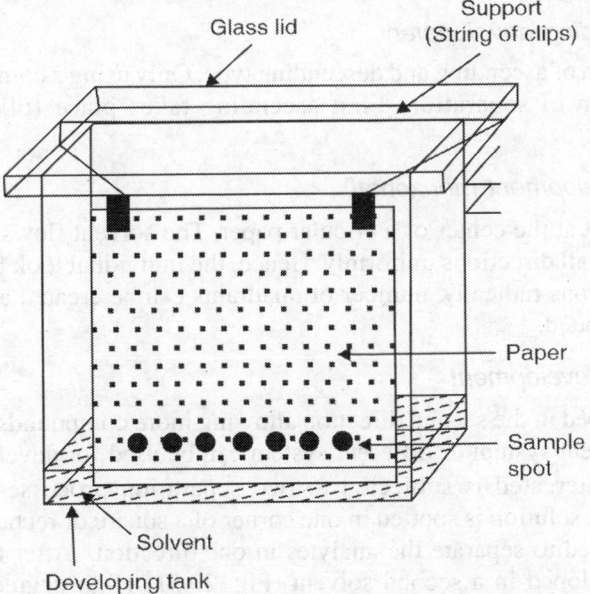

Fig. 20.3: Ascending type paper chromatography

Descending development

This is carried out in a special chamber where the solvent holder is at the top. The spot is kept at the top and the solvent flows down the paper. The advantage is that the flow of solvent is assisted by gravity and hence the development is faster.

In a chromatographic chamber, a paper strip is hanged vertically with the spotted end up. The solvent rises up the wick and descends across the spot and down the paper. This technique permits a separation over a longer distance and allows an increase in resolution.

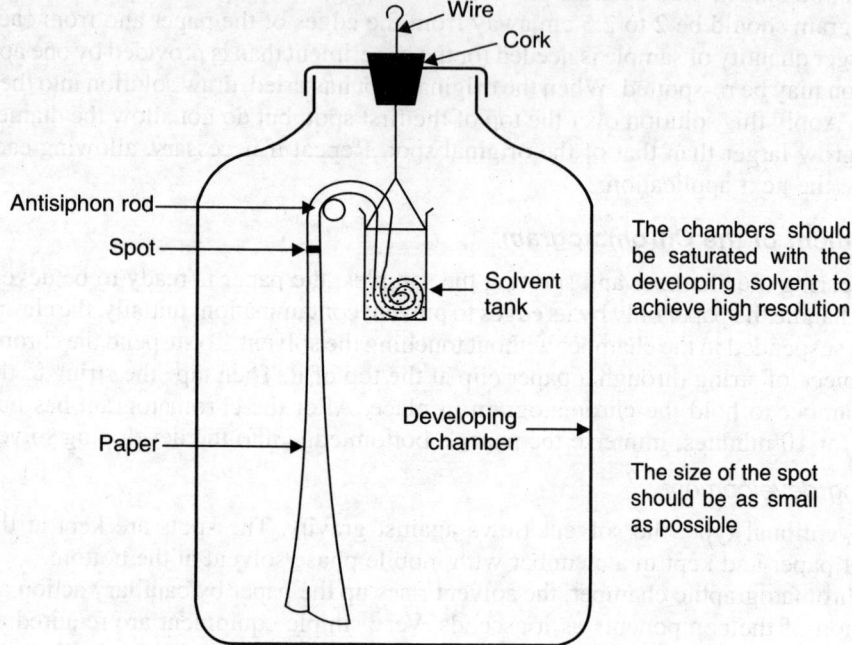

Fig. 20.4: Descending type of paper chromatography

Ascending-descending development

This is a combination of ascending and descending type. Only using a combination of techniques increases the length of separation. First ascending takes place followed by descending development.

Circular/radial development (horizontal)

Here the spot is kept at the center of a circular paper. The solvent flows through a wick at the center and spread in all directions uniformly. Hence, the individual look like concentric circles. By making perforations radically, number of quadrants can be created allowing more number of samples to be spotted.

Two-dimensional development

The paper is developed in the second direction allowing more compounds or complex mixtures, either the same solvent system or different system can be used for development.

A solution of interested is subjected to two separation processes in two-dimensional technique. A sample solution is spotted in one corner of a square or rectangular sheet of paper. One solvent is applied to separate the analytes in one direction. After the paper is dried and turned 90° and developed in a second solvent (Fig. 20.5). High degree of separation of the analytes can be achieved by this technique.

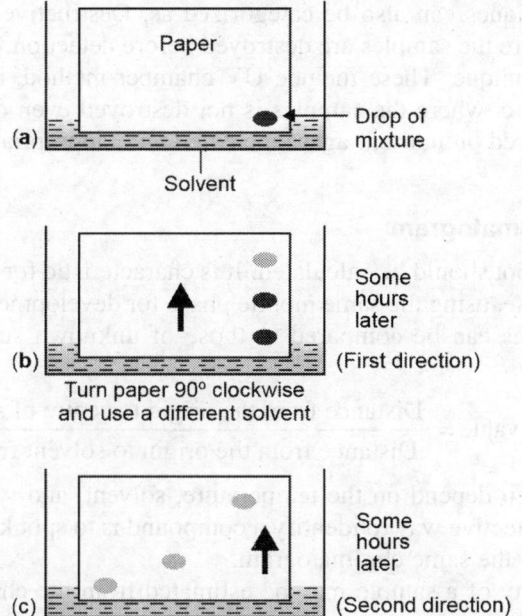

Fig. 20.5: Two dimensional paper chromatography

Removing the chromatogram

After the solvent front is within half an inch of the top of the paper, remove the chromatogram. First, open the lid of the development chamber. Then gently lift the string and the chromatogram out of the chamber. Be sure to handle the chromatogram only by the sides. Carefully mark the solvent front with a pencil and allow the chromatogram to dry in a well-ventilated area.

Visualization of the spots

After the chromatogram has dried, one can identify the spots. Detect the coloured spots visually. If the spots can be seen, outline them with a pencil. Sometimes the colour will fade over time, so the pencil outline is important. If the spots are not visible, the most common visualization technique is to hold the paper under an ultraviolet lamp. (Caution: Do not look directly into the lamp!) Many organic compounds can be seen using this technique. Outline the spots with a pencil, while the chromatogram is under the UV lamp.

Non-specific methods: In this, the number of spots can be detected, but not the exact nature of type of compound.

Examples

- *Iodine chamber method:* In this, brown or amber spots are observed when the paper is kept in a closed jar containing a few iodine crystals at the bottom.
- *Specific methods*: Specific spray reagents, detecting agents, or visualizing agents are used based on the nature of compounds for identification purposes. *Examples*:
  - Ferric chloride—for phenolic compounds and tannins.
  - Ninhydrin in acetone —for amino acids.
  - Dragendroff reagents—for alkaloids
  - 3,5-Dinitro benzoic acid—for cardiac glycosides
  - 2,4-Dinitrophenyl hydrazine—for aldehyde and ketones.

The detecting techniques can also be categorized as: Destructive technique, e.g. specific spray reagents, etc. where the samples are destroyed before detection, e.g. Ninhydrin reagents.

Non-destructive technique: These include UV chamber method, iodine chamber method, densitometry method, etc. where the samples is not destroyed even detection. For antibiotic, the chromatogram is layed on nutrient agar inoculated with appropriate strain and the zone of inhibition is compared.

Interpreting the Chromatogram

The R_f value for each spot should be calculated. It is characteristic for any given compound on the same stationary phase, using the same mobile phase for development of the chromatogram. Hence, known R_f values can be compared to those of unknown substances to aid in their identifications.

$$R_f \text{ value} = \frac{\text{Distance from the origin to centre of spot}}{\text{Distance from the origin to solvent front}}$$

Note: R_f values often depend on the temperature, solvent, and type of paper used in the experiment; the most effective way to identify a compound is to spot known substances next to unknown substances on the same chromatogram.

In addition, the purity of a sample may be estimated from the chromatogram. An impure sample will often develop as two or more spots.

Experiment 20.4: Identify the sugar molecule with the help of ascending paper chromatography. Calculate its R_f value

Reagents required

(i) Preparation of sugar solution

Prepare a 0.5 or 1% solution of standard sugar like glucose, fructose, sucrose, etc. in water or ethanol. Similarly prepare a solution of unknown sugar which is to be identified.

(ii) Developer (mobile phase)

Prepare a mixture of *n*-butanol, pyridine and water in a proportion of 6 : 4 : 3 by volume.

(iii) Spraying agent

Dissolve phthalic acid (1.66 g) and aniline (0.9 ml) in *n*-butanol (48 ml) and mix with ether (48 ml) and water (4 ml).

Procedure

1. Cut a strip of Whatmann No. 1 chromatographic paper (30–40 cm × 5 cm).
2. Draw a line of about 2″ from the top of the paper with pencil and draw four small circles on the line with pencil on the lower side of sheet and mark these as G for glucose, F for fructose, S for sucrose and U for unknown sugar.
3. Touch the tip of a clean drawn-out capillary tube to the solution of glucose and let about 3 mm of the solution rise into the tube. To spot the sample, touch the capillary to the marked circle on the chromatogram. Make sure the spot does not exceed 1 cm in diameter. Allow the solvent to evaporate. Similarly, spot the other solution including of unknown sugar at respective circle. However, all spots on the chromatogram should be 2 to 2.5 cm away from the edges of the paper and from each other.
4. Fill the chamber with developer (mobile phase), close the chamber with cover and allow to remain undisturbed for 15 minutes for proper saturation. After preparing the chamber and

spotting the samples, the paper is ready to be developed. Be careful to handle the paper only by its edges to prevent contamination. Initially, suspend the chromatogram in the chamber containing mobile phase without dipping the spotted marks.

5. Allow the paper to develop till the mobile phase just reaches the other end of the paper.
6. Take out the paper gently, carefully mark the solvent front with a pencil and allow the chromatogram to dry in a well-ventilated area.
7. Spray the chromatogram with spraying reagent and dry in oven to visualize the brownish spot.
8. Calculate the R_f value of each sugar molecule.

Observations

Sugar	Distance travelled by standard sugar	Distance travelled by unknown sugar	R_f value
1. Glycine			
2. Aspartic acid			
3. Glutamic acid			
4. Unknown			

Result

On the basis of R_f value, the unknown sugar is found to be.

Experiment 20.5: Identify the amino acid with the help of ascending paper chromatography. Calculate its R_f value.

Reagents Required

(i) Preparation of amino acids solution

Prepare a 0.5 or 1% solution of standard amino acid like glycine, aspartic acid, glutamic acid, etc. in water or ethanol. Similarly prepare a solution of unknown amino acid which is to be identified.

(ii) Developer

Prepare a mixture of 70% ethanol and 30% water.

(iii) Spraying agent

Prepare a 0.2% ninhydrin solution in ethanol.

Procedure

Adopt the same procedure as in experiment No. 20.4.

Result

On the basis of R_f value, the unknown amino acid is found to be ......

Experiment 20.6: Column chromatographic separation of pigments from green leaves

Introduction

The word 'chromatography', formed from the Greek word 'Khroma' meaning colour and 'graphein' meaning to draw a graph or to write, was coined by the Russian botanist MS Tswett

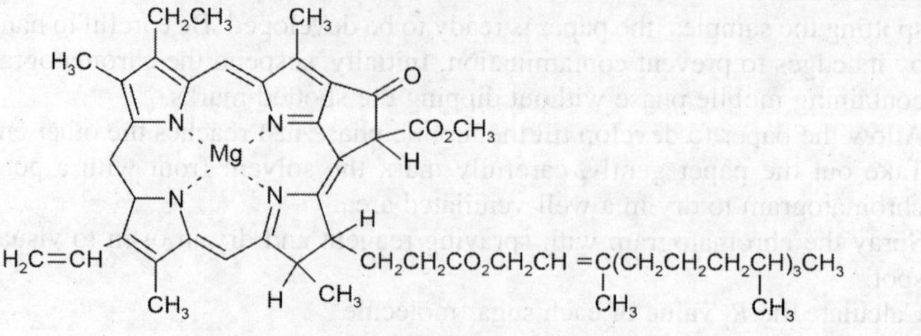

Chlorophyll a (Natural green 3)

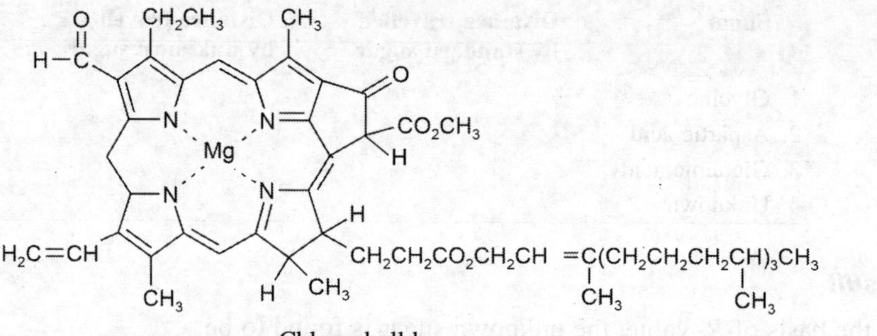

Chlorophyll b

Fig. 20.6: Structure of chlorophyll

around 1906, to describe his process of separating mixtures of plant pigments. Column chromatography is a technique which can be applied to the separation of many complex mixtures. The sample solution is applied to the top of the column. The mobile phase flows down through the column filled with the stationary phase material. Photosynthesis in plants takes place in organelles called chloroplasts. Chloroplasts contain a number of coloured compounds (pigments) which fall into two categories, chlorophylls and caretenoids. Carotenoids, yellow pigments, are tetraterpenes (eight isoprene units). Lycopene, the compound responsible for the red coloring of tomatoes and watermelon and beta-carotene, the compound that causes carrots and apricots to be orange, are examples of carotenoids. In addition, chloroplasts also contain several oxygen containing derivatives of carotenes called xanthophylls.

Chlorophylls are the green pigments that act as the principal photoreceptor molecules of plants. They are capable of absorbing certain wavelengths of visible light that are then converted by plants into chemical energy. Two different forms of these pigments found in plants are chlorophyll a and chlorophyll b. The two forms are identical except that a methyl group in a is replaced by an aldehyde in b. Pheophytin a and pheophytin b are identical to chlorophyll a and b, respectively, except that in each case the magnesium ion Mg^{2+} has been replaced by two hydrogen ions $2H^+$.

Principle

A plant pigment is any type of coloured compound produced by a plant. A chemical compound which absorbs visible radiation between 380 nm (violet) and 760 nm (ruby-red) is considered as a pigment. The general principle employed in all kind of chromatography is movement of a mixture of compounds by a mobile phase, which passes over selectively adsorbing surface, the stationary phase. In column chromatography, the components to be separated, are distributed between two phases, one of which is stationary while the other moves in a definite direction. The stationary phase is packed in a cylindrical tube (column).

The separation of plant pigments by column chromatography depends on the choice of the stationary and mobile phases. The stationary phase material is filled in a column. Any of the three possible mechanisms: partition, adsorption or ion exchange can be employed by the use of a particular type of the stationary phase inside the column. For example, for the separation based on adsorption an adsorbent is packed in the column. The choice of the mobile phase depends on the nature of the substance and how strongly it is adsorbed. In a number of cases such as alumina and silica gel as the adsorbent, the mobile phase is generally a non-polar solvent such as hexanel and benzene because polar groups such as hydroxyl–(OH) group in water and in ethanol would cause desorption. Eluents containing two or more solvents may be used for better results. In such cases the polarity is increased by adding a polar solvent with a nonpolar one.

Requirements

Apparatus

Chromatography column, glass wool, cotton wool, beaker, conical flask, separatory funnel, graduated cylinder, wash bottle.

Chemicals

Silica gel, anhydrous sodium sulphate, hexane, acetone, ethyl alcohol.

Procedure

Proceed according to the following steps:

1. **Preparation of the extract:** Take 5–10 g of fresh grass (or leaves of a green plant) cut it up into fine pieces in a mortar, grind for about 30 seconds, add 10 ml of ethyl alcohol and 20 ml of petroleum ether, grind again. Decant the liquid into a separatory funnel after filtering through glass wool placed in an ordinary funnel. Add 10 ml alcohol and 20 ml petroleum ether again to the mortar containing grass, grind and transfer the liquid after decantation to the separatory funnel containing the first fraction. Shake gently. A light green emulsion may form, if shaken vigorously. Allow to settle the layers. The bottom layer is water–ethanol layer and the upper layer of petroleum–ether contains grass extract. Remove the bottom layer and wash the petroleum layer with water for 3 or 4 times until the layer is clear. Remove the aqueous layer. The extract is now free from alcohol but contains water in very small amount. Transfer the upper layer containing the extract to a dry conical flask. To this, add anhydrous sodium sulphate (dried by heating in an oven/hot plate before use), shake the flask and leave it over for about 15 minutes to remove any water present with the extract. Transfer the extract to a clean and dry test tube, cover it and take it for chromatography.
2. **Preparation of column:** Column is packed by wet pack method. Take a cylindrical glass column and plug in a small piece of cotton. Mount the column on the stand. Take sufficient quantity of fresh silica gel (for column chromatography 60–120 mesh) in a 250 ml beaker. Pour sufficient quantity of hexane into the beaker and stir well using a glass rod to make slurry of the silica. Pour the slurry into the column. Place a conical flask below the mounted column and drain out the excess solvent (hexane). Close the stopcock when the level of the solvent reaches just above the settled silica gel.
3. **Loading of sample:** Take 1–2 ml of dried extract of leaves, drip into the column in the form of a thin layer of solution, allow to run evenly into the adsorbent until a green zone 3–4 mm deep is formed at the top of the column. This is known as the loading of the sample.

4. **Running the column:** Add the developer (hexane) to the column and allow to move the developer through the column packing until separate bands are observed.

5. Note the colour of different bands and their order.

6. Continue filling the column with hexane and elute it until the yellow coloured β-carotene runs down the column.

7. As the elution progresses, β-carotene will elute out of the column, collect this in a conical flask.

8. After collecting the yellow pigment, fill the column with column with either hexane: acetone (70 : 30) or acetone.

9. Place another conical flask below the mounted column.

10. As elution with acetone progresses, the green pigments start moving down the column.

11. Collect this compound in the another conical flask.

12. Removal of solvent.

The yellow and green pigments collected from the column are then concentrated by removing the solvents using a rotary evaporator. The pigments left behind in the round bottomed flask after rotary evaporation are transferred into watch glasses using spatula.

Result and discussion

The bands observed on the column are of different colours. The carotenes are least adsorbed by the adsorbent and can be easily washed out of the column. The green zone is due to green pigment, chlorophyll—chlorophyll a and chlorophyll b. Three main interactions are to be considered in column chromatography: The activity of the adsorbent, the polar behaviour of the substance and the polarity of the eluting solvent. This experiment is based on the results of the inventor of the technique of chromatography, MS Tswett, who applied the technique to separate various plant pigments using calcium carbonate as the stationary phase packed in a column.

Index